The Handbook of
Great Italian Perfumery

Fifty years
of exceptional scents

Marika Vecchiattini

SilvanaEditoriale

Accademia del Profumo is pleased to present *The Handbook of the Great Italian Perfumery*, the book revealing the history, wisdom, creativity and passion of the whole field engaged in the creation of Italian perfumes in the last fifty years: a period rich in tradition and innovation, in which Made in Italy scents were the protagonists.
In this same period, precisely in 1990, Accademia del Profumo was born to enhance perfume as an essential element of wellbeing, promote its creativity, increase its culture and diffusion in Italy. Thus in 2020 we are celebrating the thirtieth anniversary of this all-Italian initiative.
Perfumes are part of everyone's life: we wear them and take them to our homes, but they are not simple accessories. Perfume is an essential element to feel good with oneself and with others. Through an alchemy of fragrance notes, it knows how to convey and instill emotions, sensations and memories.
Perfumery has always played a prominent role in cosmetics: it is the confirmation of an industry of excellence and of the extraordinary cultural and social heritage of perfume, whose history still sees our country as a reference today.
Traces of perfume were already present in Etruscan and Roman times, thus demonstrating the importance of this element which has always been an integral part of daily life. Italian perfumers

were the most famous in the world during the Renaissance. It was the great Leonardo da Vinci, in search of sweet smells, who suggested the infusion in brandy and the modern technique of extraction or enfleurage. It was another Italian, Caterina de' Medici, who introduced the perfume to the French court in 1533. Again, in the late 1600s, the street vendor Gian Paolo Feminis moved from Novara mountains to Cologne, Germany, where his creation Aqua Mirabilis became the Eau de Cologne...

The book analyses the multiple aspects of perfume, from the ingenuity of its creators to the exclusivity of packaging, to the language of communication or the ability of producers of raw materials, components and finished products, which writer Marika Vecchiattini has explored thanks to the interesting conversations with some of the main protagonists of our perfumed world.

Each perfume is a heritage of culture, research, skills and talents, but the real magic is given by the emotions, desires, memories and dreams that each fragrance can arouse.

Happy reading and good perfume to all.

Ambra Martone
President, Academy of Perfume

Accademia del Profumo is the Italian association gathering and representing the perfume industry, from raw materials suppliers to packaging and production companies, from the most prestigious cosmetics companies to communication and distribution experts.
It is an initiative of Cosmetica Italia – the personal care association – in collaboration with Cosmoprof Worldwide Bologna.

Contents

Introduction

The idea of writing this book came to me while I was preparing the lecture on Italian Perfumery that I gave in 2018 at the Italian Cultural Institute of Madrid. The poet Laura Pugno, who manages the Institute, had contacted me for the purpose of giving a group of Italian language and culture students some pointers towards understanding the essence of Italian perfume.

"What sets it apart from the perfume products of other countries?" she had enquired.

And also: *"Does it make any sense to speak about 'Italianness' in perfumery?"*

Studying for that lecture was really fun, but the deeper I delved in my research, the more perplexed I became. I've got dozens of books on perfumery, and all of them mainly comment on or analyse French perfumes: only a few Italian perfumes are even mentioned. And yet, a quick browse at Ebay or at websites specialised in vintage perfumes makes it quite clear that some are very much in demand and the public is willing to pay several hundreds of euro just for a single bottle. Many Italian perfumes, often discontinued and even forgotten here in Italy, have impassioned multitudes of people all over the world, and their disappearance has been long lamented by more than one generation.

So... why is so little attention dedicated to Italian perfumery? Why are we unable to celebrate and promote our olfactory heritage as it deserves?

Many people think that perfume is a purely French matter and are unaware of the fact that modern perfumery actually originated in Italy, only spreading to France in the 1500s, when Caterina de' Medici married the Duke of Orleans. Here in Italy, at that time, the dozens of independent Seigneuries, Duchies and Republics into which the territory was divided continued to wage war against one another, and perfumery continued to be limited to the individual territorial areas.

But let's focus on the present, more specifically, on the last forty years. The 1980s and 1990s marked the golden age of Italian perfumery, a period in which the great Italian couturiers launched perfumes that were acclaimed all over the world for their extraordinary ability to convey, in a fragrance, the brand's exclusivity and unique appeal. These were years of sublime perfumes, cutting edge marketing and ultra-sophisticated bottle designs. Italian perfumes were selling like hot cakes, not only in Italy but also abroad, boosting the passion for products made in Italy.

With the advent of market globalization and the founding of large multinationals possessing the wherewithal to market their products worldwide, perfumes in the 2000s had to be reworked from a new perspective that would meet the requirements of consumers from every continent. On the one hand, thanks to the substantial investments of the multinationals which had acquired them, Italian brands became available to a vast, previously inaccessible, public, as a result of which they were able to develop further, increasing the appeal of Italian-made products throughout the world. On the other, however, the cultural peculiarities of the various countries – Italy included – lost importance, in favor of a globalized taste able to appeal to anyone at any latitude.

But not all is lost, and there are excellent reasons for not losing heart. The first is that Italian brands are still making excellent fragrances; sometimes these products are still a display of Italian taste to a greater or lesser degree; other times they are "just" well-crafted, fine creations whose beauty deserves recognition.

The other reason lies in the success of the so-called artistic perfumery, a handful of visionary brands envisioning perfume as a tool of self-expression, who continue to innovate with their revolutionary ideas and creativity.

The public, however, particularly the younger or more inexperienced, tends to view the Italian perfumery panorama in a disjointed manner, on a case-by-case basis, without acknowledging their origins of the compositional richness, the exceptional *savoir faire* underlying them, the love of Beauty permeating every note.

However, these origins are certainly there, like sturdy roots well planted in a soil that has been irrigated by centuries of research, masterly craftsmanship, and an unmistakably Italian style.

I hope these pages will inspire further research, leaving the feeling that finally there is a basis from which to start, a collection that will help you approach Italian perfumery in a more structured and rational way as for what it has been in the past, what it is today and what it is destined to be in the future.

Note

I have been lucky enough to have experienced the adventure of contemporary Italian perfumery in real time, as a consumer.

In the 1980s, I was little more than twelve years old but I already had such a passion for perfumes and such a well-trained memory that I either wore, owned, collected or gave away the majority of the most famous perfumes launched from 1980 onwards, either in the form of whole bottles, samples, testers or collector's miniature, remembering almost all of them.

Naturally, not being able to include all of them in this publication, I was compelled to make choices.

The three criteria I used when choosing which perfumes to write about concern:

1. the significance of the fragrance itself, of its bottle or other characteristics of the product as a whole;
2. its typically Italian essence;
3. the possibility of being able to smell the perfume today. Unfortunately, some perfumes are damaged by time and I couldn't find them in good enough conditions to be able to wear them and review them objectively. In such cases I decided – albeit reluctantly – not to include them.

Actually, I should also mention the fourth criterion: perfumes had to be one hundred in order to allow each of them a full review. However, at the end of the book, I did manage to add a list of all the perfumes launched by Italian brands from the 1970s until the present day. There are thousands, so I hope that you appreciate the (colossal) effort I made.

All of the perfumes reviewed in these pages are from my personal collection and came out of my refrigerated cabinet especially to be reviewed for this book. When the sample in my possession had deteriorated or too little was left to allow a proper review, I asked for a little help from my friends, who would kindly enable me to refresh my memory.

In any case, it was easier to find vintage masterpieces themselves than it was to find information about them. This particularly applied to the authors' names. Until the year 2000 the name of the fragrance composer was not considered an important detail to disclose, and it was often omitted. With regard to the design and creation of the bottles, the situation was even worse: they were rarely even mentioned.

In order to obtain the information that I needed, I had to speak directly with those who had produced or commissioned the perfumes, consult half a dozen technical volumes and plumb the depths of the internet, cross-referencing data from at least 5 sites including international discussion forums and specialised webpages.

If the name of the fragrance composer, the essence company or the designer of the bottle does not appear in the book, this means that I have not been able to retrace this information, and if any of my readers should know these data, I would be delighted to add them in future reprints.

As far as the categorization of fragrances into olfactory families is concerned, I am aware that some readers may not agree with my attributions.

In addition to my capacities to classify a fragrance correctly (acquired through time, experience and long training courses) I also made use of various professional tools: first and foremost, the *H&R Genealogy of Fragrances* charts by Leffingwell; then the *Fragrances of the World* volumes by Michael Edwards and the *Arbres Généalogiques des Parfums* charts by Osmothèque, based on the classification made by *Société Française des Parfumeurs*.

This has meant comparing completely different methods of classification: the H&R charts categorizes fragrances into three large families subdivided into thirteen sub-families, Osmothèque defines six families and thirty-four sub-families, while Michael Edwards is the author of a fantastic "fragrance wheel" with fifteen olfactory families, each of which is divided into four facets. For example, "Cerruti 1881" is classified as a fresh fougère, as an aromatic chypre or as a lively citrus, three interpretations capturing three different aspects, among which it is difficult to choose which one prevails. In cases where no classification completely satisfied me, I trusted my instinct. For example, I put "Cerruti 1881" among the aromatic citruses, in an attempt to capture as many nuances as possible.

Perfume in Italy

The art of mixing aromatic essences with the purpose of creating body and ambient fragrances was born and developed in times too distant to pinpoint an actual starting date; as for the place, Middle Eastern countries might be considered the cradle of perfumery. The North African countries and those located on the Red Sea are, in fact, the ideal habitat of many fragrant plants, such rose, spikenard, benzoin, olibanum, myrrh, and labdanum, and the inhabitants of those places soon learned to use them, both for hygienic purposes and for their special aroma.

In historical times, Arab merchants used to trade with countries even further East, coming into contact with other aromatic materials, such as cinnamon, black pepper, cloves and precious musk, obtained from the glandular secretions of the Tibetan musk deer, and began using them to enrich their already refined recipes for the body and the environment.

The use of steam to extract fragrant essences from flowers and plants is due to the Iranian doctor Ibn-Sinna, who added the cooling coil to the still around the year 1000, thus perfecting the extraction technique and allowing it to be used in the production of fragrances.

Perfumery came to the West in three distinct waves, two of which represent important moments in our history.

The first wave coincides with the Roman Empire campaigns, which brought the trend of body perfume to Rome. The Romans were already fond of going to the Thermae (Roman baths) to enjoy massages with traditional scented oils and ointments. With the arrival in Rome of people and merchandise from exotic countries, the possibilities increased and the interest in perfumes became a veritable craze. To extract oils from flowers, the Romans already used enfleurage, an olfactory technique in use until a few decades ago, which consisted of covering a fatty substance (obtained from the pig or ox) with fragrant flowers in order to saturate it with their perfume.

The "Unguentariae Tavernae" (as the ancient perfumers' shops were called), attracted a large audience of men and women who, in addition to ready-made perfumes, could purchase raw materials such as cinnamon, spikenard, saffron, costus, to be used at home to scent rooms and prepare recipes with which to enhance

1.
Ointment bottles, late Roman production, from the 4th century AD, glass height 12.5 cm, 11.5 cm, 9.5 cm. Turin, Palazzo Madama – Museo Civico di Arte Antica (Civic Museum of Ancient Ar)t, inv. top. 31, top. 2381, top. 32

2.
Blue glass stick with filaments, Roman production, mid 1st century AD, glass length 25 cm. Turin, Musei Reali – Museo di Antichità (Museum of Antiquities), inv. 3553

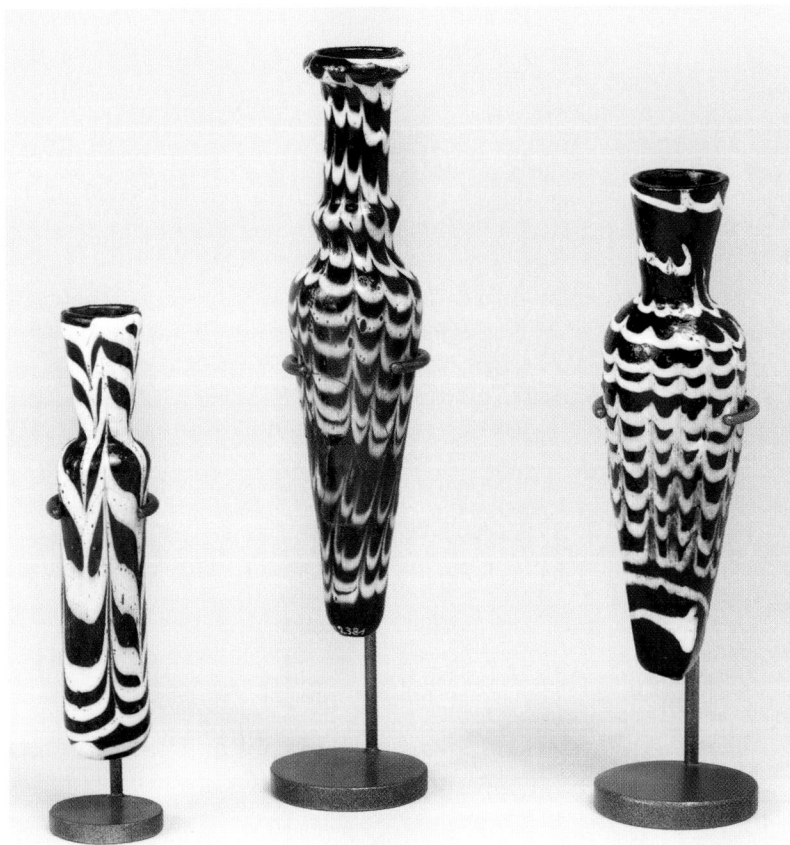

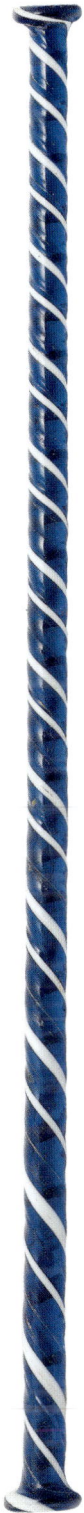

the person's well-being and charm. Rhodinum was among the most popular recipes, a mixture of rose petals, saffron, calamus, honey and wine.

But every special occasion required the use of a different perfume, from the wedding to the birth of a child, up to the funeral rituals. As an example, during the funeral ceremony of his wife Poppaea, Nero burned an amount of incense higher than what Arabia could produce in ten years.

The Romans' great interest in perfumes is testified both by the many detractors who wrote against this expensive and "useless" accessory (Martial) and by those who, like Pliny the Elder, meticulously reported several fragrant recipes.

The second wave came at the time of Alexander the Great's military campaigns, which extended as far as the mouth of the Indus River, making it possible to intensify not only trade but, even more important, cultural relations between the East and the West, (whose entrance gate was the Roman Empire).

The third wave was the conquest of Spain by the Umayyad dynasty (923-1031). In a matter of decades, the Arabs improved the territories that they had conquered, transforming small rural towns such as Toledo, Seville and Granada into luxurious modern cities. Around the year 1000, Cordoba had already half a million inhabitants and a prestigious University that welcomed illustrious scholars from all over the world. As we have already seen, perfume had been part of the Arab culture since time immemorial. The Umayyads also brought to Spain their knowledge of how to process essences, spreading their custom of generously perfuming their surroundings, their clothes and themselves.

When the Arabs left Spain, the task of consolidating the use of perfume in the West fell upon the Crusaders returning from the Holy Land (1100-1300). They succeeded in circumventing the Catholic Church's ban on fragrances (considered as emissaries of the Devil), by introducing new, "hygienical" customs such as the daily cleansing of the body and the sprinkling with curative waters made with fragrant plants.

The officinal herbs used to make these aromatic waters were not difficult to find. In addition to growing wild throughout Italy, herbs such as rosemary, sage, lemon balm, lavender and verbena were also grown in hundreds of Monasteries and Abbeys throughout the country, inside their so-called "Giardini dei Semplici" (Herb gardens). Using medicinal herbs and plants, the pharmacist monks made decoctions, ointments and scented waters to heal the most common ailments of the time... and to enhance love, fertility and beauty as well.

Only two the monasteries dating back to the Middle Ages are still in business today: the Officina Profumo-farmaceutica di Santa Maria Novella (founded in 1200) and the Farmacia SS. Annunziata (founded in 1561).

The apothecary-monks were endowed with a certain dignity and undisputed sacredness, but they were not the only ones who used herbs, flowers and plants to make remedies.

At a more "institutional" level, there were the Speziali and the Apotecari (Apothecaries) also called Aromatari (Aromataries). The first were licensed to sell medicinal herbs directly to their customers, as well as ready-made medications for curing health problems; the latters were able to prepare mixtures of herbs, salves and waters to be used for hygiene, health and aesthetic purposes. The differences between these trades were not so clear-cut, and the existence of intermediary figures such as "herb sellers" and "aroma sellers" contributed to creating problems of law and order. From 1200 onwards, the need to safe-guard and regulate the specific activities of these professional figures led to the creation of craft guilds in Venice, Bologna, Genoa, Florence and in many Municipalities, Seigneuries

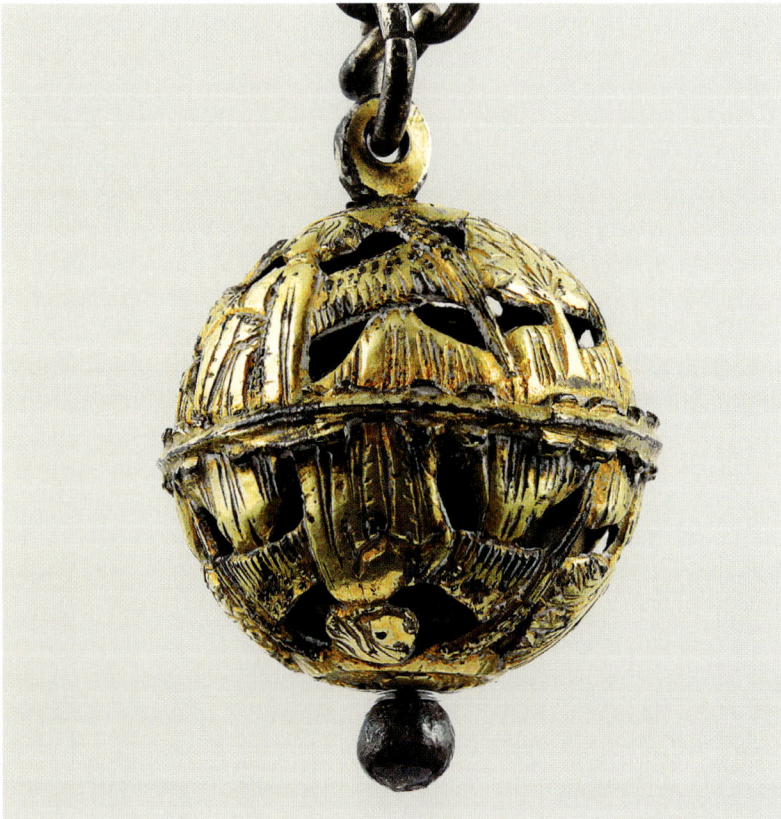

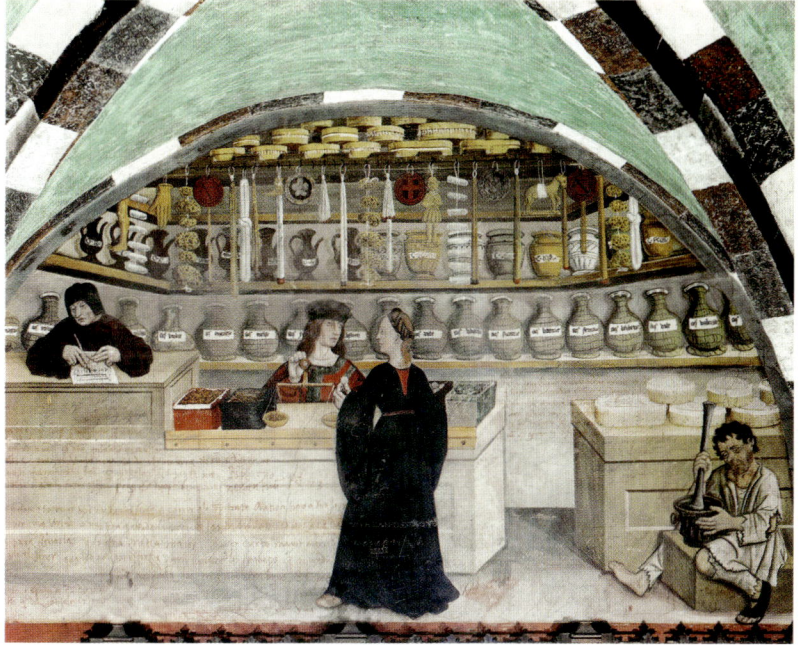

4.
Unknown artist, Interior of a pharmacy, 15th century, fresco. Val d'Aosta, Issogne Castle
The pharmacy is run by lay people; on the counter are visible blocks of soap and baskets of loose herbs, on the shelf containers of ready-made medicines. At the top left some "soporific sponges" are hanged, to be imbued with anesthetic (opium, mandrake) in order to narcotise patients undergoing surgery

and Republics chiefly situated in the North of Italy (but also in other European cities). In some cases, such as Florence for example, their economic power grew to such an extent that they gained the power to govern the city directly.

In 1498 the Collegio dell'Arte of the Medici family published the "Ricettario Fiorentino" (Florentine Recipe Book) in Florence, which collected and illustrated the most requested medicaments and antidotes, together with the most suitable practices to prepare them. The Florentine recipe book, which all apothecaries were required to know and respect when composing their recipes, represents the first example of a "public pharmacopoeia" written by an Authority with the aim of protecting public health. The majority of people, however, mainly relied on Healers, women well- versed in herbal medicine whose knowledge had been handed down from generation to generation for thousands of years. Their medical art, fruit of the observation both of Nature and of humankind, found useful remedies in all that the territory placed at their disposal: herbs, flowers, roots... enriched and "activated" by prayers, magic and spells rooted in an ancient natural sensibility.

But let's return to the Middle Ages. Throughout the Middle Ages, the Italian peninsula was a natural stopping place on trade routes back and forth from the Oriental countries. Venice in particular was

PERFUME IN ITALY

the port through which every kind of precious merchandise from the East reached the Western world. Exotic and expensive materials such as pepper, musk and benzoin arrived at the port and were stored in warehouses. Part of these stocks were used locally and part were shipped on, to every corner of Europe.

After twenty years of wanderings across the Far East, Marco Polo came back to Venice in 1296, introducing in Europe new knowledge, new uses and a completely new taste for oriental perfumery.

Still during Mediaeval times, the prestigious University of Salerno succeeded in perfecting alcohol distillation, a technological innovation which led to the transformation of traditional oil-based perfumery – the plants would release their fragrant properties when macerated in oil – into modern alcohol-based perfumery, thereby enabling the production of lighter, fresher perfumes, with a wider range of fragrances.

The habit of taking hot baths was still popular in Italy in the period between the Middle Ages and the Renaissance. People used to bathe quite frequently at the public baths (a habit deriving directly from the Roman Thermae), in hot water aromatised with flowers and herbs. The aristocracy could also bathe privately in heated rooms especially built inside their opulent homes. The soap they used when bathing was mainly produced in Genoa, Bologna and Venice, in balls or cubes, which were also used for washing laundry.

Unfortunately, the habit of bathing, was abandoned prior to the Renaissance: the Church did not approve of the physical proximity of people bathing together and decreed that all public baths should be closed.

Even the habit of bathing at home was abandoned. In fact when the plague spread to Italy (1347), Spice Merchants and Physicians advised against bathing, since hot water opens the skin pores, and doctors thought this facilitated the spreading of the disease. At that time, in facts, it was believed that diseases were caused by putrid air getting inside the body... the existence of bacteria was discovered only several centuries later.

Bathing was then replaced by the less efficient "dry toilet" carried out sprinkling perfumed waters in body areas not covered by clothes, such as hands and face.

From the Renaissance to the 17th century

Although the cleansing of the body was no longer considered a priority, perfumes continued to play a leading role in rituals for preserving health and beauty. Spices, resins and other strongly scented

5.
Renato Bianco,
Caterina
de' Medici's
personal
perfumer. In his
shop in Pont St.
Michel
dozens of new
perfumers were
formed, who in
the following
decades spread
the art of
perfumery in
all of France

6.
Unknown artist,
*Caterina de'
Medici, Queen
of France*.
Florence,
Palatine Gallery.
Catherine has
been a loved
Queen also by
virtue of her
culture and the
refined habits
she introduced
to the French
Court, which
allowed France
to recover
part of the
cultural gap that
separated it
from the Italian
Renaissance
Courts

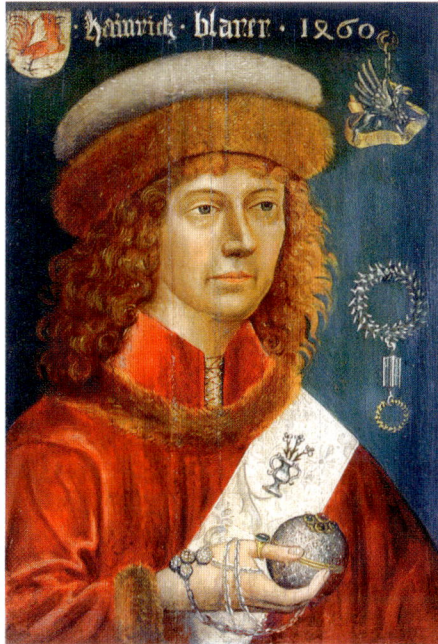 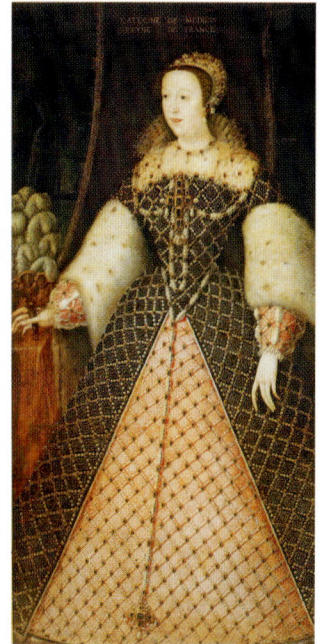

herbs such as rosemary and bay leaf were used to freshen rooms and dampen floors, and their water was sprinkled on clothes and fabrics. Herbs considered healthy were also worn, in the form of little bags hidden under clothes, or scented balls (the so-called *pomanders*) inserted inside necklaces, earrings and external belts.

Renaissance perfumers we know about were chiefly Spanish and Italian. In many cases, Italian noblewomen disclosed their beauty secrets by writing books full of recipes for fragrances, creams and lotions (*Experimenta* by Caterina Sforza and *Secreti* by Isabella Cortese are two examples). At the refined Italian Renaissance Courts it was common to find Princes – who were also poets, musicians, philosophers and scholars of a wide range of scientific subjects – creating perfumes for themselves and for the members of their entourage.

In 1533, Caterina de' Medici, great-granddaughter of Lorenzo the Magnificent, travelled to Paris to marry future King Henry II of Valois (1533), bringing with her an immense cultural heritage including many different arts. The admiration of the French aristocracy was most aroused by two of them: cuisine and perfumery. Caterina brought a wide variety of innovations to the table of the French Court: from the habit of eating with a fork to a number of traditional Tuscan recipes (omelette, onion soup and crêpes, which, of course, had different names in the Florence of yore), which the Queen had prepared for her when she felt homesick for her native city.

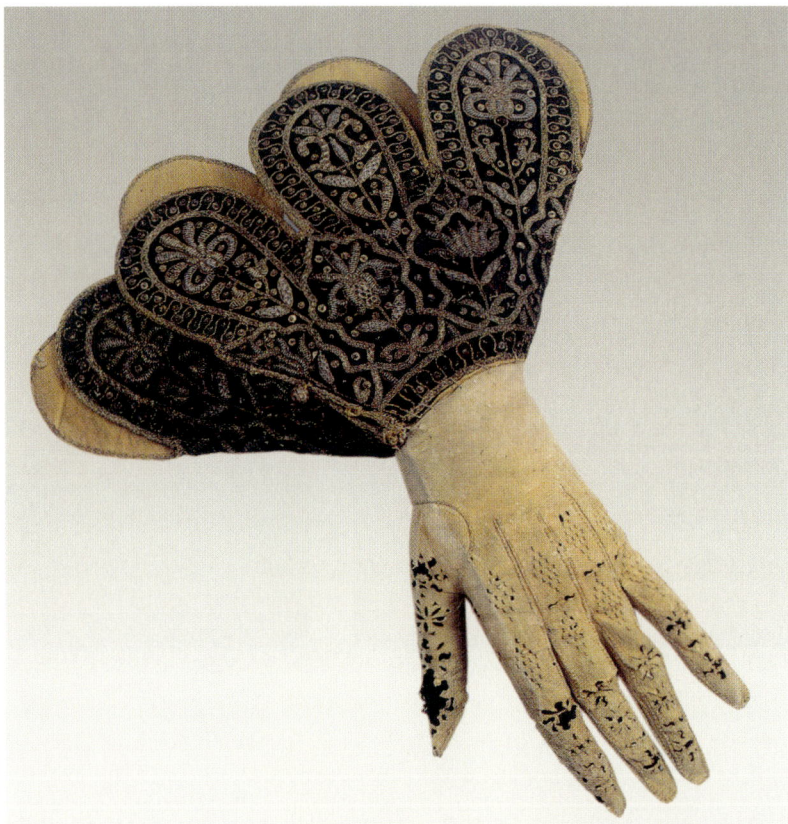

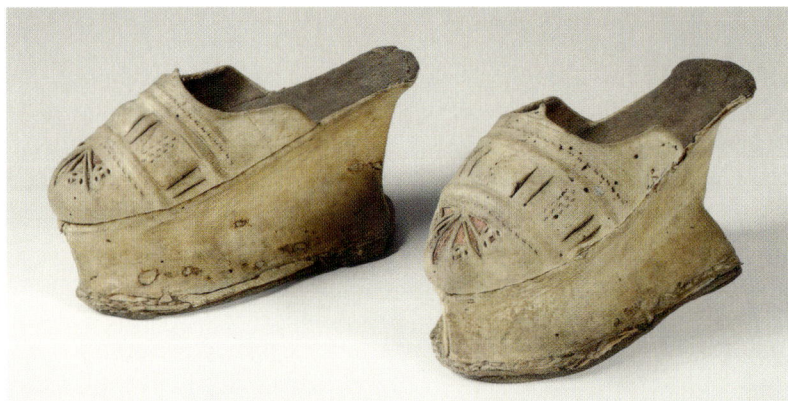

Caterina arrived in Paris accompanied by her personal perfumer, Renato Bianco (re-named René le Florentin) who learned perfumery at the Spezieria of Santa Maria Novella. Caterina used to wear perfumed necklaces and pomanders, as well as fine white embroidered leather gloves, which she anointed - together with her hands - with oils prepared by Renato according to her tastes. The

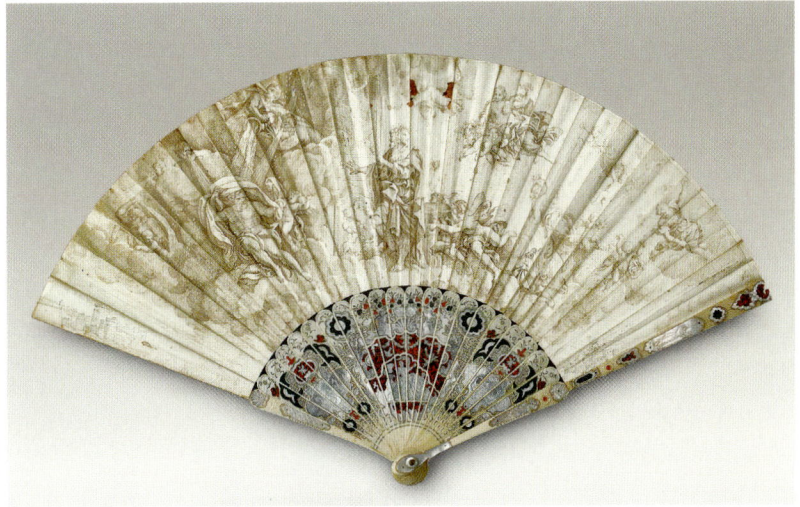

use of perfumes and scented cosmetics, which for Caterina and the other refined Italian noblewomen was a daily ritual contributing luxury, pleasure and facilitating social relations, had an explosive effect on the French, who were unused to such sophistication. The French aristocracy instantly fell in love with perfume, and the shop that René le Florentin opened in Paris was submerged with such a backlog of orders that he was hastily forced to train dozens of new perfumers. Some of these settled in Paris, while others scattered in other parts of the country, laying the foundations for the perfume industry of the centuries to come.

Seventy years after Caterina, Maria de' Medici, daughter of the Grand Duke Francesco I, also travelled to Paris to marry a King (Henry VI). She too brought with her an entourage of over three hundred people, who reinforced the Italian predilection for a certain kind of refinement of the senses.

At the start of the 17th century, the elegant leather gloves made in the Provençal town of Grasse were were highly sought-after by Courts all over Europe. This fact, together with the arrival in town of many new perfumers trained in Paris, acted as a propeller for the glovemaking industry, allowing Grasse to build a success story that lasted for two centuries. When the glovemakers gained the technical knowledge required for extracting the odorous properties from plants, they began to use this to enhance their products with simple essences (rose, tuberose, jasmine which grew wild in the areas surrounding the city) which gradually became more complex and sophisticated as time went on.

Success was worldwide and even in Italy the noblewomen started competing to flaunt their perfumed clothing from Grasse: in addition to gloves and belts, dressing gowns, footwear and fans were also perfumed with all the wonderful fragrant essences local to the Provençal town.

By the end of the 1600s, the glovemakers-perfumers of Grasse had become an extremely impressive corporation, with the power to stipulate trade agreements with the Company of the Indies for the direct procurement of the raw materials they required, and to start growing locally some of the species they had been importing, such as tuberose from Italy and jasmine from India.

10.
Perfume vials, Venice, 18th century blown glass, gilded, length 13.3 cm, 14 cm, 16 cm. Turin, Palazzo Madama – Museo Civico di Arte Antica (Civic Museum of Ancient Art), inv. 86, 87, 88 / VE

11.
Perfume bottle, Murano, Brussa workshop, mid-18th century, painted glass, silver, height 7 cm, width 5 cm. Turin, Palazzo Madama - Civic Museum of Ancient Art, inv. 318 / VD

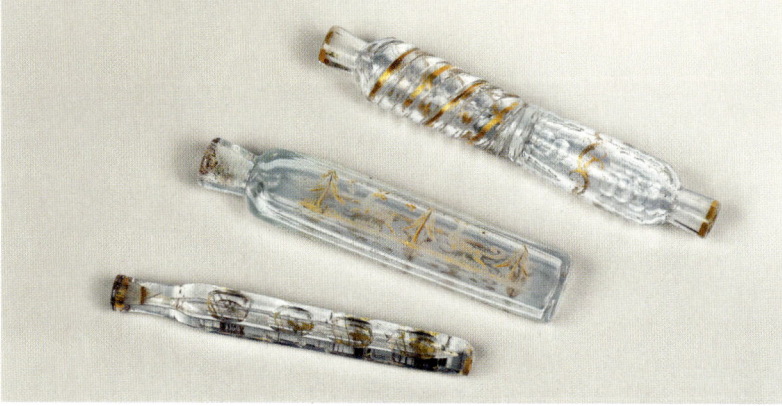

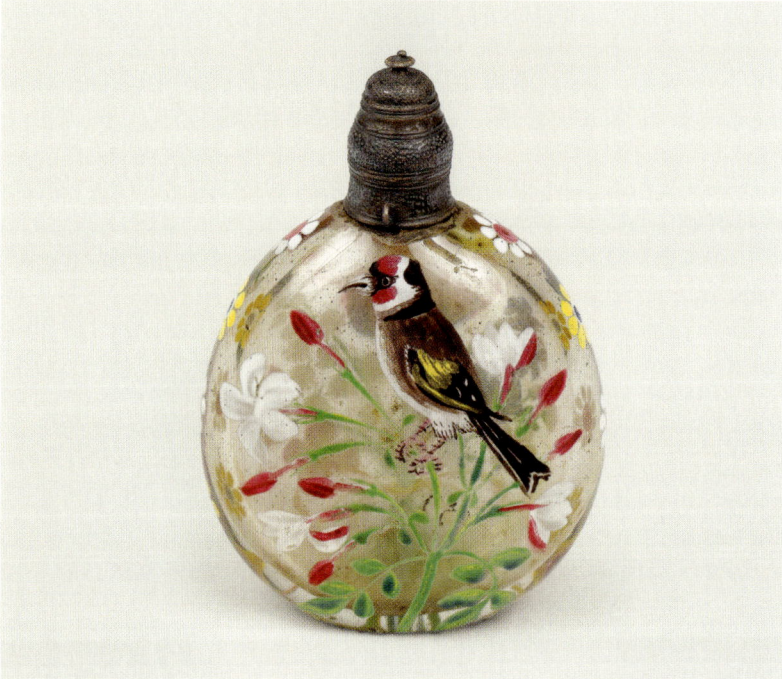

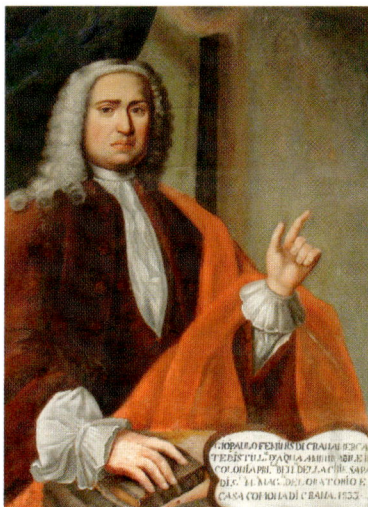

12.
Unknown artist, *Giovanni Paolo Feminis*, Crana (Val Vigezzo), church of San Rocco. On 13 January 1729 the "Aqua Mirabilis" obtained certification from the Cologne Faculty of Medicine, which in fact authorized Faminis to sell it to the public

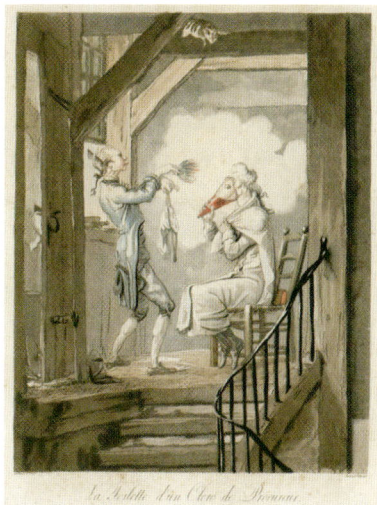

13.
Philibert-Louis Debucourt from a drawing by Carle Vernet, The toilet of an assistant prosecutor, Paris, 1816, etching with tempera elevations, 35.5 × 27.1 cm. Grasse, Musée International de la Parfumerie, inv. 9455

The 18th century

In the 18th century, Western perfumery was shaken by an event rooted in Italy: the creation of Eau de Cologne. The story begins with Gian Paolo Feminis, from Val Vigezzo (in the province of Novara) moving to Cologne, in Germany, at the end of the 1600s. Gian Paolo Feminis had come into possession of a very old recipe for a medicinal beverage that an old acquaintance of his, a herbalist monk, used to treat the various ailments of his patients. After opening a small distillery/essence laboratory in Cologne, Gian Paolo Feminis perfected the recipe, gave it the name *Aqua Mirabilis* and began producing it with excellent results. In 1729, given the success of his product, Gian Paolo Feminis obtained the approval of the Faculty of Medicine of the University of Cologne, and changed the name from *Aqua Mirabilis* to *Eau de Cologne*. Thirty years later, his cousin Giovanni Maria Farina, who had also moved to Cologne, joined Gian Paolo in the management of the company. When Gian Paolo Feminis passed away, Giovanni Maria Farina took over the company moved to Paris and continued to produce Aqua Mirabilis under a new name: *Eau Admirable de Cologne*.

At this point, the developments of story become difficult to follow, due name thefts, destruction of public archives, heirs baptised with the name Jean Marie to confirm their direct descent from the original Giovanni Maria... It is difficult to understand what really happened, since everyone involved in this affair claimed to be the owner of the formula; the fact remains that from this recipe various world-famous Colognes are still produced today: "Echt Kölnisch Wasser 4711 Original Eau de Cologne", "Original Kölnisch Wasser" by Farina Gegenüber, and "Eau de Cologne Jean Marie Farina Extra Vielle" by Roger & Gallet. In any case, the success of Gian Paolo Feminis' Eau de Cologne was so great and so widespread that his formula found a place of honour in the perfume classification, creating a well-defined olfactory structure, which over the centuries has been revamped, acclaimed or blatantly imitated hundreds if not thousands of times.

The 18th century, the "Age of Enlightenment" rekindled interest in personal hygiene practices, not only for the sake of health but also as a private pleasure. Only when the body was clean and did not emanate unpleasant odours was it possible to enjoy to the full the fresh, light fragrances of Eau de Cologne and its innumerable variations. From this moment on, the unmistakable Cologne whiff distinguished the more modern and "fashionable" aristocrats, who could afford a bathroom, from those who could not.

The 19th century

Throughout the century, perfumery continued to develop thanks to constant innovations in material processing techniques and to the discovery of the first synthetic molecules. Molecules produced in laboratories accelerated an across-the-board dissemination of perfumery: their synthetic nature gave stability to perfumes, and their practically infinite reproducibility made them much less expensive than their natural counterpart.

While, in France, the city of Grasse was establishing itself definitively as the centre of French perfumery, numerous small companies were springing up all over Italy. Many of these were extensions of barber shops, which had started by producing perfumes

14.
Bottles of *Acqua di Felsina* and *Acqua di Felsina Rossa* by Pietro Bortolotti, late 19th century. Collections: Francesca Faruolo / Smell Olfactory Art and Culture, Barbara and Pierpaolo Corazza / Authentica di Felsina

15.
Bottles of *Acqua di Felsina* with shipping box Pietro Bortolotti, late 19th century and 1970. Collections: Francesca Faruolo / Smell Art and Olfactory Culture, Barbara and Pierpaolo Corazza / Autentica di Felsina

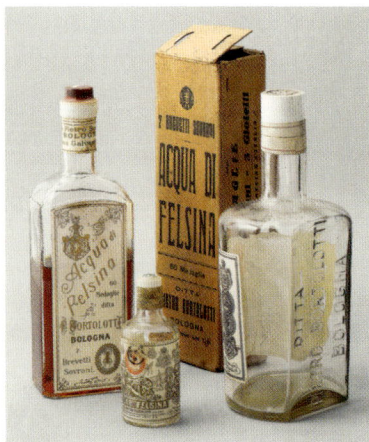

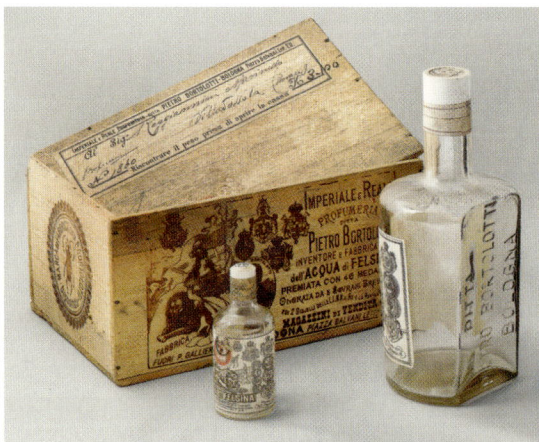

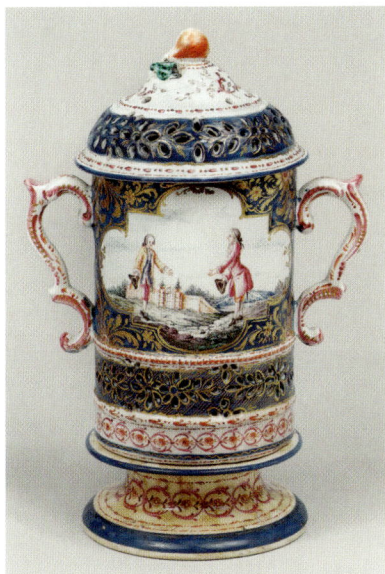

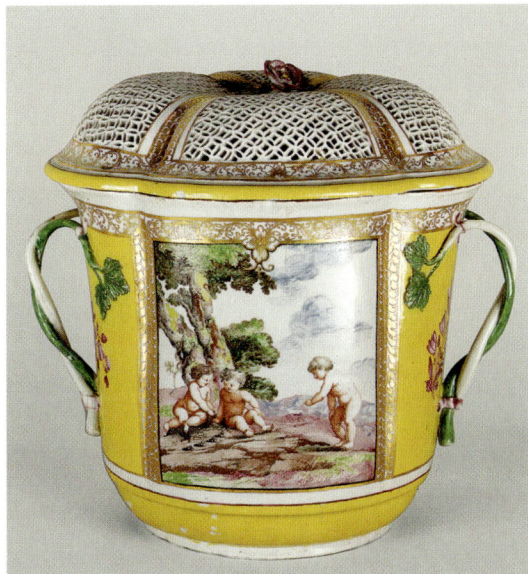

and lotions exclusively for their own customers, and had been so successful as to become known nationwide.

In Milan the "Casa di Profumo, Saponi e Articoli da Toeletta Angelo Migone", founded back in 1778 and specialising in the production of perfumes, face powder, soap, shaving and hair care products, was experiencing so much commercial success throughout the Mediterranean countries that it evolved into a soap and perfume manufacturing factory.

In Bologna in 1827, Pietro Bortolotti, representing the fourth generation of a family of aromataries/spice merchants, submitted an application to his city's Health Board requesting permission to manufacture and sell a preparation of his own making, which he claimed had curative properties. This led to the creation of the famous "Acqua di Felsina", a Cologne with a rich amber base that was a resounding success not only in the city, of which it became the olfactory emblem, but also internationally, receiving awards at exhibitions throughout Europe and earning itself a legitimate place in the history of Italian perfumery. Celebrities such as Guglielmo Marconi, Alfredo Testoni, Mario Praz and Italo Calvino liked and used it, and spoke about it in their works. Then "Acqua di Felsina" slipped out of sight for a century. Fortunately, the heirs of the Bortolotti family unearthed the documents and formulas in an attic and managed to recreate it in 2017, under a new name "Autentica di Felsina".

In 1853, Stefano Frecceri, a perfumer and distiller from Genoa, successfully launched his "Acqua di Genova" for the Royal House of

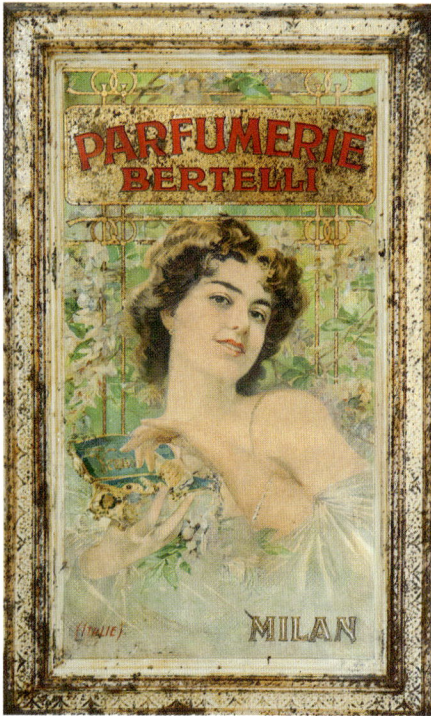

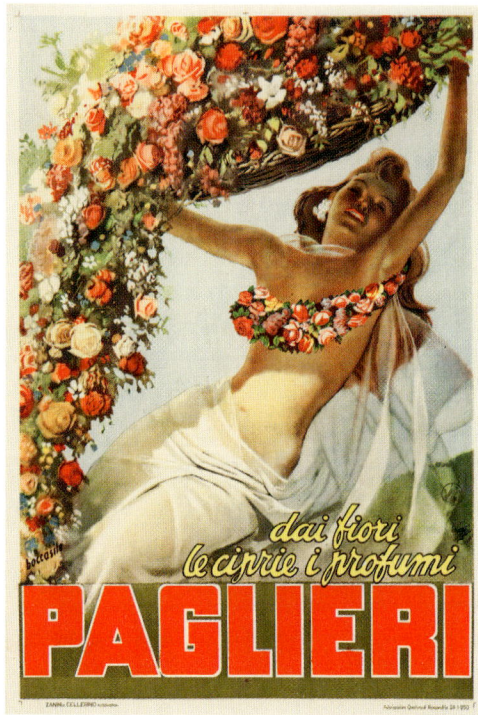

Savoy, the production of which still continues today. The fragrance, which received as many as twenty-four gold medals at the Universal Exhibitions held in Europe from the middle to the end of the 19th century, was the "olfactory signature" of Virginia Oldoini, Countess of Castiglione, dubbed by Gabriele d'Annunzio "The Divine Countess" and one of the most beautiful and elegant women in Europe (favourite of King Vittorio Emanuele, who, loving the woman, also became enamoured of the fragrance).

In the decades straddling the mid-19th century and the turn of the 20th century, some of the historic Italian companies were established: "Profumerie Igieniche Puglisi e Manara" in Palermo; in Milan "Valsecchi & Morosetti", "Ai Colli Fioriti", "A. Bertelli & C." and "Satinine" founded by Lorenzo Usellini in 1883, which initially imported toiletries mainly from France.

In Alessandria, Lodovico Paglieri took over the perfume factory from his father and decided to produce perfumes and cosmetics with a brand of his own.

Parma saw the founding of the O.P.S.O. (Officina Parmense Sostanze Odorose) and "Saccò & Borsari", a barber shop founded by Dario Saccò and Lodovico Borsari.

18.
"Parfumerie Bertelli", circa 1910, 50 × 33 cm. Marco Gusmeroli collection

19.
"From flowers, powders, perfumes Paglieri", Gino Boccasile, 1950, Zanino & Cellerino, Alessandria. Alessandro Bellenda Collection, L'Image Gallery, Alassio

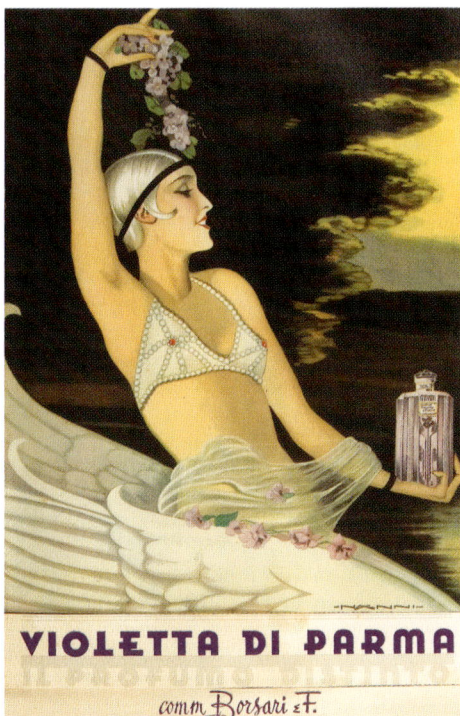
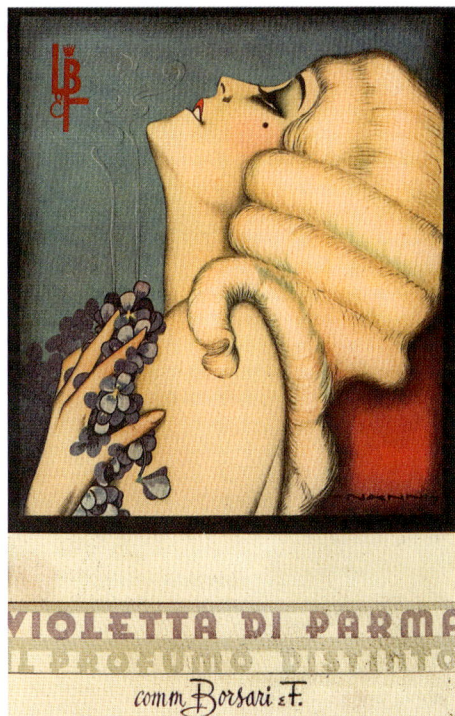

VIOLETTA DI PARMA

comm Borsari &F.

VIOLETTA DI PARMA
IL PROFUMO DISTINTO

comm Borsari &F.

20.
"Violetta di
Parma Borsari",
Nino Nanni,
1933,
40 × 30 cm.
Parma Color
Viola Collection

21.
"Violetta di
Parma Borsari",
Nino Nanni,
1933, 40 × 30
cm, Grafiche
Berardi, Milan.
Parma Color
Viola Collection

Italian perfumes of the early 20th century: Parma

If ever it existed an Italian centre of perfumery – a sort of Italian Grasse – it would unquestionably be the city of Parma, its perfume vocation would be rooted in this century and in the entrepreneurial acumen of the companies mentioned above.

Italian perfumery was given its strongest boost by a person who was brought to Parma on the wings of History: Duchess Marie Louise of Austria, Empress of France and second wife of Napoleon Bonaparte. Marie Louise was, in fact, enamoured of a shy but charming flower: the violet.

It is not known precisely how and when Marie Louise grew so fond of the violet's fragrance, but it was, in any case, long before she came to Parma: numerous invoices testify that during her stay in France she had bouquets of violets delivered by the florists who supplied the court. Perhaps it was her husband who had kindled in her the passion for this flower: Napoleon himself used to wear a violet-based perfume created especially for him and packaged in long, narrow bottles, that could be stowed inside his battle boots. And perhaps Napoleon, in turn, had grown to love violets thanks to his first wife, Josephine de Beauharnais, who loved it so much to have it featured also at her wedding, in her bridesmaids' bouquets, and in the embroidery of her wedding dress.

Whatever the case may be, when Marie Louise moved to Parma (1816) following Napoleon's deposition and exile, she became forever associated with her love of violets. She used to wear them in a perfume especially created for her by the monks of the Convent of the SS. Annunziata, and it is said that she would give lavish alms to anyone who approached her offering her a bouquet of violets.

This passion inspired some long-sighted local entrepreneurs, who founded companies that were to become famous. The first of these was Lodovico Borsari.

Having separated from his partner Saccò, with whom he had opened a barber shop/artisan's laboratory, Lodovico Borsari founded the "Borsari" company, which was renamed "Borsari e Figli" (Borsari and Sons) few years later. The same extraordinary foresight that was driving François Coty's entrepreneurship in France was also driving Lodovico Borsari in Italy. He too had understood the importance of creating original, sophisticated perfumes, contained in exquisitely shaped bottles with coloured, golden, embossed labels decorated with fanciful Art Nouveau and Art Déco designs. The boxes were unusually shaped like the bottle they contained, and they were covered with paper produced using sophisticated techniques, and embellished with avant-garde graphics.

In order to obtain such refined products, Lodovico Borsari applied to the craft workshops that had been set up during Marie Louise's time in Parma. The presence of a Court governed by no less than the former Empress of France had made it necessary to develop a series of skills (boxmakers, glassware makers, printers) which, after half a century were still up-to-date and ready to support Borsari in the packaging of the most beautiful and refined products he could create. For the manufacturing of the glass bottles the choice fell on the "Bormioli" family company. The Bormiolis had settled in Parma a few decades earlier, founding a modern factory for the production of glassware. Actually, Bormioli had over two hundred years of experience in the glass sector, but it was only in Parma that it began focusing on perfume bottles, with rich, sophisticated, exquisitely ornated designs. The lucky partnership between Lodovico Borsari and Luigi Bormioli contributed enormously to the success and democratization of perfume, allowing both perfumery and glassware crafts to grow in the following decades. The "perfume+glassware" partnership was launched in the very same years in France, too: Francois Coty and René Lalique were joining forces gaining tremendous international success.

The perfumes themselves were composed personally by Lodovico. He had refined his artistic sensitivity in the years spent in the workshop attached to the barber shop, where he had been creating perfumed waters, lotions and talcum powders for a demanding

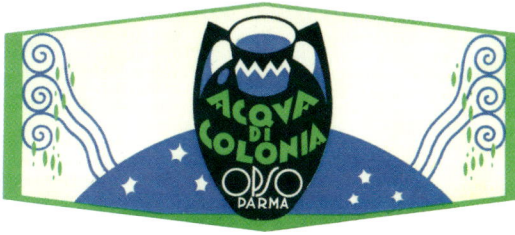
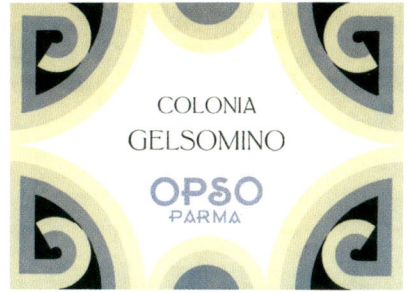
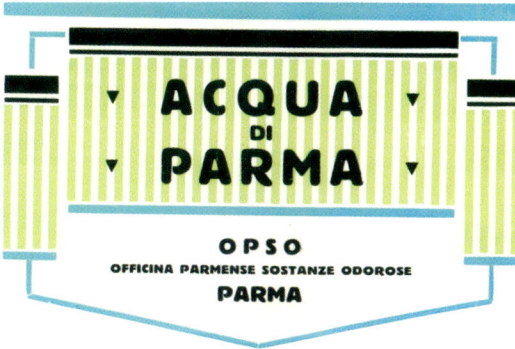
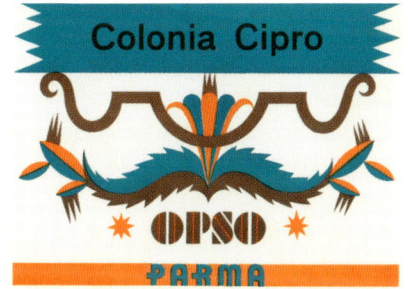

public, eager to replicated at home the pleasure of the treatments received at the barber's.

Borsari composed its perfumes from natural essences and ready-made synthetic bases, which made them more stable and persistent, but also more distinctive and "modern".

Eager to extend his clientele abroad, Lodovico Borsari decided to invest in the flower that was the symbol of his city: the violet. He managed to retrace the recipe for the essence that the monks in the Convent of the Annunziata used to make for Marie Louise. The recipe was then up-to-dated with the addition of innovative materials obtained in the laboratory –including ionones and irones. The result was simply named "Violetta di Parma". An entire line of toiletries was then created, including water, powder, soap, perfume. The "Violetta di Parma" permeated everything that could be fragranced, spreading around the distinctive essence of a brand, of a city, of a country.

Its success was so immediate and so overwhelming that, just a few years from its foundation, "Borsari", became the symbol of Italian perfume abroad, and one of Italy's most famous companies.

While Borsari was enjoying this success, another Parma-based company was following suit: O.P.S.O.

Founded at the end of the 19th century, O.P.S.O. distinguished itself right from the outset by producing perfumes inspired by Marie

Louise of Austria. O.P.S.O. was one of the first companies to invest in advertising as a commercial strategy, putting its faith in the illustrator Erberto Carboni for the creation of beautifully designed coloured plates perfectly conveying the creativity of its products to the international public.

Count Carlo Magnani, heir of an aristocratic family from Parma had a fresh, elegant cologne created under the name "Acqua di Parma". Acqua di Parma received numerous awards at the International Exhibitions and O.P.S.O. soon won the favour of the Royal House, which appointed it "Supplier of Her Majesty Queen Mother Margherita of Savoy". In the years that followed "Acqua di Parma" became a classic, receiving acknowledgements from Hollywood stars such as Ava Gardner and David Niven, who used it and spread its simple and discreet charm throughout the world and soon the bright-yellow oval cardboard box signed "Cavalieri & Amoretti" became an icon.

The existence in Italy of these worldwide famous companies acted as a driving force for the perfume industry as a whole. Not only for perfume manufacturers but also for their partners: raw materials producers, glassmakers, box factories, printers, paper mills, graphic designers and advertising agencies, followed by manufacturers of bottle tops, spray caps, subcontractors and distributors.

Thanks to the success of its entrepreneurs at the turn of the 20th century, Parma and its surrounding area became a fertile ground with the energy to sustain the development of the sector for the entire century.

The 20th century

During the 20th century, perfumery benefited greatly from the technical progress made in chemistry. French and Swiss laboratories discovered and patented hundreds of synthetically obtained odour molecules, which made perfumes not only more modern and abstract, but also less expensive.

Additionally, the technological innovations in the glass industry positively affected perfumery: the bottles began to be produced in series, at lower costs.

Thanks to these two factors, perfume became accessible also to less affluent population segments and the number of perfume brands on the market continued to grow.

At the 1901 Exposition Universelle in Paris, the atomizer (the spray) was presented, making it easier to dispense the fragrance directly from the bottle, thereby facilitating its use. But since raw materials particles tended to get trapped inside the nozzle, it often got blocked. So the ladies began diluting the essence with alcohol, and noticed that the perfume became lighter and fresher. And this is how the Eau de Parfum concentration was created!

The beginning of the 20th century witnessed the creation of two iconic Italian cosmetics products: "Borotalco" (produced since 1904 by a Florentine perfumer named Henry Roberts, who had entered into partnership with his colleague Roberto Manetti through the foundation of the "Manetti & Roberts" company) and "Felce Azzurra", which the company Paglieri from Alessandria began to produce in 1926, following the success of the Cologne with the same fragrance. Both of them are talcum powders, but have different fragrances: sweet/powdery the "Borotalco" bouquet, green/fougère the "Felce Azzurra". From then until well after the period following the Second World War, these two fragrances became entrenched in the cultural DNA of at least three generations.

In the meantime, the panorama of Italian perfumery was undergoing a fast development, with the founding of "Trionfale" and "La Ducale" in Parma, "Vidal" in Venice and "Carlo Erba" and "Gi.Vi.Emme" in Milan.

Vidal was founded in 1900 by Angelo Vidal, a Venetian operating in the production and trading of soap, lye and colonial goods from Oriental countries. In 1937 Vidal acquired an old perfumes and lotions manufacturing plant called "Longega", thereby diversifying its product range to include perfumes.

Carlo Erba, founded in Milan in 1853 as a pharmaceutical industry, was handed down from the father, Carlo, to his son, Luigi, around 1900.

Luigi set about broadening the Carlo Erba's product range – which already included articles for childcare and baby foods – by adding perfumes and toiletries. For the composition of the fragrances, Luigi Erba was assisted by his son-in-law, Giuseppe Visconti di Modrone, a cultured and refined Milanese gentleman with eclectic interests. This collaboration led to the creation of the iconic fragrances of that time such as "Contessa Azzurra", "Subdola" and "Dimmi di sì", which soon stole the hearts of the Italian ladies and kept them for many decades to come.

For the choice of the names of his perfumes, considerably more evocative and impactful than those of its competitors, Giuseppe could count on an excellent copywriter: his friend Gabriele d'Annunzio. The great poet was very interested in perfume. He wore perfumes,

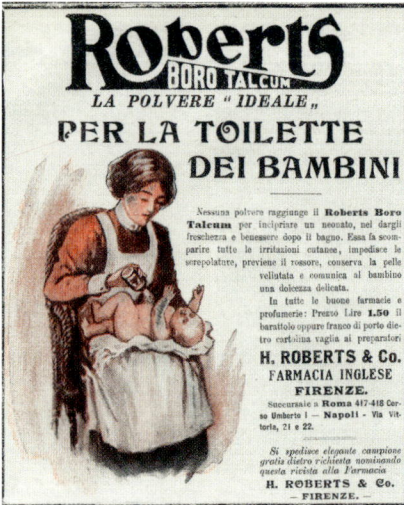

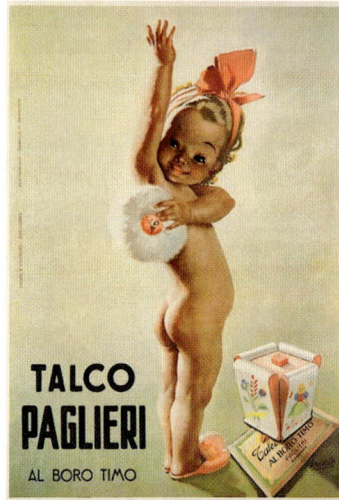

he collected them, considering them as much a delight for the senses and an expression of his own aesthetic sensitivity. He expressed his creative talent also in this field, not only by inventing names for his friend's perfumes, but also by creating fragrances of his own. Among these, "Aqua Nuntia", an elaboration of a formula found in an 18th century recipe book. Although the Poet had thought of everything – he even designed the bottle – "Aqua Nuntia" never managed to reach the public, remaining his own exclusive privilege. Its production was only launched eighty years later, at the initiative of the company Mavive, which admired the great poet and decided to pay him homage through the perfume that he himself had composed.

By the 1930s, Giuseppe Visconti di Modrone, now an accomplished perfume composer of great renown, had the wherewithal to pursue his adventure in perfumery without the support of his father-in-law. He acquired the fragrances composed for him and used them to found a company of his own: Gi.Vi.Emme.

Yet again, his refined aesthetic sense succeeded in producing memorable fragrances, such as "Giacinto Innamorato" in 1930, the first perfume to be composed on the basis of market research (the Gi.Vi.Emme laboratories had conducted a survey in order to discover the values and desires of the Italian women of the period). "Giacinto Innamorato" also owes its name to the Poet and, like many other perfumes produced for Carlo Erba before it, its success was staggering. In the 1930s, "Contessa Azzurra" and "Giacinto Innamorato" were two of the perfumes that Italian ladies loved and wore most.

Gi.Vi.Emme went on to produce other delights such as "Tabacco d'Harar" and "Acqua di Selva" as well as luxury face

28.
Perfume-sprayer
(20 cent coin),
in use in the
halls of cinemas,
around 1930.
Parma Color
Viola collection

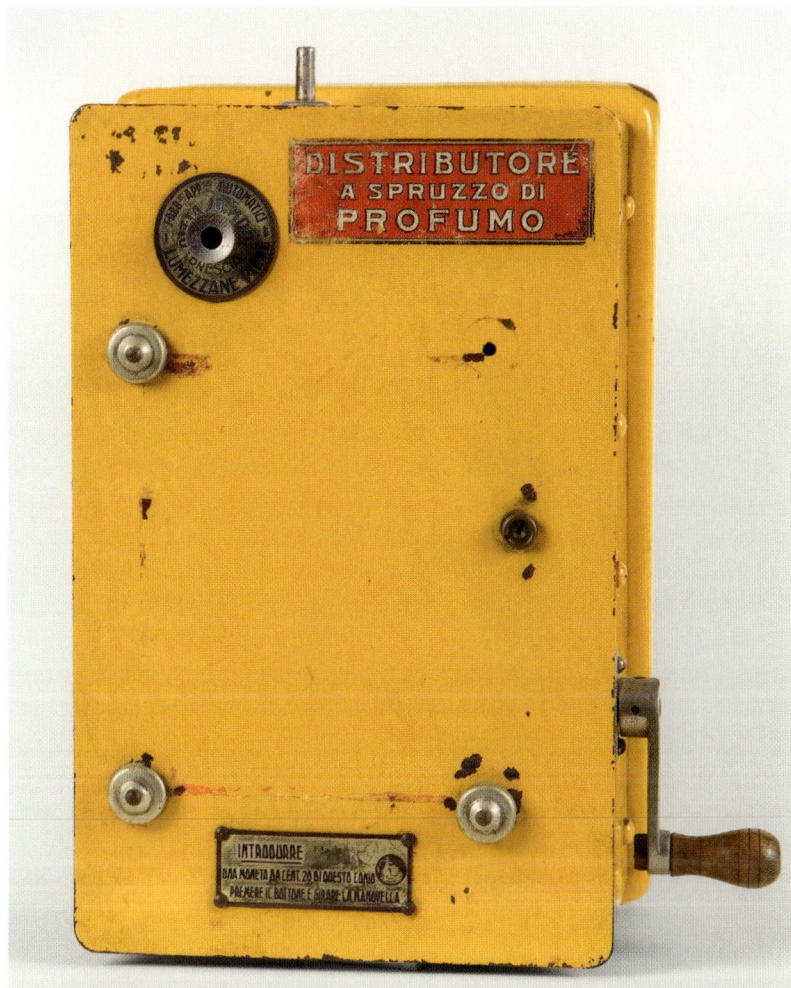

powders, lotions, brilliantine and other cosmetics perfumed with its most successful fragrances.

For the advertising campaign, Giuseppe sought out talented illustrators such as Loris Riccio, Edina Altara, and Marcello Dudovich, who masterfully interpreted many of the perfumes produced under this brand.

In 1949, in order to continue the activity launched by Gi.Vi. Emme the brand Victor was created, and acquired some historic perfumes (such as "Fresco" and "Victor"), which still exist today.

At the end of the First World War, Dario Usellini, founder of the brand Satinine, undertook a parallel perfume production activity under the name "Satinine Officina Odoraria", which he was to continue to develop in the following decades, also involving his three children.

In the 1930s, Satinine launched some successful perfumes, such as "Orchidea Nera" and "Caccia alla Volpe", packaged in precious glass bottles designed by "Vetrerie Bormioli".

By the 1940s, perfumes had practically become a part of everyday life for a large percentage of the Italian population, given the fact that distribution was widespread and prices affordable. But if an occasion required the wearing of perfume and the Lady were to find herself temporarily in need, a solution was at hand. Automatic perfume dispensing machines had begun to spring up at cinemas and theatres, containing a selection of two or three perfumes that, for a few cents, would be sprayed to the Lady's wrists and neck.

The perfumes made in that period contained those new synthetic molecules which were becoming increasingly more popular with perfume composers thanks to their greater stability, lower costs and the possibility to further expand the creators' expressive possibilities. So the simple, standardised recipes for traditional perfumes became more structured, more evocative. The figurative approach so dear to the 19th century, with its flowering gardens and dewy violets, had, at this stage, run its course, and perfume was heading towards the abstract dimension typical of contemporary perfumery.

While the use of perfume, cologne, lotions, scented water and such like was spreading fast among ladies of all social backgrounds, the masculine relationship with perfume was still limited to two modes of interaction; the use of brilliantine and aftershave.

Brilliantine was an oily product which kept unruly hair under control while perfuming it and giving it a glossy finish; brillantine guaranteed the gentlemen a well-groomed, reassuring look (e.g. before going out my grandfather would invariably oil his comb in brilliantine and run it through his hair – still jet black despite his being over eighty).

Some particularly famous brands of brilliantine smelt of lavender, while others had a fougère scent. It was, in any case, always a fresh, rustic, grassy scent which, with daily use, became a root of the olfactory culture of Italian men and women: still today in Italy lavender, rosemary and other herbs are unquestionably associated with men's perfume!

The second mode of interaction was a consequence of the Gent's visit at least once a week to the barber's shop. After shaving, the customers' skin would be disinfected and perfumed with Eau de Cologne, which might have a citrus scent or the same aromatic or fougère fragrance of the most fashionable brilliantines. The aftershave fragrance attested, beyond a shadow of a doubt, to a visit to the barber's, and hence to its wearer's interest in being well-groomed and his consideration for other people.

Even after so many decades, elderly gentlemen still tend to call men's perfume "aftershave". It has taken many years to separate the idea of men wearing perfume from that of applying a scented after shave product, and in fact, it has only come about in recent years, with the younger generations.

Another thing the barber shops used to do was to give men of all ages the gift of a scented almanac each year. These almanacs were made with a special kind of paper that would absorb perfume and release it gradually into the environment. The subjects depicted in the almanacs were mostly Hollywood actresses, theatre starlets, opera singers and... pin-ups portrayed in mischievous poses, which made them a little "spicy", and reserved for adult clients. But they also contained news on sport, music, history and literature. In some cases the drawings were done by the most famous illustrators and artists of the period. These almanacs gained pride of place in the hearts of the Italians, withstanding the test of time, so much so that they are still ardently sought after by collectors today (although, of course, the fragrance is long gone!).

In 1950, the company Vidal, capitalising on the acquisition of Longega some years earlier, launched a fragrance that soon entered the collective imagination of the Italians like none other before it: "Pino Silvestre". To advertise this perfume a testimonial was used for the first time: the movie star Amedeo Nazzari, who appealed to men and women alike, arousing the former's admiration and the latter's lovesick sighs. But the real stroke of genius was the advertisement created a few years later for the bath product line, showing the famous white horse galloping wild across the prairie. This image penetrated deeply into the collective imagination of Italy, contributing immensely to the commercial success of the product, which is still on the market today.

The period from the 1950s to the 1970s saw the founding of a number of companies that played a strategic role in the worldwide success of the Italian perfumes of the 1970s, 1980s and 1990s: ICR owned by the Martone family in Milan, and Adam, Morris, Italart and Florbath in Parma.

Among Adam's first successes was "Schu", the perfume that Emilio Schuberth commissioned in 1955 for his fashion house. With "Schu" (which was followed by "Coquillage" and "Taffetas"), the stylist's intention was to make ladies smell as elegantly as they looked. His success made him so famous that he appeared, together with Sorelle Fontana, among the costume designers of the most iconic film of the time: Federico Fellini's *La Dolce Vita*. Schuberth commissioned the great Italian-French illustrator René Gruau to create the promotional image for his iconic perfume. That was Gruau's more prolific period; the illustrator was at the height of his artistic production and talent, working for international brands such as Christian Dior.

In the 1970s, other Italian fashion designers began to realise the potential of perfume as a generator of business and a strategy for gaining visibility: Nino Cerruti, Gucci, Genny, Fiorucci and Mila Schön were the first to venture into the perfume market.

Morris Profumi was founded in 1946 by Giuseppe Borri. Among its most successful fragrances was "Ingrid" (1948), inspired by Ingrid Bergman's voluptuous beauty.

Italart was founded in 1957 by Attilio Tanzi, while Florbath was found in the 70s from the merger of two historic companies from Parma: "Trionfale" owned by the Sanguinetti family and "Ducale" owned by the Bordi family.

Their first partnerships with Italian designers for the creation and marketing of perfumes were the result of the foresight of these companies. The first agreements were signed between ICR and Trussardi; between Florbath and Krizia and then with Sorelle Fendi; between Morris and Mila Schön and then La Perla. Within a few years, all the leading Italian fashion houses had placed their trust in these companies to launch fragrances intended as olfactory extensions of their *couture*.

From the 1980s till the end of the 1990s, the main licensees of fashion brands were:

- Angelini Beauty (founded in the 1990s); it acquired from ITS and from the Spanish company Idesa the manufacturing licences for Blumarine, Mandarina Duck, Laura Biagiotti, Gianfranco Ferré and Angel Schlessler.
- Copra-Satinine (later merged with Lancetti) held the manufacturing and sales licence for Borsalino and Ferrari.
- Diana de Silva (Gianfranco Ferré, Genny).
- Eurocosmesi (Les Copains, Mariella Burani, Iceberg, Brooksfield).
- Euroitalia (Moschino, Naj Oleari, Coveri, Dolce & Gabbana).
- Florbath (Krizia, Fendi, Fiorucci).
- ICR/ITS (Trussardi and Gianni Versace, who after a few years decided to take over the production of the perfumes themselves).
- Italart (Battistoni and RoccoBarocco)

- Morris (La Perla and Grigioperla, Sergio Tacchini, Mila Schön, Ducati, Ferrari and Breil; Fendi and Krizia were later acquired by Florbath and Genny by Diana de Silva).
- Proteo (Romeo Gigli and Alberta Ferretti).
- Schiapparelli-Pikenz, later renamed Pikenz-The First and then The First (Arrogance, Annabella, Parah and Lancetti).
- Sirpea (Benetton, Basile, Pomellato).
- Weruska & Joel (Capucci, Renato Balestra, Roberta di Camerino, Nazareno Gabrielli).

This list does not include Valentino and Giorgio Armani, whose licences were already foreign property.

The companies that kept the perfume production in-house, or transferred it to companies under their direct control were: Borsari, Bulgari, Etro, Ferragamo, Gianni Versace (through Giver), Pupa (through Micys), Rancé, Trussardi, Vidal (later renamed Mavive).

The licensee companies (such as Morris, ICR, Florbath and the others) would work alongside the brands studying perfumes with the power to express their aesthetic vision, values and desires. Then they would evaluate the perfume drafts made by the international fragrance companies (Firmenich, IFF, Quest, etc.) and sign the one they consider most suitable. The real creative work would begin at this stage, with the creative team of the fragrance company on the one hand, the brand on the other and the licensee in the middle, directing the perfumer's creativity according the requests made by the brand. What made the Italian fragrances of this period so extraordinary was the surprising consistency of style between fashion and perfume – no mean feat – achieved thanks to the harmonious combination of talented composers and brands with strong ideas. The whole ensemble being orchestrated by the licensees' esperience.

Thanks to this level of cooperation, in the course of ten years the economic success of the entire Italian perfume industry reached heights, in terms of both appreciation and revenue, that were not so far removed from the French. Many of the companies involved capitalised on their results, becoming attractive partners also on an international scale.

For example, the ICR group is, today, the most important subcontractor in Europe, producing eighty-five million bottles per year for all the most prestigious brands, such as Angelini Beauty, Blumarine, Bulgari, Collistar, Eau d'Italie, Emanuel Ungaro, Gai Mattiolo, Gianfranco Ferré, Intimissimi, Laura Biagiotti, Lord, OVS, Salvatore Ferragamo, Shaka, Tezenis, Trussardi, Altaia.

Another success story is that of Bormioli Luigi: still firmly in the hands of the Bormioli family, the company controls almost a quarter of the world's glassware market for the fine perfumery sector, with extremely innovative bottles being produced for brands in every continent.

The 2000s

At the turn of the century, the top fashion brands were acquired by large foreign groups.

The companies holding production and marketing licences for their perfumes were also acquired by large groups – mostly investment funds, multinationals specialising in pharmaceuticals, detergents or the food sector. The new owners, with no firm grounding in the perfumery industry (nor were they interested in fully understanding what they had purchased) focused on growth targets – usually short-term. Managers of these multinationals treated perfumes in exactly the same way as all the other products in their *portfolio*.

The cultural features that had previously generated extraordinarily creative fragrances, real ambassadors of good taste, conveying the essence of Italian-ness, were set aside, in favour of a "taste globalisation" imposed by the need to sell products in dozens of different countries throughout the world.

From the late 1990s on, perfumes had to be developed in a matter of months, launches followed on each other's heels in order to keep the public's attention high and capitalise on the initial investment.

In this new standardised market, major consumers of perfumes began to feel nostalgic for the interesting and distinctive perfumes that they had been used to. They began to venture outside of the "traditional" perfumery in pursuit of fresh inspiration and new vibrations, and they were welcomed by a handful of small craft enterprises, which still saw perfumes, first and foremost, as a means of expression. Their founders were dissatisfied with the dominant role played by marketing, and with the overwhelming power of the multinationals, having created their own small companies with a very different approach in mind. Thanks to their compact dimensions and strong personal imprint, these companies managed to fill the creative niche that industry had vacated, attracting droves of customers who had finally found that freedom of expression and "Italian-ness" that was difficult to find elsewhere.

Among these new, "niche" brands there were the mediaeval apothecaries of Santa Maria Novella and Farmacia SS. Annunziata, some other successful "historic" brands, such as Borsari and Acqua di Parma, together with a bunch of pioneers who opened business in those years, such as Bruno Acampora, Etro, Lorenzo Villoresi, Carthusia, BOIS (Bottega Italiana dello Spigo), Nobile 1942, Eau d'Italie, Laura Tonatto, Calé, followed a decade later by Xerjoff-Casamorati, Maria Candida Gentile, Nasomatto, Antonio Alessandria, Meo Fusciuni, Nobile 1942, Laboratorio Olfattivo, Nu_Be, Homoelegans, Masque Milano, Orto Parisi, Francesca Bianchi, Gabriella Chieffo, Uermì and many more, who are still successfully conveying the traditional values of Italian perfumery, sometimes modernising them, other times taking them to extremes, but always following the cultural path that sets us apart.

The olfactory delights these Companies created and launched to an international public of enthusiasts may be seen as the ideal prosecution of a rich and captivating cultural history lasted over a millennium. The soil in which these works are rooted nourished the ancient Romans, too, as well as the mediaeval Spice Merchants, the perfumers of the Renaissance Courts, the 19th century Parma, the great fashion designers of the 1980's, and it is a soil fertilized by creativity, daring attitude, communication skills and joie de vivre. And by a culture of Beauty that will never lose its appeal.

The Italian-style essence

When it comes to perfume, words can only go so far: the best solution is always to test it first-hand.

When we sniff, our brain recognises concepts that it would not be able to grasp through words alone. So I suggest that you seek out and smell the perfumes presented in this book, so as to become aware that there actually are attributes characterising Italian perfumes and differentiating them from those produced by other cultures.

And that these are not even so difficult to recognise, if you know what to look for.

In order to better understand the characteristics shared by perfumes composed for Italian brands, it is essential to keep in mind some fundamental elements of Italy's culture and aesthetic sensitivity:

- a distinct sensuality, i.e. the pursuit of sensations that can gratify the senses;
- a complex aesthetic, refined during hundreds of years of a visual culture bringing together Giotto, Leonardo, Caravaggio, Brunelleschi, Donatello and all the great geniuses of the past, whom Italian children study at school and whose work surrounds them as they stroll in any city of the Peninsula;

• a propensity for communication and social relations, man- ifested in the pleasure of meeting, talking and convivial interaction.

Each of these elements is the result of a sensitivity evolved over the course of centuries and which has a direct effect on many aspects of our lives and our preferences, whether we realise it or not.

Gratifying the senses

Italian perfumes all share the mission to gratify their wearer's senses. Although Italians love challenging, eccentric or unconventional fra- grances, the ones we find most congenial are those that are instantly captivating. Too cerebral scents, taking too much time to be deci- phered are not in line with the expectations of a nation that wears perfume for the sake of pleasure... what Italians like about wearing perfume is the pleasure that the fragrance itself can covey. And this pleasure must pop up as soon as possible and last as long as possible.

The materials triggering an immediate pleasure are vigorous and exhilarating citrus notes such as orange, bergamot, mandarin, lemon, ripe round fruity notes, rich, opulent flowers such as jasmine, rose, carnation and orange blossom.

Also aromatic notes such as lavender, rosemary, sage, basil and juniper are close to our taste: they are part of our daily land- scape and, above all, of our Italian gastronomical culture.

The texture: i.e. roundness, fullness, three-dimensionality

Anything diaphanous, flimsy, whispered, evanescent or rarefied does not reflect our tastes. It may surprise us momentarily, for a change, but we inevitably tire of it. Even the "white musk/clean fragrance" Gender of perfume could never have originated in Italy: we are a people accustomed to the sumptuous naked flesh of Michelangelo, to the velvety complexions of Raphael's women... We love rotundi- ty, full breasts and buttocks, like those of Sophia Loren or Monica Bellucci, generous embodiments of Italian beauty, generous, full and sensual. You look and you are tempted to touch. And we Italians like to touch. A lot.

When it comes to perfume, we are seduced by sensations of "living", pulsating three-dimensionality, an unparalleled tactile quality that can also be defined "texture". Perhaps the fact that the bright- est stars in the Italian perfume industry have been predominantly fashion designers for so long, has led to the development of an olfactory culture characterised by strong textural elements.

The fragrances express this trait with their rich floral tones such as rose, jasmine, carnation, tuberose, orange blossom, hyacinth, freesia and honeysuckle, which, already through their honey scent, reveal the sumptuousness of the fleshy petals. But also with rich, sensual animalic notes, such as civet, castoreum, natural musk, grey amber and the modern note of oud, woody but endowed with a powerfully animalic nuance.

The notes must be orchestrated in a complex, well-structured manner to create a well-defined tactile sensation, resembling the touch of a soft, voluptuous material like fur, or the dry roughness of tweed or the fluid slipperiness of satin, or the clean crispness of a freshly ironed linen shirt.

But there are fragrances that are even more abstract, the materiality of which recalls the texture of a cold rock, or a cloud of primitive gas. In any case, on smelling an Italian perfume, the word that often comes to mind, is in fact "texture".

Taste as inspiration

Many Italian perfumes draw inspiration from gastronomy. When I use the term "gastronomy", I am not referring to high-calorie desserts, but to complex taste sensations: exotic spices, candied citrus peel, fine liqueurs, elaborate cocktails, black olive pâté, basil ice cream, rose liqueurs, shellfish salads, precious smoked teas, spicy panforte... Only a nation with a visceral love of food, a nation that has always experimented with its infinite expressive possibilities, elevating it to unattainable cultural heights, can add it to its perfumes in such an audacious and convincing manner. Our fragrances are enriched by many notes reminiscent of food or wine, offering original slants and surprising sensations, without deteriorating into the "sweet, dull, boring" cliché typical of perfumes composed for other populations with less complex taste.

The visual aesthetic: a richly detailed sfumato

Leonardo da Vinci had observed how demarcating the surfaces of things with too sharp lines tended to render them almost caricature-like in their lack of nuance. So with the intention of rendering the outlines of his portrays less clear-cut, Leonardo made the outlines disappear, replacing them with an infinite number of delicate, overlapping chiaroscuro strokes. Thanks to his sfumato technique, his figures emerge from their background with a kindly friendliness, not with the violence of sharp lines, but revealing – or concealing – their innermost essence. Sfumato – whether it be in perfumery or in painting – is the exact opposite of the strictly dualistic school of thought, which sees everything either all black or all white, all right or all wrong, cleanly axe-cut, and without second thoughts. Dualistic thinking is perennially seeking absolute certainties and if on the one hand this could make life simpler, on the other it prevents an authentic representation of more complex realities.

Italians, on the other hand, love complexity. We have it in our DNA: we are intricate, individualistic, our hearts are capable of accomodating all the opposites; and so are the perfumes that most represent us. The contours of Italian fragrances are rarely clear-cut, so much so that at times it is difficult to classify them in a distinct olfactive family. The accords of which they are composed dissolve into one another, slowly and deliberately, or sometimes they lie in layers one on top of the other in a web of sensations that make the perfumes dense, structured, rich with a thousand nuances and interesting details which literally "pull you in".

Occasionally, complexity becomes apparent as an under-current, a colour or an olfactory sensation passing through the fragrance, creating a contrast with all the rest of the composition, acting in the same way as a wacky detail – seemingly out of place, but which attracts attention – upgrades an outfit that would, otherwise, be boring or dull.

Effervescent communication

One of the things that most strikes foreign visitors to Italy is the spectacular beauty of our squares. From the Roman Forum on, our squares have always represented the beating heart of our civilisation, the place where Italians of every era have come together to communicate: to celebrate, to listen, to learn, to rebel, to plan and nowadays, even just to have a seat and enjoy a long aperitif in the company of friends. These town squares and the love of lively communication have coexisted for centuries in our DNA, benefiting from a mild climate and gentle Nature. And it could not be otherwise, given that Italy is a peninsula facing – literally stretching out into – the sea, which has always been open to welcoming different stimuli and cultures.

And in fact the perfume that best represents us is full of vibrant, sparkling top notes conveying their message immediately and bringing to mind relaxed, informal outdoors encounters, friendly chats and good cheers.

Even the very structure of the perfumes expresses a propensity for exuberance, through pyramids in which the top and heart accords account for almost the entire fragrance and the base accord often serves only to support and give structure to the dialogue established between the top and the heart.

Far from being delicate and evanescent, Italian fragrances radiate with confidence, spreading their message around their wearer for several hours. Most of the time the scented bubble they create is not large enough to bother others... but it is certainly present.

Open, exuberant, sunny, immediate, communicative, sensual, exquisite, sparkling... what makes the fragrances produced for Italian brands recognizable are the same characteristics that make any expression of our civilization sound "Italian": openness, communication, sensuality, love of Beauty, but first and foremost, a vibrant complexity, capable of conveying all the infinite facets of the human soul.

70

The Great Italian Perfumes
of the 1970s

The social and cultural background

In the 1970–1980 decade, Italian society was engaged in a historic transition, on several fronts. One of these concerned the progressive abandonment of the rural areas: a third of the Italian population moved to the cities to work in industry and the tertiary sector, transforming a traditionally agricultural nation into an industrial one.

The second transition concerned the role of women in society: the introduction of divorce (1970), of the voluntary interruption of pregnancy (1978) and the reform of family law (1975) endorsed, also from a legal standpoint, the sweeping changes that were taking place in society and that were to bring about, notwithstanding difficulties and resistance, the identification of women as political subjects and their emancipation from the roles traditionally assigned to them by patriarchal society.

The 1970s were years of instability and crisis also from an economic perspective. Due to austerity policies, the population was subjected to energy consumption measures which, although non excessively invasive, made the people aware nonetheless of the fragility of an economic and production system entirely dependent on oil.

This already precarious social context was then further jeopardised by the terrorist activities of the Brigate Rosse, which fomented a climate of uneasiness and suspicion.

Notwithstanding the feeling of uncertainty that was pervading Italian society, its businesses began to gain unprecedented success on foreign markets: from clothing to design objects, from food to jewellery, from shoes to sports cars, Made in Italy labels began to be coveted all over the world, as a symbol of style and elegance.

Fashion took on the task of reflecting the strongest social demands of the moment, and clothing became a way of standing out from the crowd and communicating one's own essence. Some fashion trends bore eloquent witness to the social changes in progress: the feminism of the multitasking working woman, the neo-romantic style of the romantic woman, still attached to traditional values, the iconoclastic punk of the younger generation, the rowdy, off the wall vitality of the newly-founded gay movement.

International perfumery

The fashionable perfumes of this decade were strongly influenced by all these styles: some featured green, floral notes typical of the Flower Power movement (Chloé, 1975), others evoked sensations of freshness and cleanness aimed at the romantic dreamer ("White Linen" by Estée Lauder, 1978, "Anaïs Anaïs" by Cacharel, 1979), rich floral notes alongside aldehydes, gave some fragrances great personality and structure, ideal for career women with clear ideas and little time to spare ("Rive Gauche" by Yves Saint Laurent, 1971, "Charlie" by Revlon, 1973, "First" by Van Cleef & Arpels, 1976).

Still others tended towards citrusy notes, evoking the natural, fresh sensations of outdoor life ("Ô de Lancôme", 1969, "Eau de Rochas", 1970).

Last but not least, the impact of disco music, the discovery of drugs and a predilection for the forbidden, for the Orient and for a sensuality bordering on the illegal, was the inspiration behind perfumes such as "Cinnabar" by Estée Lauder, "Magie Noire" by Lancôme, "Opium" by Yves Saint Laurent, "Mystère" by Rochas (all released between 1977 and 1978) and other floral Orientals with a strong spicy imprint.

Men too began to show interest in perfume, learning to distinguish aftershave from true perfume. Marketing strategies bombarded these new potential consumers with products such as "Monsieur Rochas" (1969), "Gentleman" (Givenchy, 1974), "Capitan" (Molyneux, 1975), the names of which evoked an indisputable masculinity, entitling the European man to take care of his own well-being and his own image in an unprecedented manner.

Between 1969 and 1977, some new synthetic materials were discovered that were to leave an indelible imprint on the perfumes launched twenty years later: in 1969 Ethyl Maltol (the sweet milk note in "Angel" by Thierry Mugler, 1992), in 1973 Helional (the aquatic/floral note in "L'Eau d'Issey" by Issey Miyake, 1992); in 1976 IsoESuper (the floral/musky note with a strong grassy nuance of Dolce&Gabbana "Light Blue", 2001); in 1977 Floralozone, the floral, crystal clear, aquatic note in "Acqua di Giò" (Giorgio Armani, 1996).

In Italy

Perfume was widely available in Italy; Italians tended to use perfumes of Italian production (Paglieri, Gi.Vi.Emme, Borsari, Capucci, Schubert etc.); French, English and American perfumes (Chanel, Christian Dior, Fabergé, Rochas, Atkinson's, Revlon) were equally acclaimed and sought after, but not everyone could afford them.

Feminine fragrances belonged first and foremost to the floral aldehydic and chypre families, while masculine fragrances tended to opt for classic, reassuring fougère notes.

Towards the end of the decade, a group of well-established fashion designers decided to introduce perfume as an olfactory ambassador of their brands: Gucci, Mila Schön, Nino Cerruti, Fiorucci were among the first to discern, in perfume, the path to visibility and economic success.

Their entrepreneurial audacity will give rise not only to interesting fragrances – the perfect Made in Italy ambassadors – but will also pave the way to the great successes of the following years.

Gucci N° 1

Brand: Gucci
Gender: feminine
Year of launch: 1974
Status: discontinued
Analyzed version: original Eau de Toilette
Author: Guy Robert
Classification: floral aldehydic

"Gucci N°1" is the perfect example of the rich, complex 1970s structure, characterised by rich floral notes such as carnation and and jasmine, associated with the lustrous brilliance of aldehydes and a green accent running through, and contrasting, all the main accords from top to base.

"Gucci N°1" opens with an explosion of white, rarefied aldehydes, sparking off a floral bouquet with a tender heart graced with green notes of hyacinth, lily of the valley, lilac and geranium. As the minutes pass, a carnation-jasmine-ylang ylang accord of great personality and impact emerges from the centre of the bouquet. This accord lasts powerfully for half an hour; it is gradually joined by a dry, austere oak moss note and the softest ever amber base, which takes a good hour to fully express itself, and then last indefinitely.

The three phases during which this fragrance develops (bright opening, floral heart, ambery base) are well stitched together, the fragrance glides smoothly from one to the next with extreme naturalness.

"Gucci N°1" shows a complex and resounding personality – anticipating the great sculptural fragrances of the 1980s – and yet, it is not intrusive, thanks to a formula balanced to the finest degree to achieve richness and sophistication, without the pomp and circumstance generally associated with it. Real luxury, no ostentation.

This perfume is a creation of the legendary Guy Robert. "Gucci N°1" exemplifies his predilection for structured, multifaceted and yet exquisitely delicate formulas: a rare and precious feature which has become a new trend in these modern times. Perfumes authored by Guy Robert are declarations of formal elegance, achieved through raw materials of exquisite beauty, such as bright aldehydes ("Calèche" by Hermès) exuberant floral bouquets rich in personality ("Madame Rochas", "Amouage Gold"), natural, delicate green notes ("Chanel N°19").

"Gucci N°1" perfectly illustrates his famous mantra: *"Un parfum doit avant tout sentir bon"* (a perfume should first and foremost smell good). Although it was discontinued some time ago, "Gucci N°1" can still be found, usually in good conditions. If you love classic floral aldehydics such as "Calèche", "Amouage Gold" and refined, feminine bouquets immersed in liquid gold, definitely seek it out!

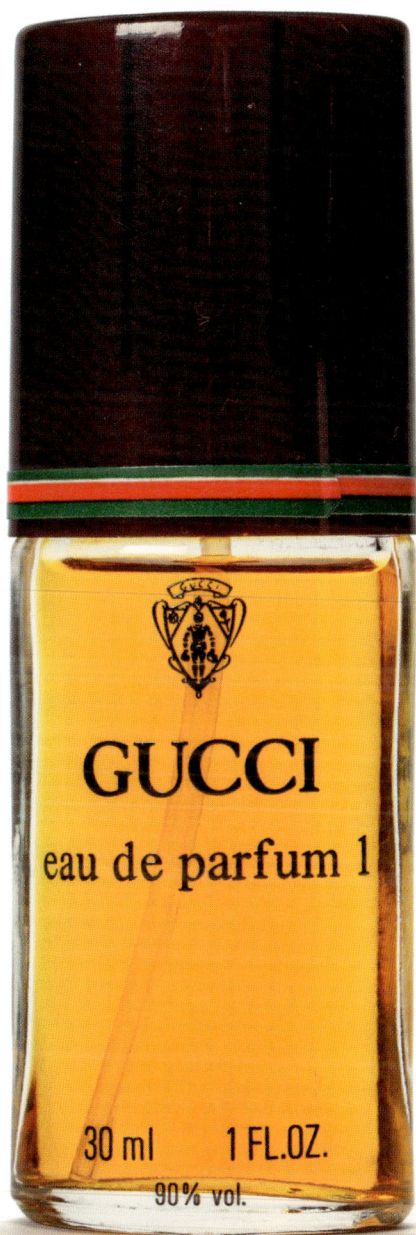

GUCCI

eau de parfum 1

30 ml   1 FL.OZ.

90% vol.

Yendi

Brand: Capucci
Gender: feminine
Year of launch: 1974
Status: discontinued
Analyzed version: original Eau de Toilette
Classification: floral chypre

Roberto Capucci, a pioneer of Italian Haute Couture, was among the first to consider perfume as complementary to his *couture* launching, as far back as the 1960s, a range of fragrances for men and women, that were very successful. "Yendi", released in 1974 for a female target, is a surprising hybrid of floral with green nuances, a descendent of "Vent Vert" (Balmain, 1947) and a classic example of the typically 1970s lush green chypre ("Chanel N°19", 1971; "Diorella", 1972 and "Alliage" by Estée Lauder, 1972). Green chypres share a compositional structure of great charm and delicacy that was to continue until the 1980s with "Ivoire" (Balmain, 1979) and Jean Louis Scherrer (1980) and which, unfortunately, was ultimately discontinued due to international restrictions on the use of certain raw materials.

With respect to its above-mentioned forerunners and successors, "Yendi" plays the role of the younger sister: naive, fresh, sincere and full of promise. Characteristics which, for a chypre, are by no means obvious, and make "Yendi" totally unique.

"Yendi" opens with a bouquet of emerald-coloured flowers (hyacinth, cyclamen, lily of the valley, rose) ushered in by bergamot and cloves and ignited by the brightness of clean aldehydes (among which the peach-scented C-12). A honey note develops around the flowers half an hour from application, contributing gracefulness and "gentleness" to the whole green bouquet. Amber notes emerging from the base (benzoin, iris and oak moss), bring "Yendi" towards a rounder, more mature chypre, without marring its adorable, innocent brio. This evolution makes "Yendi" a lesson in balance; it evolves smoothly and without contrasts for its entire length (six full hours), with a satisfying sillage enveloping the wearer in a sophisticated, green, retro aura. Today, "Yendi" may sound rather dated, even if surprisingly less so than other perfumes released in the following decades.

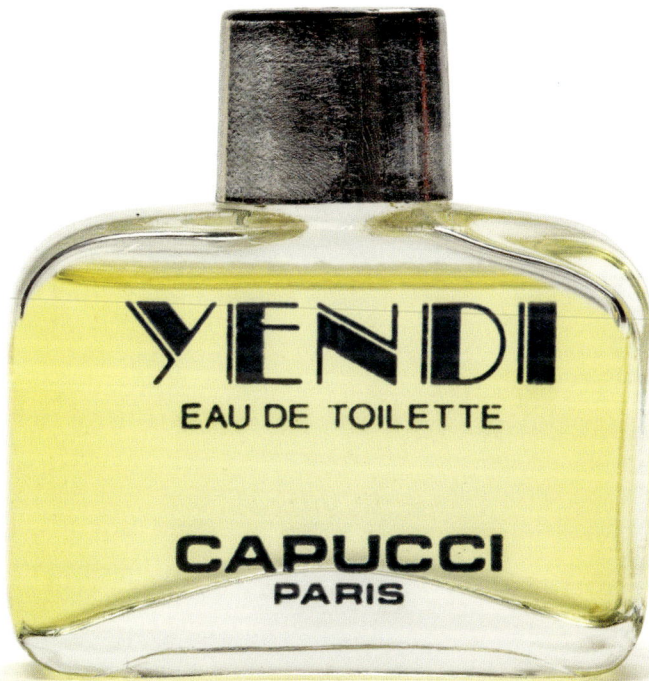

Musc

Brand: Bruno Acampora
Gender: unisex
Year of launch: 1975
Status: in production
Analyzed version: original perfume oil
Classification: floral oriental

Anyone convinced that "niche" concept was created in France needs to have a closer look at Bruno Acampora's story, because the same idea of "alternative perfumery" that led the great Jean Laporte to found L'Artisan Parfumeur in the late 1970s, had already been realized by Bruno Acampora a few years earlier. It was 1975 when Bruno Acampora, an eclectic Neapolitan gentleman founded the company, and composed the first seven perfumes (among which "Musc") in order to share the memories and emotions of his trips around the world. As the years passed, the production continued without any other fragrances being added, and without any advertising, since Bruno preferred the real Luxury of "handmade" products and a very small production, reserved for those who sought genuine emotions. During the early 2000s, Bruno's son Brunello took over the brand and decided that the time had come to develop it. Meanwhile, "Musc"'s appreciation had been increasing over the decades. In addition to the enthusiastic reviews of its aficionados, who kept raving about it until they had made it famous throughout the world, in 2016 the Christmas edition of the "Sunday Times" published it among the five most sensual perfumes of all time. And "Musc" is not, by any means, a fragrance for the faint of heart: generous, exuberant to the point of audacity, it works by adding layers, which stratify to form a thick and impenetrable lattice, in which the notes melt into one another and are no longer singly perceptible. It opens with an imposing musky vegetal note bringing to mind the scents of a wood. In the still, silent dimness, the trees exhale a sweet, warm scent of wet earth, rotting leaves, newborn mushrooms. A rose note develops inside this sensation from the heart onwards, reaching heights of three-dimensionality never explored before. A dry note of clove adds a - very mild - contrast. When all this richness reaches its peak, the base notes begin to emerge: warm, amber, velvety sandalwood and patchouli, enhanced with resins and with an animalic note that recalls civet musk. The base notes envelope the floral heart and the perfume, as a whole, resonates as opaque, earthy, erotic, vibrant for hours, for days... forever.
The pure oil essence is the ideal way to envelope the wearer into a magnificent sillage. its projection is powerful, instantly recognisable, making an unforgettable scented signature.

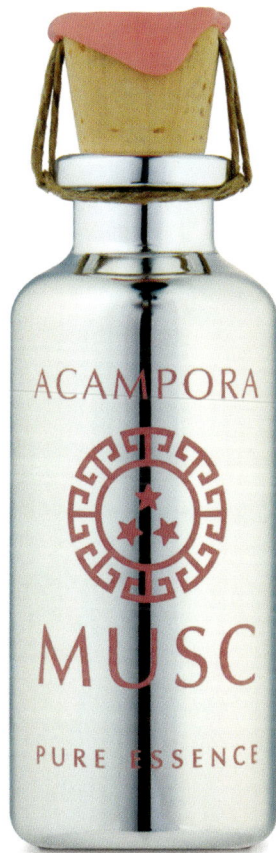

Valentino

Brand: Valentino
Gender: feminine
Year of launch: 1978
Status: discontinued
Analyzed version: original Eau de Toilette
Classification: rich floral
Author: Givaudan
Bottle design: Atelier Dinand

The stylistic consistency between perfume and couture shown by Italian fashion designers in the 1970s and 1980s never ceases to amaze me, and Valentino is no exception. The first perfume launched by this worldwide-venerated designer is a textbook example of the heights that can be attained when the artist's personality is strong enough to permeate all of his creations. "Valentino" – the perfume – is, to all intents and purposes, the son of Valentino – the designer –, and this is immediately evident from the red V printed on the box ("Valentino red", of course), the splendid frosted glass bottle designed by Atelier Dinand and, last but not least, the perfume itself, graceful, feminine and elegant, especially crafted to turn Women into Goddesses. Valentino opens delicately, with a splash of citrus and green notes which welcoming a very traditional floral accord of jasmine and rose, caressed by a gentle, exhilarating, almost summery breeze of neroli with a fruity note of melon. The floral bouquet is further refined by aldehyde c-12, whose peachy tang adds roundness and a velvety feel to the whole fragrance.

The amber and woody notes (sandal and cedarwood) of the base cling to the skin delicately yet decisively. Valentino is not intrusive, neither is it "fur-clad": the "Grande Dame" effect that we might expect from a floral fragrance launched in 1978 is light-years away from this gem, still delightful today, both in formal occasions and leisure time.

The intrinsic quality of the perfumes that acquire the status of "Great Classics" resides in measure, and in the wise use of raw materials to evoke harmony and good taste. Such fragrances have interesting stories to tell in any period: "Valentino", like "Amazone" (Hermès, 1973), "1000-Mille" (Patou, 1972) and a few other classics with a floral bouquet, simple refuse to grow old. If you get the chance, don't miss it.

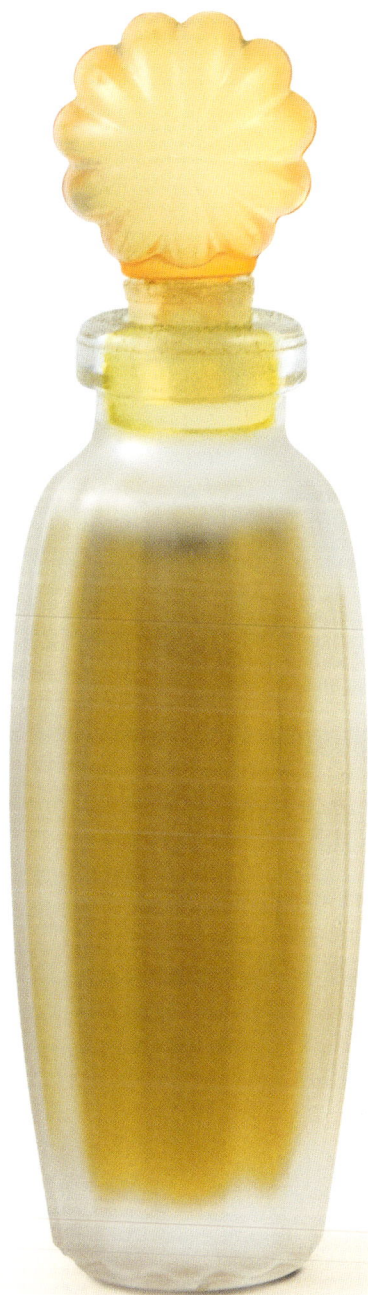

Nino Cerruti

Brand: Nino Cerruti
Gender: masculine
Year of launch: 1979
Status: discontinued in 1999
Analyzed version: original Eau de Toilette
Author: Jean Claude Delville (Firmenich)
Classification: woody aromatic

"Nino Cerruti" was the first perfume launched by the former Lanificio Fratelli Cerruti, a business founded in Biella at the end of the 1800s, which, thanks to Nino's creativity and long-sightedness, was to become one of the most prestigious Italian Fashion Houses of the 1980s and 1990s.

The fact that "Nino Cerruti" is no longer in production is a real pity, because it contained the precise doses of class, style and irony that are lacking from so many of today's masculine fragrances. This was achieved through a well-balanced formula of classic structure, enriched with splendid natural notes, and with an open, relaxed feel that was quite irresistible.

A fleeting sparkle of citrus fruits gives way to a bouquet of aromatic herbs reminiscent of a summer stroll along the Italian Riviera. Basil, tarragon, artemisia, mint and thyme, make-up a traditional accord in male perfumery, still holding its own brilliantly today. The aromatic bouquet is flanked by a floral heart of carnation and jasmine, whose greenest aspects are underlined by the aromatic herbs. A dusting of aldehydes brightens and adds freshness to the whole landscape. As the minutes go by, the scent mellows, becoming more dusky and allowing its magnificent woody and resinous cedarwood, oak moss, benzoin and birch tar notes to emerge.

And perhaps civet musk too.

The fragrance, as a whole, is poised, with a fine, silky texture (particularly in the drydown), though unobtrusive, its longevity is excellent: eight hours on the skin, and longer on fabrics. Although it was composed forty years ago, "Nino Cerruti" has not aged at all, and still feels pleasantly modern (I have no doubt that it will continue to be so for the next forty years).

Watching the video clips and interviews with Nino Cerruti on the internet, the resemblance between the person and the fragrance bearing his name is indisputable. They are both lively, interesting, exuding natural elegance and a relaxed, easy-going style that is instantly appealing, and perfectly embodies the essence of *Italian chic*.

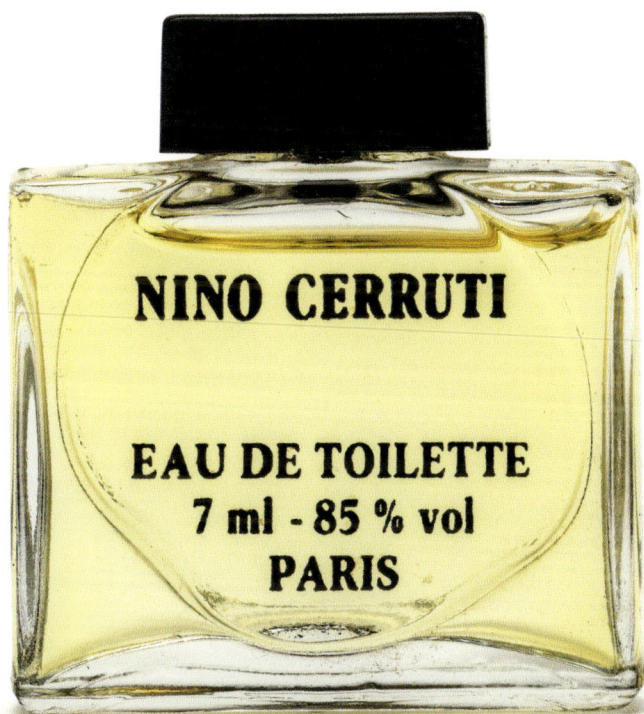

NINO CERRUTI

EAU DE TOILETTE
7 ml - 85 % vol
PARIS

Vanilla Scent

Brand: Fiorucci
Gender: feminine
Year of launch: 1979
Status: discontinued
Analyzed version: original Eau de Toilette
Classification: oriental gourmand

In the period when "Vanilla Scent" was released, the olfactory scene was dominated by showy floral bouquets, challenging notes, head-strong chypres; the taste for mellow gourmand perfumes full of creamy and sugary notes was still two decades away. And yet... And yet Elio Fiorucci decided to launch a perfume totally against the trend, showing that he was a pioneer in everything he did. And come to think of it, it could not have been otherwise. Fiorucci incarnated the essence of youth, irony, light-heartedness... he could only create a perfume like this: delicious and carefree. "Vanilla Scent" is a vanilla fragrance. Pure and simple. A warm, tender, reassuring accord of vanilla and vanillin lasting for hours without evolving an inch or gaining in complexity or depth. And this should not be seen as a limitation, because it is exactly what makes it extraordinary. At least, when we smell it again today, forty years after its launch, in an era dominated by the "extreme-gourmand" trend. Such a simple and linear scent, built on a single gourmand accord today could be hugely successful (...of course it could go completely unnoticed, for exactly the same reason). "Vanilla Scent" was an experiment, and it was short-lived. It is, nevertheless, important to point out that one of the leading Italian fashion brands of the 1980s launched a perfume perfectly in line with its aesthetic, anticipating the most important trend in contemporary perfume by over 20 years.

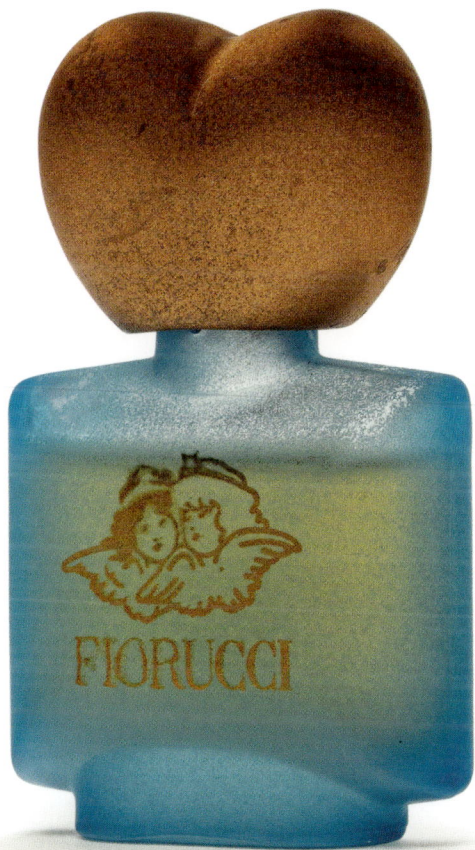

80

The Great Italian Perfumes of the 1980s

The social and cultural background

The horrifying nuclear accident in Chernobyl and the discovery of a hole in the ozone layer that protects our planet caused by the use of harmful gases profoundly impacted people all over the world, urging us to reflect on how the environment, climate and human activity are connected to one another, and leading to the creation of the first ecological movements.

The political, social and economic reform system implemented by Mikhail Gorbachev in Russia, known by the name of "Perestrojka" allowed the return to dialogue between the USSR and the United States of America, and put an end to the so-called "Cold War". At the same time, on November 9, 1989, the border between West and East Berlin was reopened, and within a few months, the Wall that had separated them for thirty years was completely demolished. The new diplomatic and economic relations between the countries of the East and West blocs will require a political reorganization on a global level, which will affect the following decades.

Personal computers like the Commodore 64, the Amiga and the Atari, mostly used to play videogames, made their entrance in many homes.

Cinema-goers were being wowed by hitherto unseen special effects, in movies such as the *Star Wars* Trilogy, *E.T.*, *Blade Runner*, *Back to the Future*, *Alien* and *Terminator*, hitting the public's fantasy and earning unprecedented money.

In Italy, the 1980s were marked by the Bologna and Ustica massacres, the Irpinia earthquake and the attempted assassination of Pope John Paul II in Rome, all of which had a profound impact on public opinion. The decade is also remembered, however, for the Italian World Cup win in 1982, the disco parties, and the famous *"Milano da bere"* lifestyle: wealthy, modern and vibrant.

US shows such as *Dallas* and *Dynasty* arrived on Italian TV screens, bringing with them a push for self-assertion and showing off status symbols that became a must for success. This was the decade of the "yuppy" phenomenon.

The trends of the decade

The materialistic aspect got important also in perfumery, with fragrances becoming a tool to underline the wearer's presence; the public was seeking power, impact and persistence. Successful perfumes had to speak intolerably loud, and required a strong, distinctive personality. This actually resulted in a number of them (such as "Giorgio Beverly Hills") being banned from use on public premises, with restaurants displaying signs inviting ladies wearing them to stay away – a risk also run by fans of Chanel's "Coco" and Dior's "Poison".

The 1980s marked the return of floral chypre fragrances with a strong personality: women wrap themselves in mystery with "Missoni Donna" (1981), "Diva" (Ungaro, 1983), "Ysatis" (Givenchy, 1984), "La Perla" (La Perla, 1985), "Parfum de Peau" (Montana, 1986).

Classic floral fragrances took on new approaches: featuring subtle notes reminiscent of face powder, like in "Ombre Rose" (J.J. Brosseau, 1981), "Paris" (Yves Saint Laurent, 1983), "Loulou" (Cacharel, 1987), "Eternity" (Calvin Klein, 1988). Fruity notes add their "zing" to traditional floral bouquets, like in "Giorgio Beverly Hills" (1981) "Boucheron" (1988) and "Jardins de Bagatelle" (Guerlain, 1983).

Oriental fragrances were the bestsellers of the decade; they started displaying more modern, original nuances incorporating floral, spicy, and woody notes like in "Poison" (Dior, 1985), "Coco" (Chanel, 1984) and "Samsara" (Guerlain, 1989). But the real novelty was the green undercurrent running through "Must" (Cartier, 1981) and "Obsession" (Calvin Klein, 1985).

In the 1980s, the ozonic/floral theme started being developed in feminine scents, the new aquatic notes accentuating the freshness of "New West for her" (Aramis, 1988), "Byblos" (1990) and later on, "L'Eau d'Issey" (1992).

As for men, the fougère family, a typical 19th century structure, witnessed a happy comeback. The traditional fougére formula –revolving around the aromatic notes of lavender, clary sage, artemisia and tarragon, as well as notes of vanilla, tonka bean and coumarin– acquired innovative woody, leathery and amber facets, with examples including "Kouros" and "Jazz" (Yves Saint Laurent, 1981 and 1988), "Drakkar Noir" (Guy Laroche, 1982), "Xeryus" (Givenchy, 1988), and "Tsar" (Van Cleef & Arpels, 1989), but also fresh, citrus and "new freshness" notes evident in "Eternity" (Calvin Klein, 1989), "Cool Water" (Davidoff, 1988) and "Cerruti 1881" (1990).

A number of men's fragrances even rose to the challenge of incorporating floral notes; among these was "Fahrenheit" (Dior, 1988), featuring a tender violet tucked away within a woody heart, and "Joop! Homme" (1989), with a strikingly evident floral bouquet.

Another theme developed in this decade is leather: offering unparalleled impact and persistence, leather is the key note in "Drakkar Noir" (Guy Laroche, 1982) and "Trussardi Uomo" (1984).

All the fashion designers of the decade embarked on the production of their own line of perfumes, and jewellers soon began to emulate them (Van Cleef & Arpels in 1981, followed by Cartier, Pomellato, Tiffany, Bulgari etc.).

Dihydromyrcenol, a molecule characteristic of functional fragrances, made its début in the world of fine perfumery, creating a new olfactory classification known as "New Freshness". The clean sensation it contributes to fragrances paved the way for perfumes featuring cool, clean, striking notes with a "detergent" smell. The success of "Cool Water" (Davidoff, 1988), the first fragrance to contain Dihydromyrcenol, persuaded perfumers to add the molecule also to feminine fragrances, teaming it with fresh floral and aquatic notes for a clean, bright result.

Headspace technology allowed for the laboratory recreation of the watery fruity notes that were to become so popular in the following decade (watermelon, plum, melon and exotic fruit). Headspace also made it possible to recreate flowers, in particular those not suitable for processing using traditional techniques. The new floral notes built with Headspace technology were more subtle, lost specific weight and presence and became pure and transparent.

Italian perfumery

The international triumph of the Italian fashion industry persuaded the most renowned stylists to take a step into the perfume business, with more than 30 of them entering the perfume industry by the end of the decade. All the taste, originality and creativity of Italian fashion items was mirrored by equally audacious, vibrant fragrances, ready to thrill consumers all over the world.

The creation of the fragrances was entrusted to experienced fragrance composers able to tune into the tastes of their clients, using powerful materials and articulated structures with a rich variety of nuances and undertones, and the results were so splendidly creative and richly expressive that they are still considered masterpieces today, like "K" (Krizia, 1981), "Trussardi Donna" (1984), "Fendi" (1985), "Roma" (Laura Biagiotti, 1988).

Most of the raw materials used were still natural: spices, flowers and woods such as rose, jasmine, carnation and sandalwood (which would become at risk of extinction in the decades to follow, compelling perfume composers to seek more eco-sustainable synthetic alternatives). The classic rose-jasmine accord was in evidence, often teamed with ylang ylang and carnation, a dry, pungent note that was used until the 1990s and has now been virtually abandoned due to its "dated" feel.

The base accords were complex woody bouquets, enhanced with vanilla, sandalwood and the bitter, salty note of oak moss.

Almost all the fragrances composed in Italy during the 1980s belonged to the chypre classification, with complex, structured bouquets that were at the same time mysterious, distinctive and powerfully feminine. The Italian chypres of this period are adorned with rich floral bouquets ("La Perla", "Genny", "V/E"), woody notes ("Missoni Donna", "Fendi"); they even dare original leathery facets ("Trussardi").

Many men's fragrances of this period also belong to the chypre family ("Hascish", "Armani Eau pour homme").

The chypre phenomenon that characterised this period was peculiar to Italy, while in other countries, oriental and floral fragrances proved more popular.

Towards the end of the decade, the oriental family was innovated by Moschino, which began the transition from the classical oriental accord (vanilla in evidence, associated with woods and resins), towards the "new generation" amber accord (resins in greater evidence, associated with ambergris and vanilla). In addition, Moschino already brings the new amber accord towards that gourmand nuance that will become one of the major trends of the 90s.

Men still favoured the fougère family, often enriched with ambery or woody undertones ("Grigioperla" and "Sergio Tacchini"), offering impact and distinction.

K de Krizia

Brand: Krizia
Gender: feminine
Year of launch: 1981
Status: discontinued
Analyzed version: original Eau de Parfum and Eau de Toilette
Author: Maurice Roucel (IFF)
Classification: rich floral aldehydic
Bottle design: Atelier Dinand
Glassware company: Bormioli Luigi

"K", the first fragrance from Krizia, is classified as a rich floral aldehydic, although it closely resembles a chypre, given the structure, complexity and the aura of mystery enveloping it! "K" revolves around a classic floral structure, created to perfection to obtain a choral harmony. "K" opens with bright aldehydes, coupled with flowers rich in character – rose, tuberose, lily of the valley, carnation, narcissus and a sullen, indolic jasmine – to form a vibrant, jubilant choir in which no single note emerges clearly above the others, coming together to sing a single word: "Temperament!".

Right from the opening, an underground current adds a rather markedly green, lush sensation; lily of the valley and jasmine of the top are accompanied to meet the corresponding green sensation in the base, created by vetiver and oak moss, while a subtle vegetable sweetness (tuberose, narcissus) acts as a mere counterpoint.

An audacious leathery note, teamed with iris, benzoin and civet musk, brings a delicate animal/powdery facet to a floral fragrance that would otherwise be all dry, green and pungent. This level of collaboration from the materials featured in the composition requires vast experience and sublime expertise, as well as premium-quality materials. It comes as no surprise that the man behind this marvellous fragrance is Maurice Roucel, the undisputed perfumery genius that has created, to mention but a few, "Tocade" by Rochas (1994), "Gucci Envy" (1997), "24, Faubourg" by Hermès (2005), "Insolence" by Guerlain (2005), "Hypnose homme" by Lancôme (2007). In "K", Roucel shows – just like his mentor Henri Robert did in "Gucci N°1" –, his love for the elegance of rich floral bouquets full of character, and for the aldehydes, which he uses with great skill to create a modern masterpiece with a foot in tradition.

"K" has a strong sillage and excellent persistence: the Eau de Parfum shows a more markedly floral personality, the generous leather/oak moss finish allows several hours of longevity, while the Eau de Toilette is greener, more transparent, bitter and almost salty, with particularly brilliant aldehydes and a more sharply focused accord of lily of the valley and jasmine. This shining star of the 1980s guarantees you won't go unnoticed even to this day.

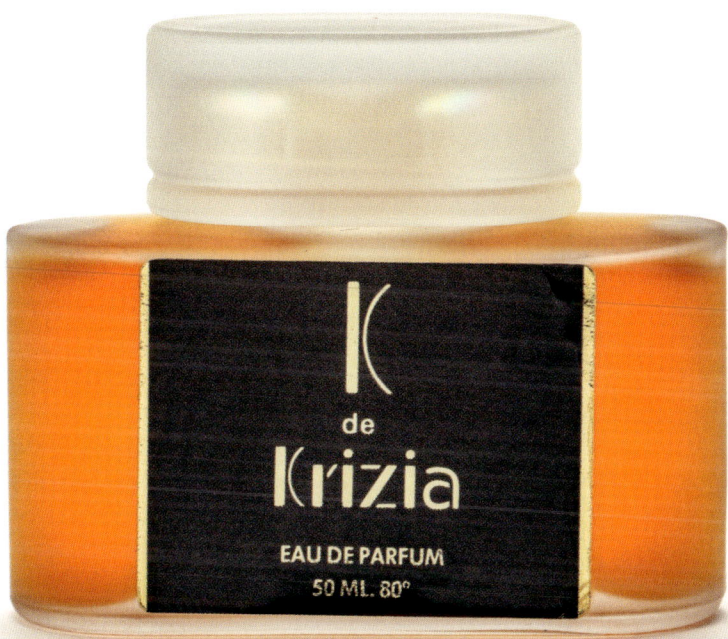

Missoni Donna

Brand: Missoni
Gender: feminine
Year of launch: 1981
Status: discontinued
Analyzed version: original Eau de Toilette
Author: Maurice Roucel (IFF)
Classification: woody chypre
Bottle design: Atelier Dinand

For its first fragrance, Missoni chose a classification that today is considered challenging, but in those days expressed the essence of femininity, class and personality: chypre. And what's more, a chypre with woody nuances. Very few woody chypre fragrances appeared in the history of perfumery, partly because obtaining such complex effects of light/shade alternation requires a level of mastery that is difficult to find. Partly because woody chypres are awkward creatures that rarely appeal to those looking for an immediately pleasing fragrance. However, if the right person can only get close enough, without being intimidated by their surly character, they'll be rewarded with a world of subtle emotions and an indomitable soul tempered by wisdom and kindness. The first to appear in this family was "Aromatics Elixir" (Clinique, 1972), followed by "Coriandre" (Couturier, 1976) and this Missoni in 1981, followed by "Diva" (Ungaro, 1973) and a handful of other courageous fragrances, all of them splendid.

After a brief opening of bergamot and red fruits, Missoni dives straight into the heart of the fragrance with jasmine, geranium and ylang ylang, peaking with a triumphant velvety, palpitating rose. The moment the typically chypre accord makes its appearance, with patchouli and oak moss, the flowers dull to a darker tone. The third transformation of the fragrance ushers in honey, civet musk and styrax, bringing with them a nocturnal, animal sensation.

Although it is a creature of the 1980s, Missoni spreads its allure quietly, with a longevity that's perfectly satisfying. Slightly dated, yet still appealing, partly thanks to the premium-quality materials, Missoni was composed by Maurice Roucel, who has always been tremendously popular with women, courting them with fragrances able to light up every corner of their soul.

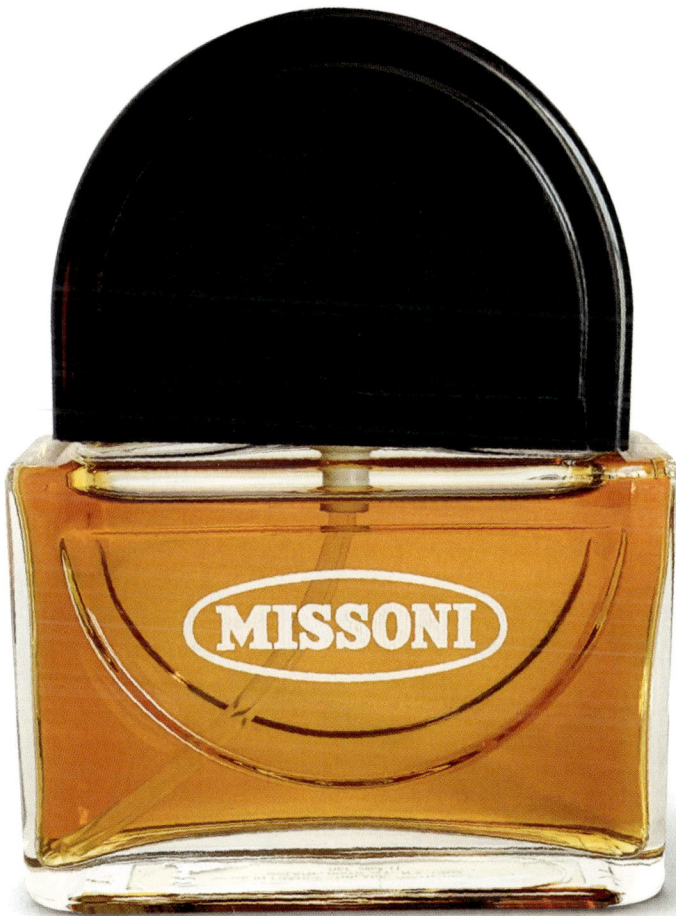

Gianni Versace

Brand: Gianni Versace
Gender: feminine
Year of launch: 1982
Status: discontinued
Analyzed version: vintage Eau de Toilette
Author: Givaudan-Roure
Classification: rich floral
Bottle design: Alain de Morgues

The first perfume launched by Gianni Versace is a beautifully rich, feminine floral *jus*: exuberant and seductive, the scent is a perfect representation of Versace's couture and tasteful aesthetic. Central to "Gianni Versace" is a splendid floral bouquet built "in the grand manner", with jasmine and narcissus, topped with an open, sunny, smiling tuberose. This precious floral bouquet is welcomed in by bergamot, while a minimum amount of aldehydes is tasked with bringing a clean finish to the flowers, drenching them in light. The base notes of iris, benzoin, oak moss and leather carry "Gianni Versace" – an hour after the spray – towards a warm, vegetable drydown that maintains a soft, elusive floral sensation, bonding with the base notes to transmit a sense of harmony and rigour that's laid-back yet sophisticated, able to make any wearer feel beautiful. Although the bergamot opening, the floral heart notes and the oak moss base would appear to identify "Gianni Versace" as a chypre, the generous floral accord places the fragrance within the classification of rich florals, leaving the chypre nuance only the task of adding structure and longevity to the marvellous floral accord. Gianni Versace's place is up there with the great rich florals that made history, in the company of Chloé (1975), "Ysatis" and "Amarige" (Givenchy, 1975 and 1983). Unfortunately, tracking a bottle down has become an arduous task; it is certainly worth the effort, however.

Although it is not one of the big, resounding perfumes in typical 1980s style, "Gianni Versace" does boast excellent sillage, with a duration of more than five hours.

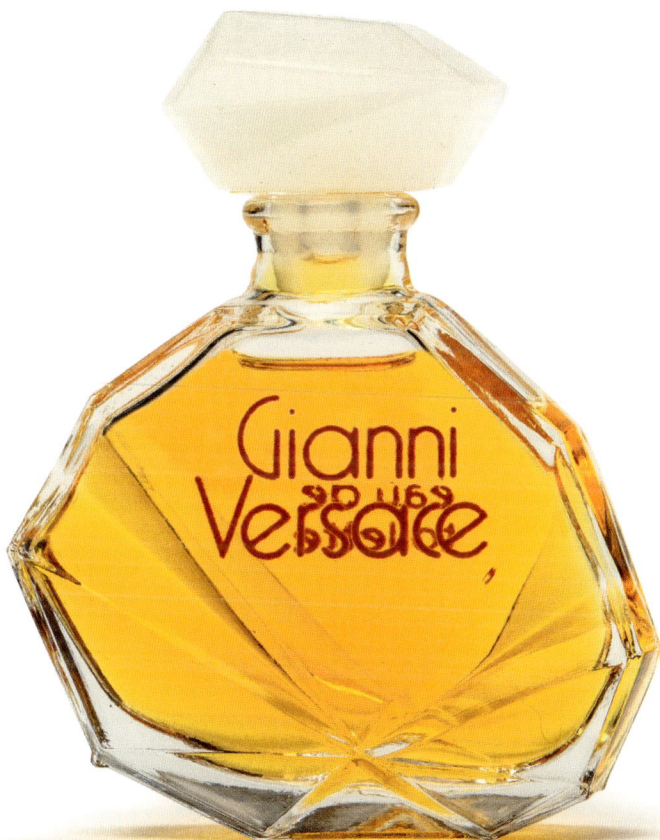

Arrogance pour femme

Brand: Arrogance
Gender: feminine
Year of launch: 1982
Status: reformulated
Analyzed version: modern Eau de Toilette, vintage Eau de Toilette
Author: Raymond Chaillan
Classification: green floral
Bottle design: Schiapparelli - Pikenz

In the past decades, Arrogance has been able to conquer a vast base of aficionados by mesmerizing them with its apparent simplicity, its clean, fresh, spring-like frivolity, and its unsurpassed technical performances (sillage, radiance, longevity).
"Arrogance" was composed by Raymond Chaillan, one of the most prolific fragrance composers of the 1970s, co-author of "Opium" (Yves Saint Laurent, 1977, together with Jean Amic and Jean Louis Sieuzac). "Arrogance"'s opening sparkles with bergamot, introducing a floral bouquet of candid, virginal purity (lily of the valley, white lily, and rose), with jasmin and neroli adding a slighlty green facet.

Over this green, spring-like floral accord a handful of cool, metallic aldehydes is gleaming: the Virgin holds a sword, and is not afraid to use it!
The base, built on sandalwood, cedar and musk, fully comes through a couple of hours after application: what is perceived for virtually the entire duration of the fragrance is a twinkle of dry, cold metallic light of blinding clarity which, in recent years, got an even drier, more sharply focused top accord.
For many wearers, "Arrogance" is a hallmark scent, given its impressive sillage and virtually endless, 24-hour longevity, announcing the wearer's presence with the clarity of a drum roll!

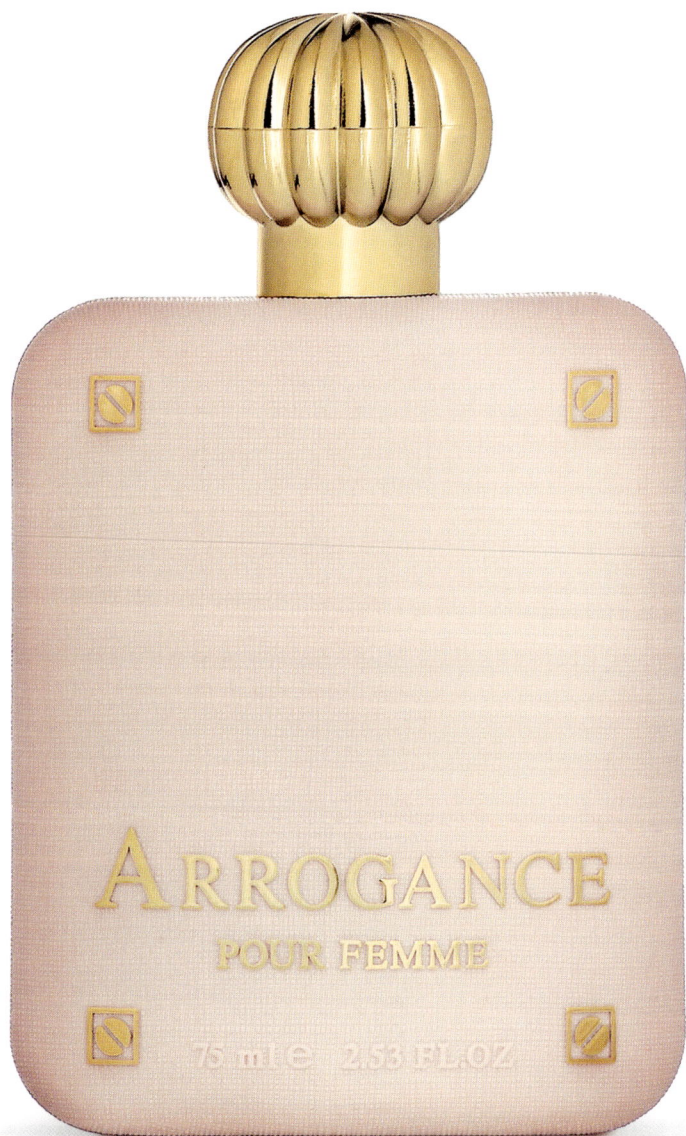

Trussardi

Brand: Trussardi
Type: feminine
Launch date: 1983
Status: in production
Analyzed version: original Eau de Toilette
Classification: leather chypre
Bottle design: Nicola Trussardi

For his first fragrance, Nicola Trussardi chose an unusual "reptile" bottle designed by himself, immediately evoking the refinement of his leather accessories. Leather is also present at the olfactory level, since the scent is a chypre leather executed with extremely refined skill: soft, welcoming and at the same time showing a great temperament. Above all, rich in every bounty that you can imagine: citrus fruits, spices, aldehydes, a triumph of fresh flowers (jasmine, hyacinth, geranium, rose, lily of the valley, ylang ylang, tuberose, iris), the green note of galbanum, solid and deep woods (cedar, sandalwood, patchouli, oakmoss), wonderful resins (benzoin, olibanum), amber notes, vanilla, musk and a bit of civet. At the heart, a very refined note of leather orders and disciplines the triumph of notes, exactly as an orchestra conductor would do during a thunderous "Tutti" at the end. "Trussardi" boasts all its dazzling beauty thanks to a flowery, dry, luminous opening, with green and aldehyde accents, lasting for a good half hour, until it is reached by the woody notes. This is the moment when also resins soar, melting the flowers into a suffused languor of unspeakable yearning, which would be all too exciting to wear. The oak moss and the leathery note take care of enveloping all this fragility into a deep and fascinating night veil. Shady light, melancholy joy, wild elegance, fragile pride. Oxymorons that can't even remotely reveal the complexity and refinement of a formula at times approaching both Robert Piguet's "Bandit" launched earlier (1944) and "Paloma Picasso", launched later (1984), while remaining smoother and more welcoming than both, more "Italian" in the meaning of being articulated and rich in nuances, yet immediately pleasant. Designed for a female audience with sophisticated tastes, "Trussardi" is great also for men. Its sillage lasts about three hours, radiating perfectly without ever being excessive. The modern version is significantly different from the original, like its male counterpart. The main reason for the restyling is not only aesthetic, but is largely linked to the impossibility of using today some fundamental components of these two formulas. The operation was not painless (the current fragrance is a very contemporary floral chypre), but the floral heart has been fortunately preserved, acquiring a more optimistic momentum and enveloping itself into a cloud of elegant white musks, which make it more "easy" and widen its wearability.

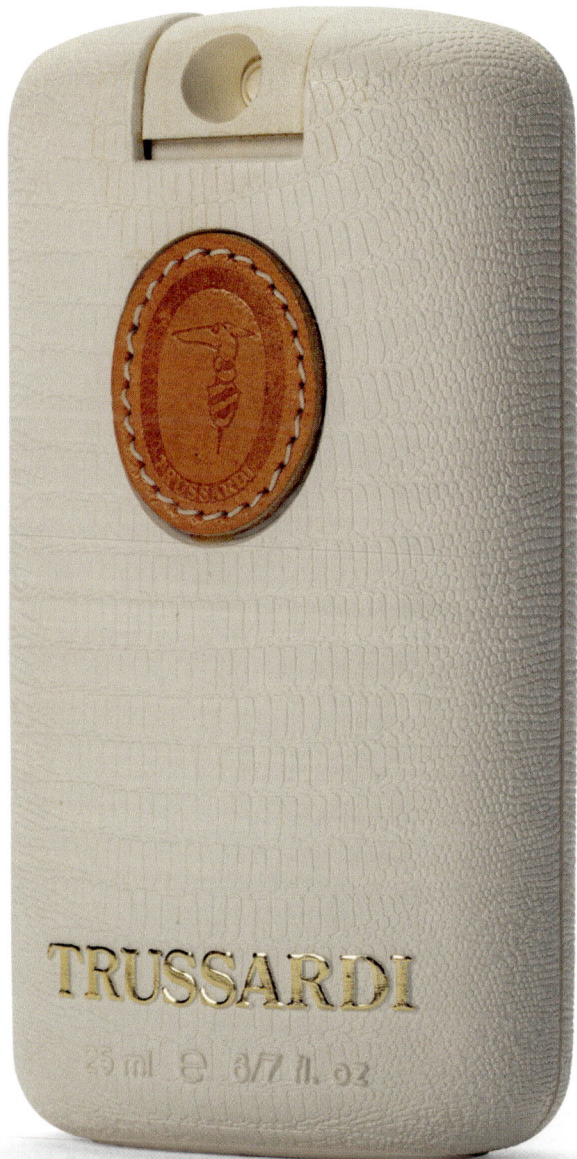

Paillettes

Brand: Enrico Coveri
Gender: feminine
Year of launch: 1983
Status: relaunched in 1993
Analyzed version: original Eau de Toilette
Classification: floral chypre
Glassware company: G. D. & P. Sironi

Enrico Coveri's style was eccentric and carefree, embellished with a cascade of colourful sequins that lit up his creations with that frivolous, tongue-in-cheek sparkle that became his hallmark. Named in honour of those sequins, "Paillettes" opens with a citrus accord, rapidly joined by a floral bouquet of rose and neroli and aldehydes; this translucent, sparkling, slightly soapy accord is reminiscent of a number of masterly creations from the 1970s and 1980s by the great Sophia Grojsman ("Paris" by Yves Saint Laurent, 1983). After a few minutes, the initial accord is enriched with two undertones: a sweet-sharp fruity one (blackcurrant) and a warm-spicy hint of cloves, creating a superbly balanced counterpoint that allows it to last and to keep attention focused. Deliciously explosive, "Paillettes" is one of those rare fragrances living up its name, since a swirl of colourful sequins is effectively the sensation it offers for the whole of the first half hour. The cloves then climb slowly in intensity, prevailing over the more fleeting fruity note and bonding with the flowers and the aldehydes, which light up once more and reclaim their central role. In the meantime, the amber base begins to come through, crowned with a marvellous vetiver. This evolution completely transforms the texture of the fragrance, which shifts from a light, transparent chiffon sprinkled with sequins towards a velvet pillow, featuring warm, golden, dusky tones. It is then that the perfume becomes a recognisable chypre, placing it clearly among the style that characterised the 1970s and 1980s. Deceptively young and carefree, this is a fragrance that boasts a fairly articulated structure, with a wealth of interesting undertones, long-lasting and able to spread with medium intensity. It is best tried on the skin; paper does not bring out the multiple nuances of the fragrance, which thus tends to remain two-dimensional.

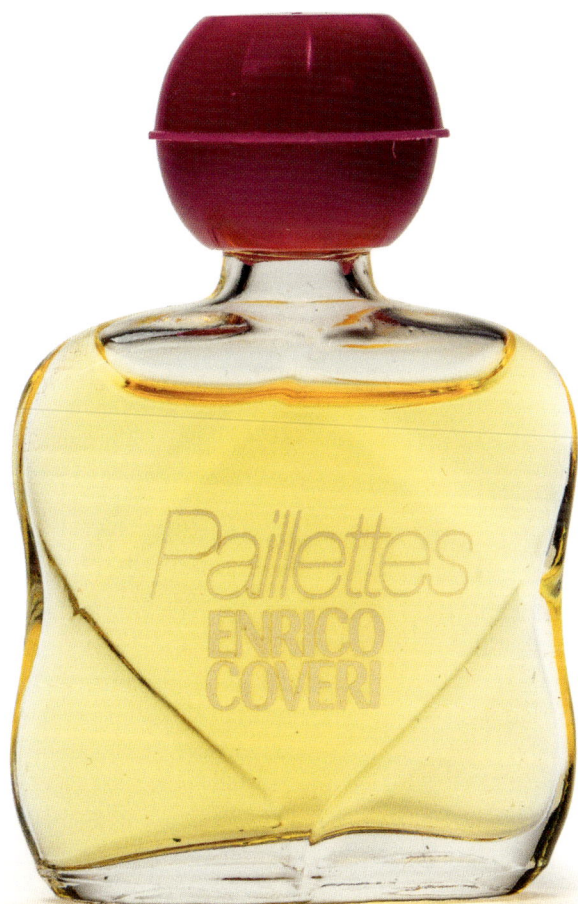

Hascish Femme

Brand: Veejaga
Gender: feminine
Year of launch: 1983
Status: discontinued
Analyzed version: original Eau de Toilette
Classification: floral chypre

This perfume is one of the many masterful Italian creations unfortunately remained on the sidelines, despite the sophisticated design of the bottle, the surprising name and one of the most interesting bouquets ever produced in Italy.
The opening accord of juicy-spiced citrus fruits (orange and bergamot) introduces a sultry bouquet of dried spices, amplified by rose and the floral/spiced note of carnation, along with green hints of jasmine and ylang ylang. The gorgeous base begins to come through minutes after application. Sandalwood and patchouli, dense, opaque resins such as benzoin and incense, musk, castoreum and an amber accord all bubble away in an enchanted cauldron to create a dark, stormy, magical potion, lit up only by subtle touches of aldehydes sparkling through the inky black sky like lightning bolts. The dry, bitter, humoral, sullen bouquet of "Hascisch" is the main characteristic of chypres, with exquisitely affable and languid notes also coming through. Masterfully constructed and featuring splendid materials, "Hascisch" is a commendably balanced fragrance that undoubtedly required extraordinary experience: it is a pity the composer is not known.

I cannot pick up the slightest note of hashish; it is likely the name was intended to evoke the same exoticism of "Mystère" (Rochas, 1978), "Magie Noire" (Lancôme, 1978), "Cinnabar" (Estée Lauder, 1978) and above all "Opium" (Yves Saint Laurent, 1977), whose iconic fruity echo resonates also in Hascish's top accord. These marvels with their ambery nuances are in fact all perceptible here, but featured in the chypre style, as if they were blended with "Aromatics Elixir"(Estée Lauder, 1971). A similar structure would later be chosen for "Must" (Cartier, 1981), with the addition of a smoky note and a marked emphasis on the green undertone.
In any case, "Hascish" belongs among the Greatest: whether they are composed in the 1970s, 1980s or later is of no importance, half the history of perfumery is concentrated into this single bottle. Can we ask for more than that?
We can, indeed. For instance, it would have been nice for "Hascish" to receive a welcome worthy of its rank. If "Hascish" had been recognised as the work of art it is, it would have become a cult object all over the world; and instead of the scant information we might find hundreds of pages of details, glossy photos and enthusiastic reviews. And we might even be able to track down a bottle to buy.

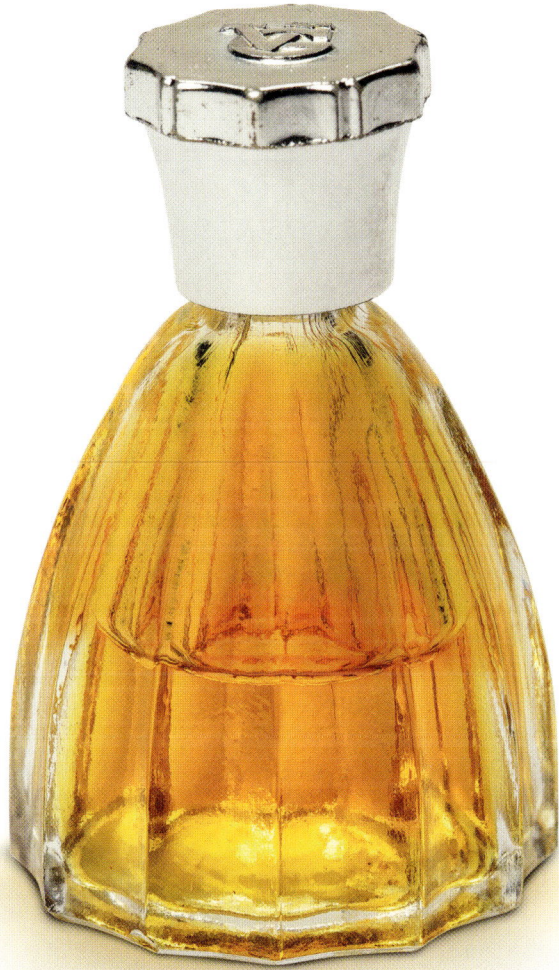

Hascish Homme

Brand: Veejaga
Gender: masculine
Year of launch: 1983
Status: discontinued
Analyzed version: original Eau de Toilette
Glassware Company: Bormioli Luigi

Just like its female partner fragrance, "Hascish" for men did not receive the attention it deserved, and remained the hidden treasure of a tiny group of sensation seekers looking for original fragrances able to awaken strong emotions with top-quality materials and a rich, satisfying sillage.

"Hascish" was launched at a time when Italian market was dominated by fougère fragrances: interesting and modern though they were, they nonetheless proved extremely successful for their well groomed, traditional, "freshly-shaved dad" aura. "Hascish" went down a totally different road, venturing into a thick, gloomy forest inhabited by creatures with hoarse, leathery voices that were far from reassuring, yet possessed irresistible magnetism.

"Hascish" opens with a fresh, dry, citrus-aromatic accord highlighted by artemisia and other aromatic notes; within minutes, a floral heart of carnation, geranium and jasmine joins in, binding the aromatic bouquet and taking a dry, green, extremely manly direction. Black pepper and nutmeg blow a heady, parched, dusty, breath over the flowers, rendering them even more austere and reserved. This is where the base note emerges, with a magnificent patchouli/vetiver/cedarwood accord that harmonises sublimely with the flowers and spices to create a dynamic, multi-faceted, fascinating effect. As the flowers and spices gradually fade away, the woods are captured by an exquisitely balanced drydown of leather, green musk, castoreum in which none of the notes prevails over the others, coming together to form a dry, dark, smoky concoction. Frankincense alone, with its mystical, unearthy note rises above the other base notes, uplifting an accord that might otherwise prove on the verge of disturbing.

"Hascish" projects with balance, powerful but never excessive, with excellent longevity.

Versatile, ultra-modern and featuring materials of outstanding quality, it occupies the middle ground of the finest leather chypre fragrances ever composed: "Gentleman" by Givenchy (1974), "Yatagan" (Caron, 1976) and "Antaeus" (Chanel, 1981). "Hascish" smells rawer than "Gentleman", more wearable than "Yatagan", more audacious than "Antaeus", and has undoubtedly influenced the creation of a number of men's fragrances that appeared after it. Although it went largely unnoticed by consumers, composers were quick to grasp its value and study it closely...

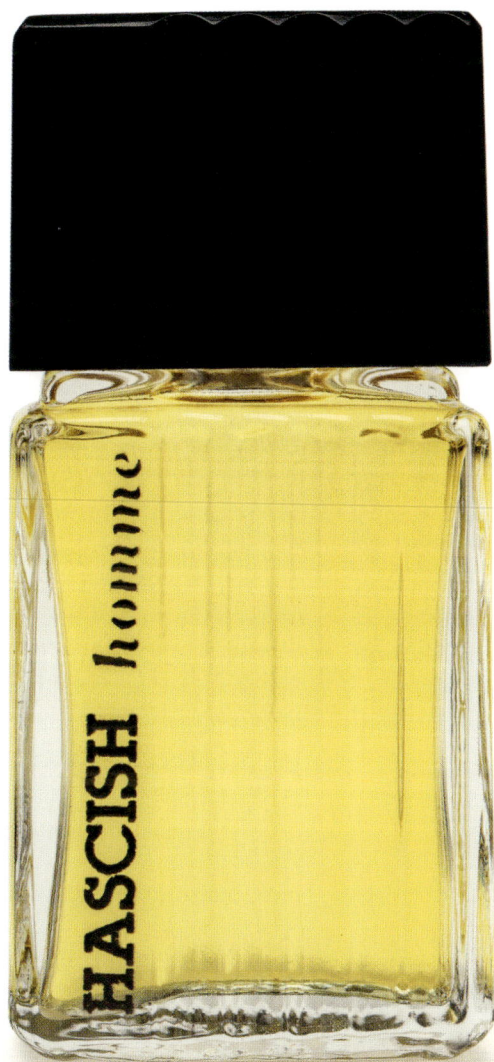

Armani eau pour homme

Brand: Giorgio Armani
Gender: masculine
Year of launch: 1984
Status: in production
Analyzed version: original Eau de Toilette
Author: Roger Pellegrino (Firmenich)
Classification: aromatic fougère
Bottle design: Atelier Dinand
Glassware company: Bormioli Luigi

In 1980, Giorgio Armani dressed a young Richard Gere in the movie *American Gigolò*, with deconstructed jackets, natural fabrics and flowing lines: outfits with an extremely sophisticated yet casual allure, designed for a man who is confident without being showy, endowed with self-awareness and presence, and with a subtle, irresistible touch of humour. The first "Giorgio Armani" fragrance for men shares this natural feel, opening with a sharp burst of sun-drenched citrus, given an injection of dynamism with lavender, rosemary and sage. When the citrus notes make their exit, the aromatic notes are joined by a handful of pungent spices (nutmeg, cloves and coriander), softened slightly around the edges by a whisper of jasmine and neroli, forming a rich heart accord with floral, citrus, spicy and aromatic facets. The magnificent base notes of oak moss and woods (vetiver, cedar, patchouli and sandalwood) rise up into the heart of the fragrance, enveloping aromatics, spices and flowers in a solid, comfortable embrace with a perfect balance and an extremely natural sensation.

The first five minutes of "Armani eau pour homme" recall the opening notes of "Pour Monsieur" (Chanel, 1955), but the real comparison is with "Eau Sauvage" (Dior, 1966). Both share the same structure, as well as many notes. Smelling them side by side is a useful exercise to understand the cultural differences between French and Italian perfumery. "Eau Sauvage" is restrained, sophisticated, très chic, inimitably French. It's Alain Delon, perfectly shaved, speeding along in a sports car with a nonchalance bordering on insolence. "Armani eau pour homme", on the other hand, is casual, relaxed, outgoing. It's a suntanned Richard Gere, with damp hair and unbuttoned shirt, approaching you with a chilled glass of Prosecco and a smile of anticipation.

Composed of essentially citrus and aromatic notes, the fragrance does not exceed three hours of longevity, remaining discreet and subtle all the time, completely bucking the trend set by the big, booming perfumes of the time. The adjustments made to this fragrance over the years to comply with IFRA directives have reduced the presence of severalraw materials, including oakmoss and sandalwood (being an endangered species, its exploitation is now subjected to extremely stringent international treaties). Despite these changes, the style of the fragrance continues to shine bright against the light.

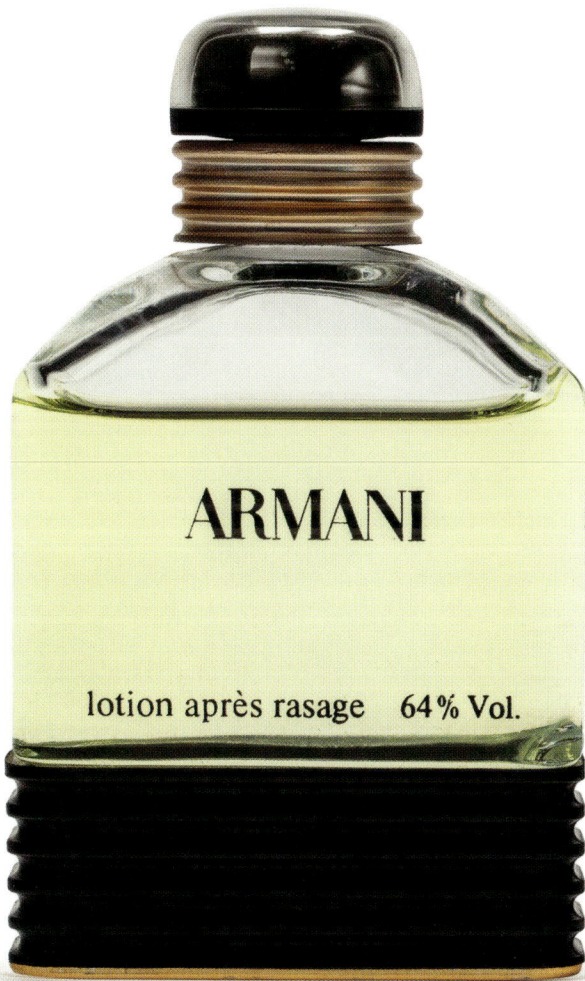

Trussardi Uomo

Brand: Trussardi
Gender: masculine
Year of launch: 1984
Status: relaunched in 2011
Analyzed version: original Eau de Toilette
Author: Givaudan
Classification: aromatic fougère
Bottle design: Nicola Trussardi
Glassware Company: Bormioli Luigi

Smelling the first men's fragrance by Trussardi is like opening a time capsule: compared with other fragrances with a more classic, timeless design, "Trussardi Uomo" has exactly that olfactory structure and intensity typical of the 1980s that make it seem "dated" today. The need to launch a new version of the fragrance thirty years down the line was perfectly understandable, although vintage fragrance aficionados would remain fond of the original.

The complex opening accord offers a prelude to the heavier base notes: bitter citrus, aldehydes and an aromatic bouquet featuring mirtle and a leathery note of sage. This fresh, clear, almost reassuring opening is typical of aromatic fougères, conjuring up an image of barber shops and country gentlemen. The beast within, the Mr. Hyde, will not emerge until later: to be precise, when the base accord of patchouli, leather, oak moss and castoreum rises up into the heart on the wings of the sage/myrtle accord, while a sharp note of incense cuts right through it all.

From that moment on, "Trussardi Uomo" takes on a whole new personality, shifting towards a leathery chypre: dark, dense animalic and dangerously sexy. This is a men's fragrance with buckets of testosterone in circulation: self-confident, exuberant, for the man who knows just what he wants and doesn't think twice about throwing out an invitation to dinner.

The drydown lasts for hours, with a perfectly composed woody/aromatic/leathery accord.

Excellent projection and perfectly satisfying duration.

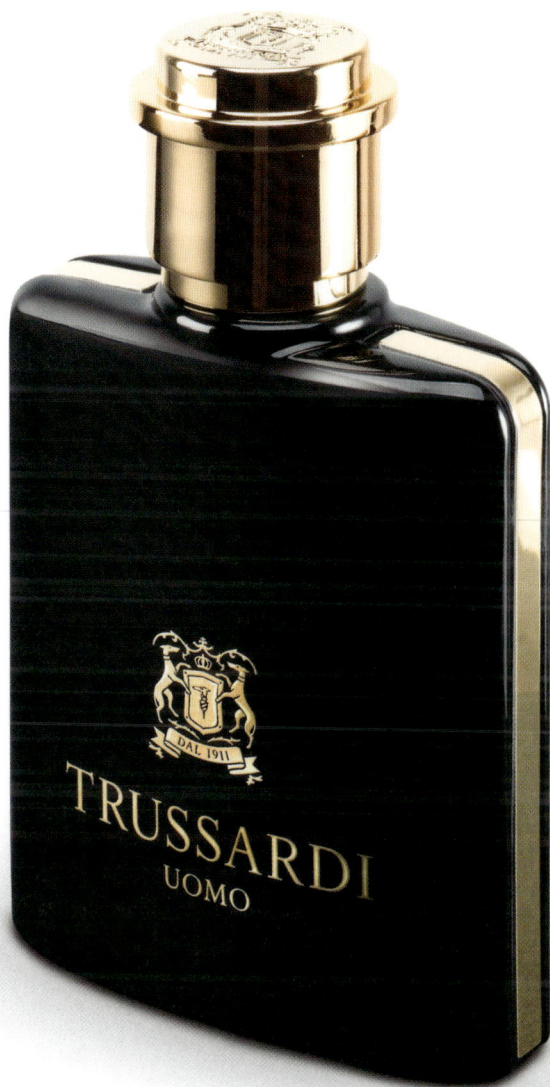

Gianfranco Ferré

Brand: Gianfranco Ferré
Gender: feminine
Year of launch: 1984
Status: discontinued
Analyzed version: original Eau de Toilette
Author: Annie Buzantian - Firmenich
Classification: rich floral
Bottle design: Atelier Dinand
Glassware company: Bormioli Luigi

1982 saw the entrance onto the Italian perfumery scene of the great Gianfranco Ferré. And a grand, stylish entrance it was, with a scintillating fragrance perfectly keeping with his exuberant couture creations. Wearing this fragrance is the best way to understand his love for women and his burning desire to make them feel beautiful. The opening of Gianfranco Ferré is euphoric, to put it mildly: the golden citrus and ripe fruit accord makes its appearance beautifully blended with a sumptuous bouquet of rose, hyacinth and white flowers with creamy and nectarine facets, while the aldehydes (in particular the peach-scented c-12) spread right throughout the bouquet the blinding white light of a summer sun shining down on the poolside. The result is an explosion of optimistic, sunny femininity.

Half an hour from spraying, the fragrance takes on a more intimate texture, with the metallic nuance of the aldehydes acting as a perfect counterpoint to the warm, ambery base accord, over which the bouquet of white flowers continues to whisper softly. A warm, golden glow spreads right across the composition, from beginning to end.

"Gianfranco Ferré" is not a particularly intricate fragrance, its classic floral structure focuses on delicacy and a carefree wearability, with a reasonably good sillage and a duration of a few hours. "Gianfranco Ferré" is the demonstration of how the generous floral fragrances of the period were taking on a sugary, fruity edge, destined to gradually evolve into the modern trend of fruity florals with a gourmand side. The hugely successful fragrances of those years that helped usher in this trend were "Giorgio Beverly Hills" (Charles of the Ritz, 1981) and "Jardin de Bagatelle" (Guerlain, 1983); but while Giorgio is a fanfare of brass instruments played as loudly as the human ear can stand, "Gianfranco Ferré" remains balanced and affable, and although it is a clean fragrance, it does not have the soapy, metallic facets that characterise "Jardin de Bagatelle".

The composer is Annie Buzantian of Firmenich, the creator of highly successful perfumes including "Pleasures" by Estée Lauder (1995). Annie Buzantian enjoys working with floral notes; whereas other composers highlight their full-bodied, shrill, rounded aspect, she prefers to work more transparently on them, capturing not so much the flower itself as the fragrance of the dew that has settled on the petals during the night.

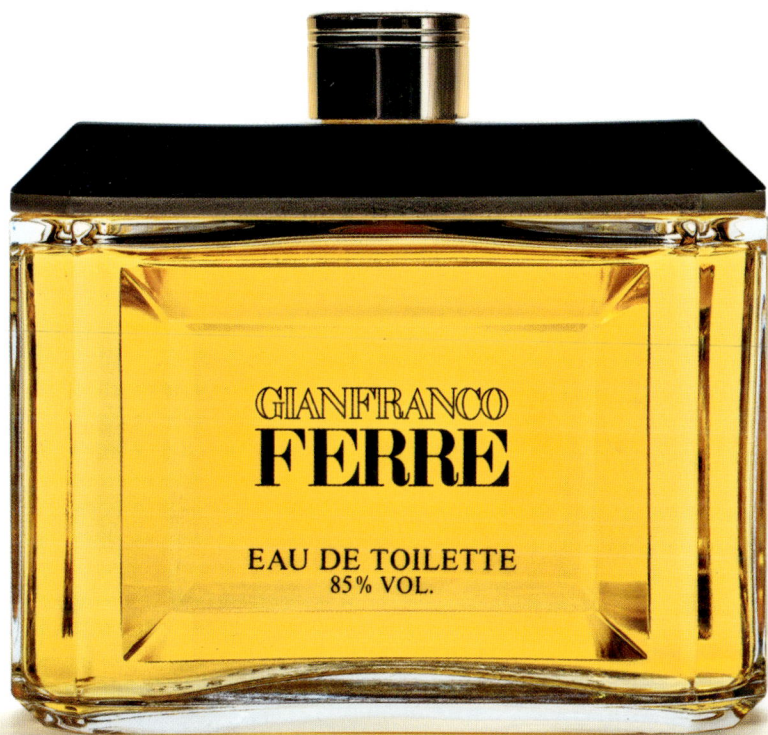

Fendi

Brand: Fendi
Gender: feminine
Year of launch: 1985
Status: discontinued
Analyzed version: original Eau de Parfum and Eau de Toilette
Author: Jean Grèget (Firmenich)
Classification: floral chypre
Author: Jean Grèget (Firmenich)
Bottle design: Pierre Dinand
Glassware Company: Bormioli Luigi

The Fendi brand obtained outstanding international success thanks to the sophisticated leather and fur models designed by the Fendi sisters, so it came as no surprise that for their first fragrance, they went for a typical "fur coat fragrance": the epitome of loud, complex, structured perfume that was big in the mid-1980s, with successes such as "Diva" by Ungaro (1983) and "Coco" by Chanel (1984).

A Baroque triumph of generosity, "Fendi" revolves around a classic aldehydic floral heart, featuring rose, jasmine, ylang ylang, carnation and orange blossom, introduced by warm, juicy citrus notes. The base is dry and severe, featuring patchouli, sandalwood, vetiver, iris, oak moss and benzoin.

A spicy bouquet raises the temperature of the whole creation, contributing expressive fullness to the flowers and accompanying the woody base up into the top of the formula. The overall effect is deep, three-dimensional, with top-class materials richly layered into a warm, luxurious, voluptuous texture to delve into with abandon to get ultimate protection from the cold, hostile world. The Eau de Toilette veers more decisively towards chypre: dryer and more restrained, bitter to the point of being almost surly, with an alluringly sexy, "wild" undertone.

The Eau de Parfum has a warmer, smoother, more liqueur-like texture which better supports both the flowers in the heart and the patchouli/resins in the base, shifting it away from chypre towards amber. This version highlights its author's signature at best, since Jean Gréget had a special talent for treating oakmoss and green notes with unusual delicacy, enhancing dynamism and transparence, a feature evident also in "Ô de Lancome" (1969).

Fendi never goes unnoticed: the wearer will often be asked for the perfume's name. But there are two requisites for this little piece of magic to work. The first one is a few harsh winters of experience: Fendi is not for young girls, but for adult women (and men) who have no fear of their own desires. The second is the ability to use just enough of it: a single spray is enough, going over the top will do nothing but distort the fragrance and make it unbearable. If you'd like to try it – and I very much hope so – you'll find reliable retailers online who will be happy to send you a bottle of this invaluable fragrance: at an exorbitant price, of course, because masterpieces never come cheap.

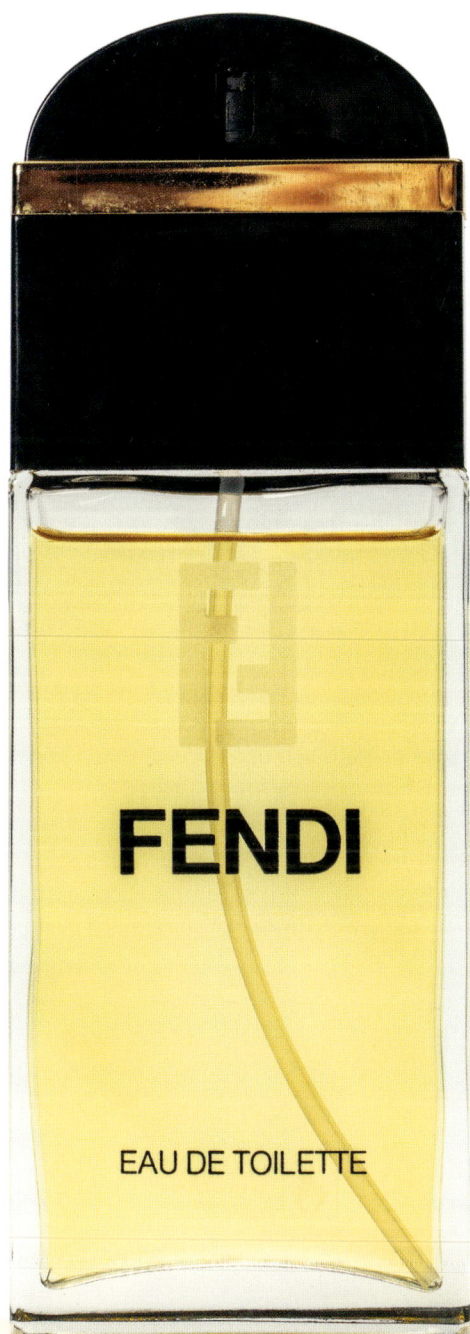

Fendi Uomo

Brand: Fendi
Gender: masculine
Year of launch: 1985
Status: discontinued
Analyzed version: original Eau de Toilette
Author: Jean Grèget (Firmenich)
Classification: spicy woody
Bottle design: Fendi Sisters

The Fendi Man turns up right on time for his date. Gentlemanly, impeccably dressed, with a white flower in his buttonhole. He gets out of an old Bugatti and stretches out his hand with a pleasant smile. You're a little disconcerted while you think: "*Help! Too old fashioned: he reminds me of my uncle!*"
With a somewhat forced smile, you get into the car, hoping the restaurant's lost your booking. With a mischievous half-smile, he takes hold of the wheel, and a shiver runs down your spine as you realise he's not heading for the restaurant. Your disconcertment increases while he smiles, presses down on the accelerator, and winks at you: "*Hold tight, baby!*" And it's then you discover that your date is none other than a Formula One world champion, and he's decided to impress you by taking you for a spin that will literally leave you breathless. You don't know it yet, but you will get out of his car with your hair unkempt and your heart in turmoil, only hoping for a kiss.
"Fendi Uomo" starts out as a classic men's fragrance with a fougère atmosphere: the citrus and lavender top notes and the floral-spicy heart notes of carnation and cyclamen, cinnamon and aldehydes combine into a skilfully drawn, if not particularly original, portrait. Just when it seems to be heading in a totally predictable direction, an extraordinary woody base emerges, with cedar, vetiver and patchouli teaming with a leathery note to compose a magnificent dry accord, with the maturity of a fine liqueur and the majesty of the Colosseum, whose sculptural beauty brings value to the whole fragrance.
"Fendi Uomo" is the very essence of 1980s Italian style: exuberant and three-dimensional, it smells expensive from the top notes right through to the base. It's the male version of the "*Grand Soirée*" concept. It sings in a tenor voice for the whole of the first hour, making it inadvisable for busy places or convivial occasions. As soon as the base begins to come through, it gets more intimate, with a longevity of a further two splendid, indescribable, heavenly hours.

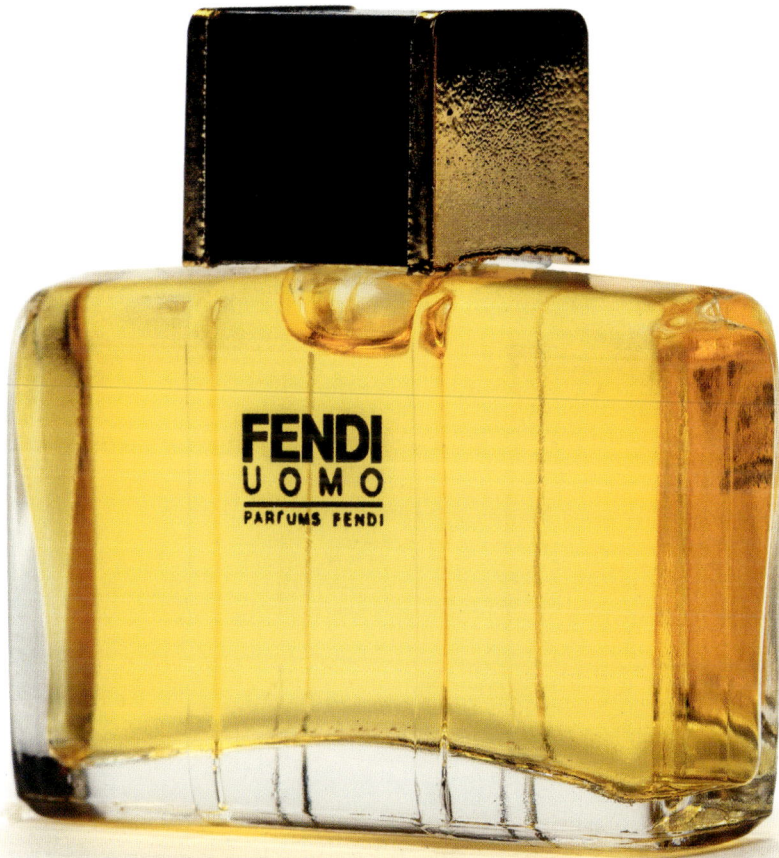

La Perla

Brand: La Perla
Gender: feminine
Year of launch: 1985
Status: reformulated
Analyzed version: original Eau de Toilette
Author: Pierre Wargnye - IFF
Classification: floral chypre
Bottle design: Pierre Dinand
Glassware Company: Bormioli

La Perla takes us on a trip through the very essence of the 10 years from 1975 to 1985 with a generous, powerfully resonating fragrance enhanced with the finest of details, able to cling to clothes and accessories for days, creating an unforgettable fragrance hallmark.

"La Perla", one of the finest creations by Pierre Wargnye of IFF ("Drakkar Noir", 1982; "l'Homme" by Yves Saint Laurent, 2006) has the classic enchantingly complex structure of the chypre fragrances of the period: the fresh, spiced opening of bergamot, pepper and coriander builds to a floral heart accord of rose, carnation, jasmine and ylang ylang. Shortly after application, the base (patchouli, vetiver, sandalwood, benzoin and oakmoss) reaches the rest of the perfume, providing structure, softness, depth and a delightful three-dimensionality. The spices, which come right through the composition adding an interesting, angular touch, are strengthened by the bergamot top, the carnation heart and the oak moss/patchouli base, forming the *trait d'union* that binds the composition tightly and lets it unravel gradually and masterfully, allowing it to last for hours on end, with a magnificent sillage.

The shift back and forth from warm to cold, bright to shadowy, sharp-edged to soft sensations conjures up an aura of mystery, creating a tantalising effect able to keep attention focused throughout the development of the fragrance and attracting endless compliments. Profound, vibrant and with a wealth of alluring details, "La Perla" is a woman with a mysterious past everyone talks about yet no-one really knows much about. With her fine black veil, scarlet lips, husky voice and slightly foreign accent, her suitors are never sure if they'll be allowed close, or she'll dash their hopes with a mere curl of the corner of her lips. It comes as no surprise that this perfume was released by a lingerie brand: it is brimming with enough sensuality to knock anyone for six. One of the greatest Italian fragrances ever composed, its place is in the Olympus of Floral Chypres, along with "Diorella" (Dior, 1972), "Aromatics Elixir" (Clinique, 1972) and "Coriandre" (Jean Couturier, 1973). After these three, nothing but one fleeting, intense thrill ("Agent Provocateur", 2000). Followed by oblivion. The new version, adapted to the restrictions imposed by the IFRA regulations has lost some of its narrative tension, nonetheless maintains the vibrant character of the original, with a softer, smoother, markedly more contemporary edge.

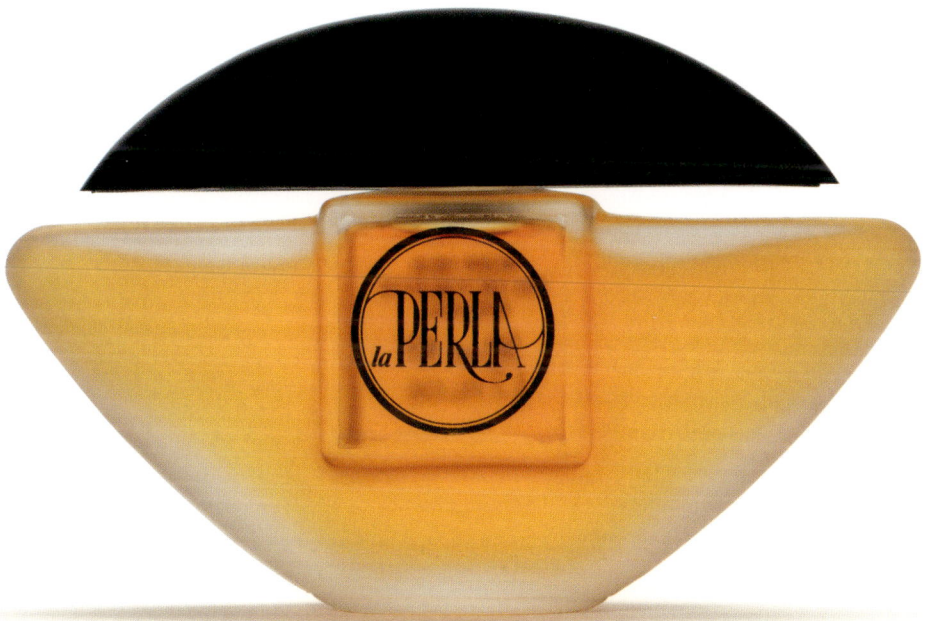

Roccobarocco

renamed Roccobarocco Uno

Brand: Rocco Barocco
Gender: feminine
Year of launch: 1986
Status: relaunched in 1988
Analyzed version: vintage Eau de Parfum
Author: Maurizio Cerizza
Classification: Rich floral
Glassware Company: Bormioli Luigi

"Roccobarocco", renamed "Roccobarocco Uno" a few years after its first appearance, is a perfectly tuned choir of floral voices (with rose, hyacinth and tuberose rising above all the others), softened by a citrus top accord of bergamot and sweet orange, and a velvety-smooth touch of ripe fruit. The heart accord, while not particularly original on today's olfactory scene, was rather surprising at the time, because floral fragrances enhanced with evident fruity nuances would not emerge powerfully until a few years later. "Roccobarocco" moves in completely the opposite direction from its resoundingly powerful contemporaries, softly caressing the skin with a graceful, gentle fragrance, whose whispered, restrained lusciousness would today be welcomed as an example of class and moderation.

Projection is kept discreet and is never invasive; a couple of hours after application, "Roccobarocco" settles down into a soft, subtle, floral languor that invites the wearer to apply it afresh. Spraying it on fabrics is the best way to make it last longer.

"Roccobarocco" has earned its place in this volume not only for the beauty of the fragrance, but also for three other reasons. The first regards the composer, Maurizio Cerizza, one of the Italian greats in his field: this was his first successful fragrance. The second is its longevity: unlike many fragrances that appeared in the same period, "Roccobarocco" is still in production – and for a perfume, thirty years is the equivalent of 300 for a human being. The third reason is the exquisite bottle, with its tall, square shape that offers a contemporary take on the spectacular cobalt blue skyscraper of "Je Reviens" (Worth) created by Lalique in the 1930s.

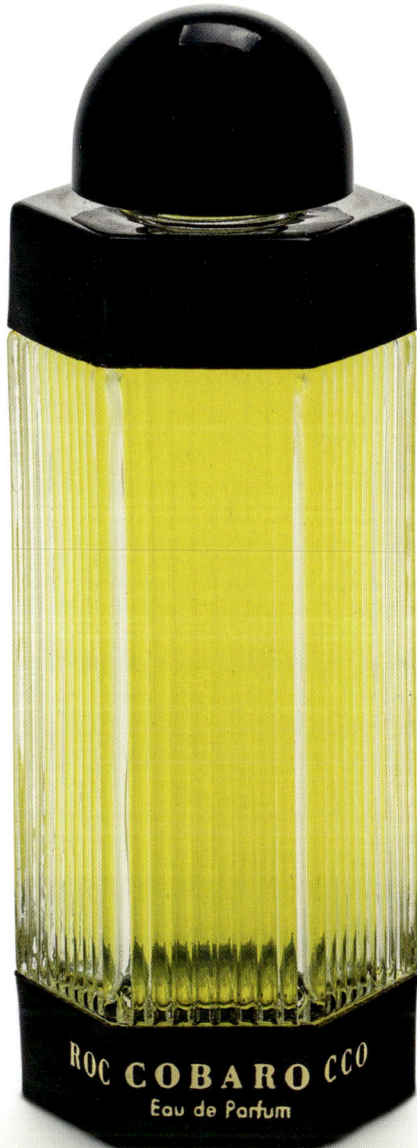

ROC COBARO CCO

Eau de Parfum

Grigioperla

Brand: La Perla
Gender: masculine
Year of launch: 1986
Status: in production
Analyzed version: vintage Eau de Toilette
Author: IFF
Classification: amber fougère
Bottle design: Pierre Dinand

For at least a decade, "Grigioperla" was one among of the most popular fragrances with Italian men. It was often a gift from their wives or girlfriends, who chose it for a specific reason. "Grigioperla"'s strength lies in the fact it is midway between a smiling, clean-shaven dad and an attractive gentleman that gets out of the car first so he can open the door for you.

A bright, clean citrus accord shines briefly upon application, before the heart accord steals the show with its floral accent of carnation and geranium and a bouquet of aromatic notes of rosemary, anise, coriander, sage and lavender.

The base notes of oak moss, sandalwood and cedar, tonka bean and a touch of ambergris envelop the aromatic notes in a long, lingering, clean, reassuring embrace that's invitingly, intimately seductive.

The aromatic fougère structure makes it similar to two iconic fragrances of the period: "Drakkar Noir" (Guy Laroche, 1982), which came before it, and "Cool Water" (Davidoff, 1988), which came afterwards. While "Drakkar Noir" is direct, open and sunny, not excessively nuanced, "Grigioperla" has a more introverted, reserved character, which shines through only towards the end. And while "Cool Water" is cold, haughty and metallic, "Grigioperla" offers a soft, indefinable caress.

Although it doesn't smell particularly original today, it certainly was when it came out, with the amber note to the fore. Pleasant and versatile, with excellent longevity and a fair sillage that invites a closer scent experience.

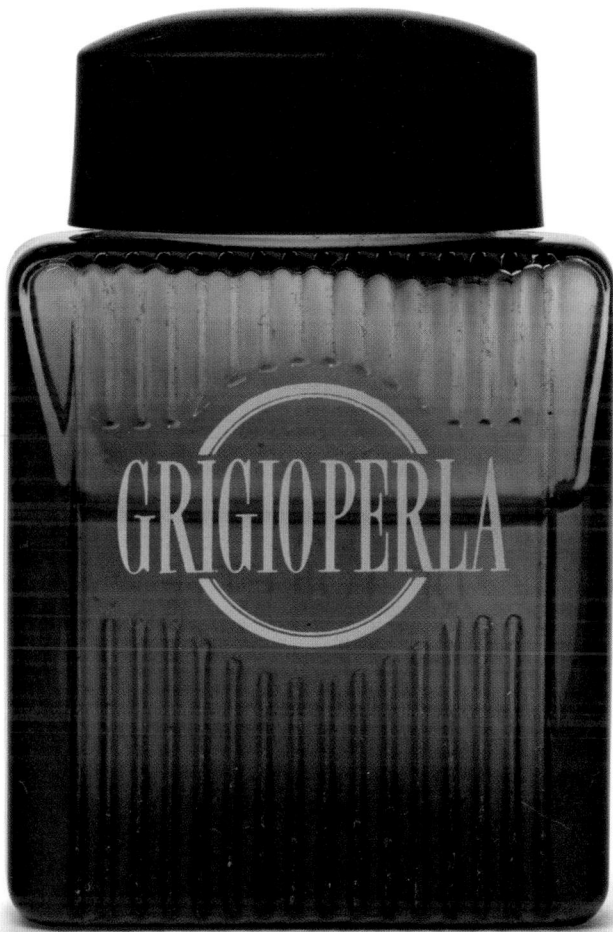

Colors

Brand: Benetton
Gender: feminine/unisex
Year of launch: 1987
Status: discontinued
Analyzed version: original Eau de Toilette
Author: Bernard Ellena (Mane)
Classification: floral oriental

The Benetton family has invested heavily in their brand communication, conveying, for at least two decades, an original, recognizable image, often ahead of its time. The United Colors of Benetton commercials of the 1980s for example, feature Nordic, African and Oriental models, and even Aboriginal Australians, all dressed, of course, in Benetton apparel. Today we live in a multi-ethnic society, but in the 1980s, Benetton was the only fashion brand that showed the variety of colours and shapes that make up our marvelous human tribe. The Benetton promotional model – the whole world united in the name of the Brand – was not emulated by international marketing strategists until many years later, when globalisation has already taken a firm hold (the famous campaign for the launch of "CKOne" by Calvin Klein is substantially the exact same idea, realized in 1994).

"Colors" shares the same extreme originality: it was, in essence, a fougère embellished with surprising floral and fruity touches. A rare, magnificent hybrid between an ultra-traditional masculine fragrance and a fruity floral with a deep, resounding feminine voice.

This mix of two classic accords, one typically masculine and the other typically feminine, makes "Colors" not so much an unisex fragrance, but a transgender one: indeed the first transgender fragrance in history, able to anticipate all gender issues of the following decades, and offer an interesting point of view even today. Evidently, at the basis of this perfume there was a very strong vision of the future, which today appears almost prophetic.

"Colors'" fougère base accord is very much "old school", with aromatic notes of lavender, sage and basil, alongside oak moss and vanilla and tonka bean. Resting on this dusty, rustic accord is a fluorescent pink lace, decorated with ultra-feminine notes of neroli, hyacinth and tuberose, and exotic fruits (pineapple, passion fruit and peach). The fruity floral accord is densely sweet, and only thanks to the fougère counterpart it is able to maintain a precarious balance, right on the far edge of excess.

Fluorescent, over-the-top and "teenage", "Colors" is not easy to wear, requiring a bigger personality than its own and a huge desire to have fun. It has an impressive projection, with a clingy sweetness that lasts a couple of hours, fading slowly over the subsequent two hours.

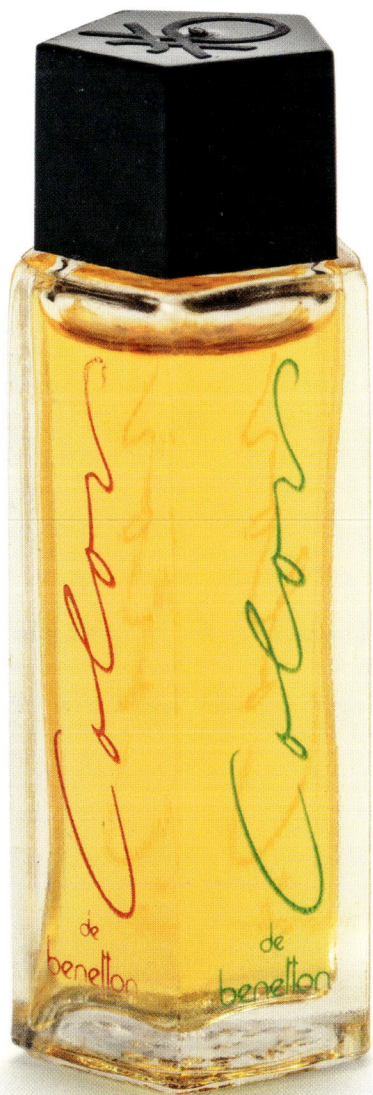

Moschino

Brand: Moschino
Gender: feminine
Year of launch: 1987
Status: in production
Analyzed version: original Eau de Toilette
Author: Firmenich
Classification: oriental
Bottle design: Pierre Dinand
Glassware Company: Bormioli Luigi

The first Moschino fragrance descends from an extremely noble lineage that began a century ago with the first two successful orientals in history: "Emeraude" (Coty, 1921) and "Shalimar" (Guerlain, 1926).

"Emeraude"'s oriental heart was very avant-garde; its angular, audacious character was toned down a little and made more affably "wearable" in "Shalimar" and all the other orientals of classic structure that followed. Sixty years later, "Must" by Cartier (1981), "Obsession" by Calvin Klein (1985) and "Lancaster" (1986) brought oriental fragrances back into fashion, shifting the focus from the classic oriental accord (with vanilla and wood, sometimes "seasoned" with resins and spices) towards a new one, with resins (labdanum, benzoin, myrrh, Peru and Tolu balsams, etc.), and ambergris (both natural and synthetic).

Moschino is poised perfectly between the most illustrious classic orientals and the new-generation ambers; perceptible in this fragrance is both the shadow of the great orientals by Guerlain ("Shalimar" and "L'Heure Bleue" in primis) and a gourmand nuance that is merely hinted at, offering a foretaste of "Cašmir" and "Angel". All this richness is enveloped by a chypre sensation that brings a more resolute edge, making it less affable than those coming before and after it.

"Moschino" opens with an unusually dry, green accord of marigold and galbanum, stretching right into the heart of the formula, featuring a whispering bouquet of sweet/green flowers (honeysuckle, freesia, gardenia, rose, ylang ylang). This floral/green bouquet is warmed by a handful of spices (black pepper, nutmeg and cloves), which team the top and heart of the fragrance with a classic base shaped by patchouli, sandalwood, amber notes, musk and vanilla.

The three accords do not so much replace one another as layer one over the other, becoming fully mature an hour after application. Despite the generous natural notes creating a myriad of nuances and undertones, "Moschino" is perfectly balanced and interesting from beginning to end, brimming with personality and drive through every note. Its place is among the crown jewels of the oriental/amber family of any period. "Moschino" is endowed with impressive sonority, yes the projection is never overpowering. Its record-breaking longevity, however, makes it perceptible even after a long day at work and a quick shower.

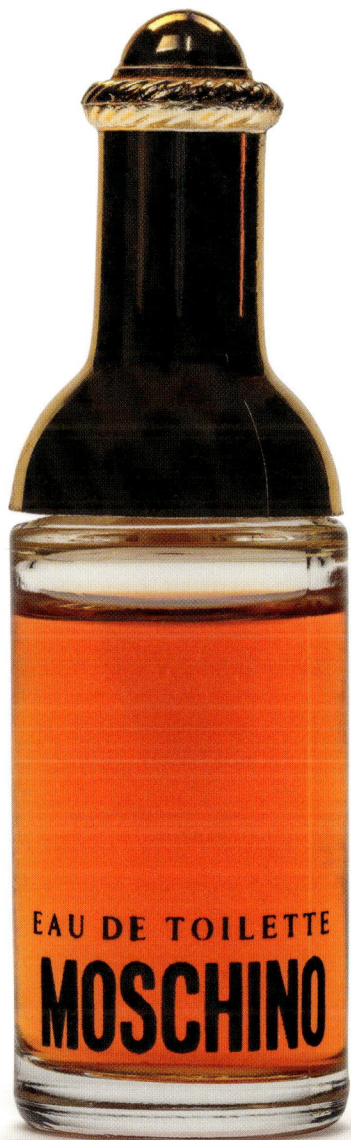

EAU DE TOILETTE

MOSCHINO

Sergio Tacchini

Brand: Sergio Tacchini
Gender: masculine
Year of launch: 1987
Status: in production
Analyzed version: original Eau de Toilette
Classification: woody fougère
Bottle design: Macchi

"Sergio Tacchini" is one of those typical understated fragrances that is not immediately, distinctively noticeable, yet helps to bring the wearer perfectly into focus (an achievement many fragrances with high-sounding names don't even come close to). It opens with a spark of bitter citrus (lemon and bergamot) and Mediterranean aromas, lit up by a minimum amount of aldehydes, making a start that although not particularly original, is lively and persistent. The aromatic component of the top accord slips into the heart/base accord, dominated by cedar and sandalwood notes and a fair amount of benzoin; this classic accord is always effective, hinting at a simple, unassuming elegance. Soundly, skilfully composed, with a fairly good sillage and endless persistence, it comes as no surprise that "Sergio Tacchini" is still in production and continues to find favour with the public. Its fine, tonifying essence makes it suitable for all hours and adaptable to all occasions: from a trip along the Riviera on a silvery motorboat to a board meeting or a game of tennis. Its linear, perfectly clean-cut olfactory structure makes it a timeless, ageless fragrance.

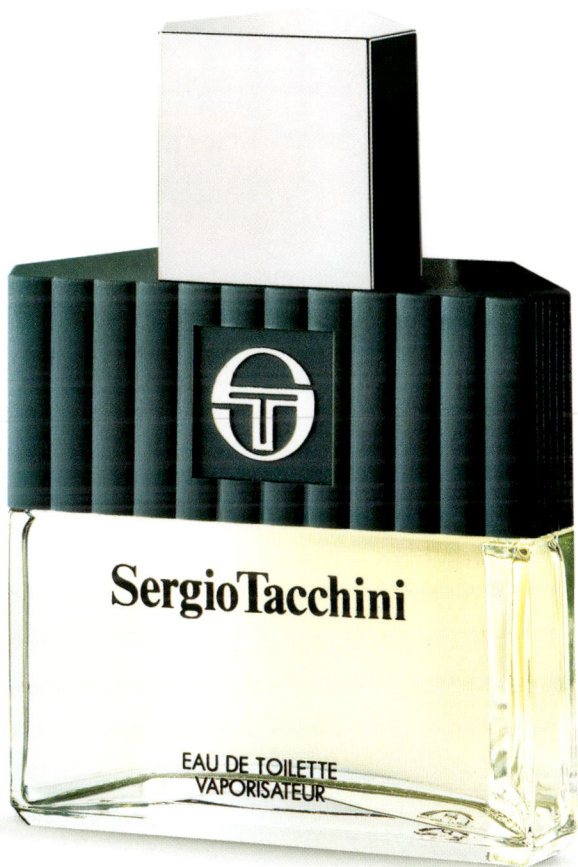

Genny

Brand: Genny
Gender: feminine
Year of launch: 1987
Status: relaunched in 1993
Analyzed version: vintage parfum de toilette
Classification: floral chypre
Bottle design: Saint Gobain Desjonqueres

If the legendary "Aromatics Elixir" (Clinique, 1971) were Italian, its name would be "Genny". It would shine like the most precious of diamonds, thanks to the crystalline aldehydes; it would be more generous with white flowers (orange blossom, jasmine and tuberose), and would be more affable, even fun at times (not all the time though, because a chypre remains a chypre, even an Italian one...). The quality of the materials and the perfectly executed olfactory structure place "Genny" at exactly the same level as its illustrious forebear, while at the same time giving it that open, generous, sunny personality that sets it apart from it.

"Genny" is a marvellous fragrance, the "parfum de toilette" concentration – less potent than a *parfum*, but stronger than an Eau de Parfum – gives it a powerful, resounding character with an audaciously feminine edge, and allows for a confident projection of up to a metre for the whole of the first hour. As the base accord comes through with the passing of the hours, "Genny" tones down and takes on woody, dry, salty, leathery, almost masculine nuances, with a duration of more than six hours. The Eau de Toilette version is more transparent, with the white flowers and aldehydes not coming through as strongly; the chypre notes are evident from the beginning, with accentuated green undertones that bring it closer to a green chypre than a floral chypre. The IFRA restrictions on the use of materials – primarily oak moss and jasmine – have altered this fragrance, as they have all its glorious siblings from the period. Many have been removed from the market; others are fortunately still available, although slightly different from the original version. If you're lucky enough to find the vintage version, make sure you don't let it get away. In any case, however, even the modern version of "Genny" merits a length trial on the skin, because fragrances with such a sparkling personality have all but disappeared. The "Genny" bottle – a triangular shape with a tall, Zen-inspired top – is a sublimely simple yet sophisticated example of design, mirroring the angular beauty of its content.

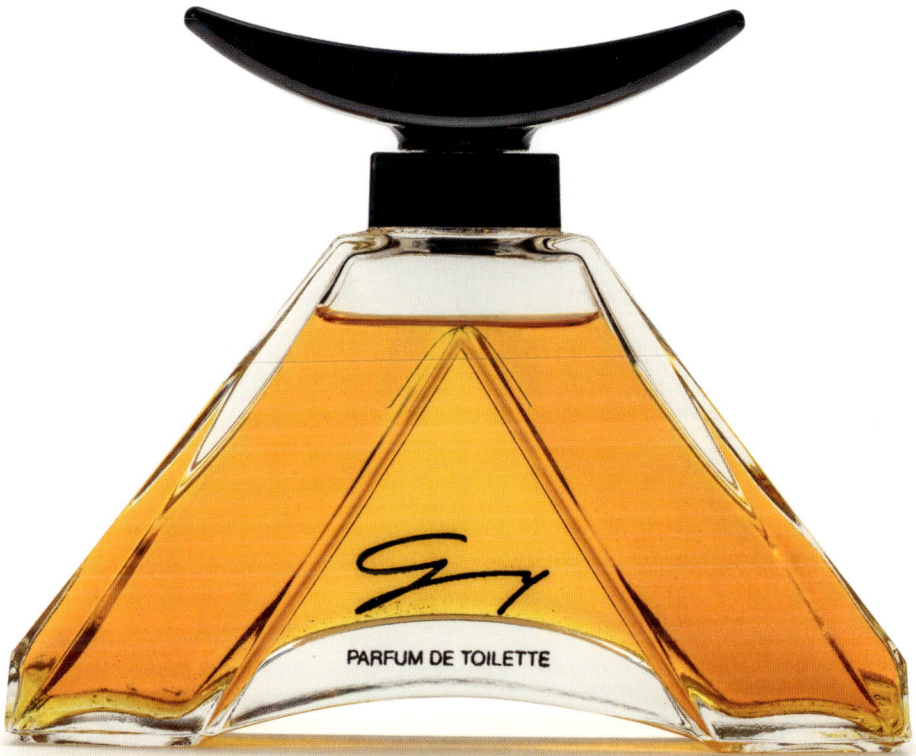

Roma

Brand: Laura Biagiotti
Gender: feminine
Year of launch: 1988
Status: in production
Analyzed version: original Eau de Toilette
Author: Jean Pierre Mary (IFF)
Classification: woody oriental
Bottle design: Peter Schmidt/Laura Biagiotti

When the first perfume for her maison was launched, Laura Biagiotti was already a leading name in Italian fashion, who introduced the Made in Italy concept into countries such as China (1988) and Russia (1995) well before they were colonised by the big multinationals. Her first fragrance bears the name of her beloved Rome, and the city's eternal allure (referred to in the tagline *a breath of eternity*) is reflected in the shape of the bottle: a section of an ancient column in satin glass. The liquid inside the bottle has a superbly romantic pink tinge. The combination of the name, bottle and colour creates a strikingly alluring effect, conjuring up images of breathtaking sunsets admired from a terrace looking out over the Imperial Fora, and undoubtedly contributed to the huge success of the fragrance.

Right from the opening, "Roma" expresses an assertive personality, with excellent structure. The top and heart accords feature fruity/floral notes of lemon, grapefruit, blackcurrant, orange blossom, rose, tuberose and lily of the valley, which could have been assembled in a less original manner, were it not for a minty note running through them, capturing the attention and counterpointing the sweetness. The base is a classically smooth, velvety ambery ("Shalimar" style, shall we say), featuring precious resins (myrrh, benzoin), patchouli and sandalwood, vanilla, and a whisper of creamy musks. This base works wonders also on men's skin, recalling the depth of "Obsession" (Calvin Klein, 1985), but with a less "stormy" construction.

The main interest of this fragrance lies in the subtle, almost imperceptible tension between the amber base and the decidedly floral heart, which attract and repel one another for the entire duration of the formula. This interplay is managed magnificently so that neither of the two accords prevails, and "Roma" remains interesting for its whole life.

"Roma" has straightforward evolution and than settles in a linear melody which lasts for several hours, with a textbook projection fading out very softly.

Both fresh and warm, with dry notes of face powder, its sculptural elegance remains timeless and thoroughly contemporary to this day: a sort of olfactory "Great Beauty" everyone should know.

"Roma" is still in production. The mint in the opening has been replaced with a hint of citrus that gives a fresher, more contemporary edge with an addition of powdery accents.

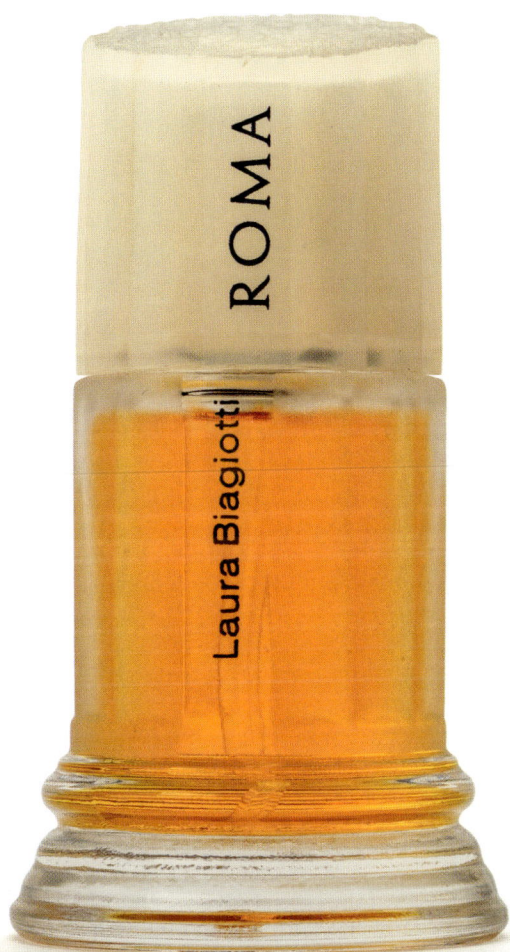

Atelier

Brand: Sergio Soldano
Gender: feminine
Year of launch: 1988
Status: discontinued
Analyzed version: vintage Eau de Toilette
Classification: gourmand oriental

"Atelier" is an opulent, sensual oriental fragrance composed in the grand manner, with a wonderfully generous, very 1980s olfactory structure that draws its inspiration from "Shalimar" (Guerlain, 1926), developed in a sumptuous, luscious direction. Italian Baroque at its best. "Atelier" features a generous opening of sunny citrus notes (bergamot, sweet orange, petitgrain), layered over a beautiful rose, strengthened by notes of geranium and ylang ylang, enhanced with a delicious raspberry nuance. The base accord rises up almost immediately into the heart of the formula, with sandalwood smoothly complementing a precious thick, sticky balm (Copaiba); the task of the vanilla is to bind all the sweet notes together and bring them to a triumphant climax. Velvety-smooth and bathed in an autumn glow, Atelier is an authentic "fur coat" fragrance, by which I mean a luxury perfume that "smells" expensive, and must be worn on the skin like a precious jewel, without any other adornments to steal the limelight from it. Its powerful, *very* diffusive fragrance gives away its 1980s origin, without taking anything at all away from its allure. Best worn in winter, when it develops slowly, allowing you to fully enjoy every single note.

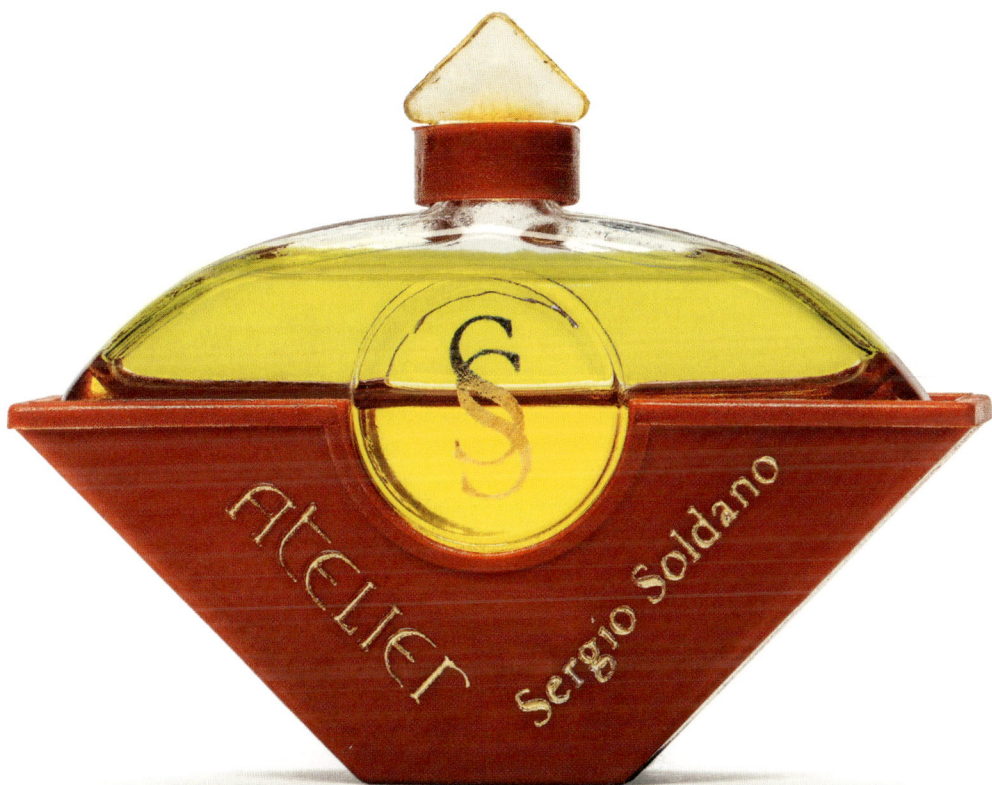

Gucci Nobile

Brand: Gucci
Gender: masculine
Year of launch: 1988
Status: discontinued
Analyzed version: original Eau de Toilette
Classification: aromatic fougère
Bottle design: Peter Schmidt
Glassware Company: Bormioli Luigi

Gucci "Nobile" is the archetypal Italian-style fougère: an aromatic fragrance with a lush freshness and a floral nuance offering a sophisticated nonchalance, perfect for those who prefer the natural scents of the woodland to the asphalt jungle. "Nobile" opens with citrus notes and a bunch of aromatic herbs such as lavender, rosemary, tarragon and mace, along with green notes conveying a vigorous, energising, outdoorsy "push". The moment the floral notes make their entrance – flowers with a hint of green and spice such as carnation, geranium, jasmine, with a touch of aldehyde – the fragrance heads in the "barber's shop" direction typical of its category.
In the meantime, the base accord comes through, offering a beautifully rich, woody bouquet of patchouli, vetiver, cedar and sandalwood, tonka bean, birch tar and vegetable musk; as well as stabilising the fragrance, it takes it in a subtly chypre direction, making it more complex and luxurious than a "simple" 1980s aromatic fougère in the style of "Eternity" by Calvin Klein (which appeared a year later, with an olfactory structure very similar to "Nobile", but without the chypre nuance). "Nobile" is a structured, dense, profound fragrance, both natural and sophisticated, with an excellent projection and a duration of a good few hours; unlike many other men's fragrances from the period – exuberant, "manly", almost insolent – "Nobile" effectively gives off an air of noble detachment.
A few bottles can still be found for sale on internet: at exorbitant prices, of course. If this kind of fragrance appeals to you, rest assured you won't be disappointed: "Nobile" is the best you'll find.

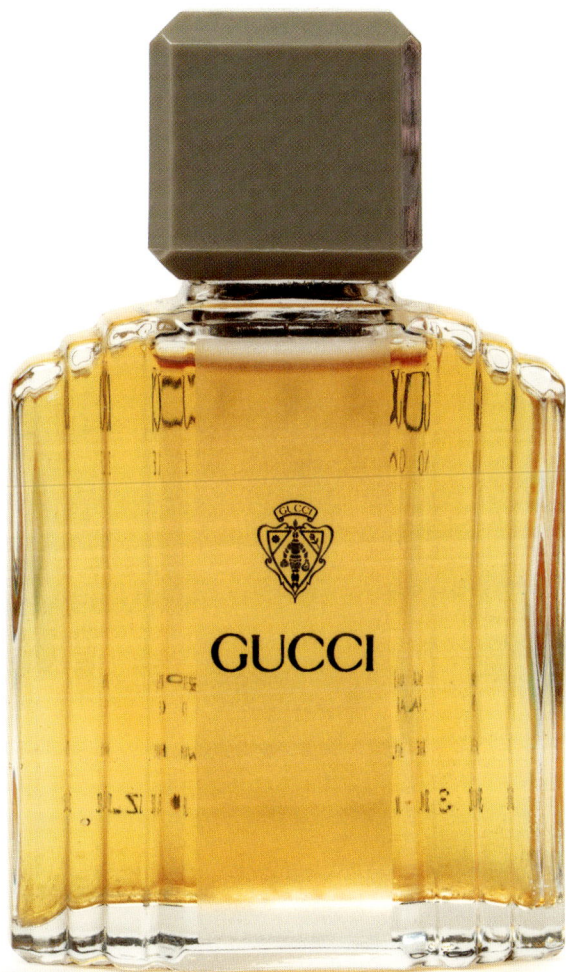

Patchouly

Brand: Etro
Gender: unisex
Year of launch: 1989
Status: in production
Analyzed version: original Eau de Toilette
Author: Jaques Flori
Classification: woody oriental

The couture designed by Etro is an invitation to travel to the most exotic and fascinating places in the Far East, populated by Maharanis dressed in long caftans of precious silks in warm, lively colors, embellished with Paisley graphics and original cuts. Even the perfumes of the Etro line play with the idea of an harmonious and seductive Orient, and their "Patchouly" is the perfect invitation to those who are not so keen on patchouli because they see it as an inflated note, its damp, grassy, musty character being a little too reminiscent of the flower power people of the 1970s. In this "Patchouly", there's no perceptible trace of hippy gatherings or strange souped-up cigarettes. Here there's just a warm, extra-dry patchouli, with all its enchanting nuances of mint, earth and tobacco. The demure vanilla and amber notes, together with end notes of vetiver and liquorice, highlight the fragrance's woody essence, while the slightest, barely perceptible touch of incense raises it up from the earth into an almost mystical experience.

In the "Patchouly" formula, the damp, ambiguous, harsh edges have been concealed to perfection, allowing for a severe, reserved sensation that's both profound and sophisticated. It's a hard act to follow!

"Patchouly" deserves a place right up among the greats in its category: "Coromandel" (Chanel), "Borneo 1834" (Serge Lutens), "Patchouli Noir" (Histoires des Parfums), "Patchouly" (Reminiscence) and "Patchouli Nobile" (Nobile 1942).

The version currently available has been mellowed further; all the edges have been smoothed, with a less reserved and more approachable effect.

"Patchouly" is an intense fragrance that spreads confidently, and although it is a cologne, it lasts for over five hours.

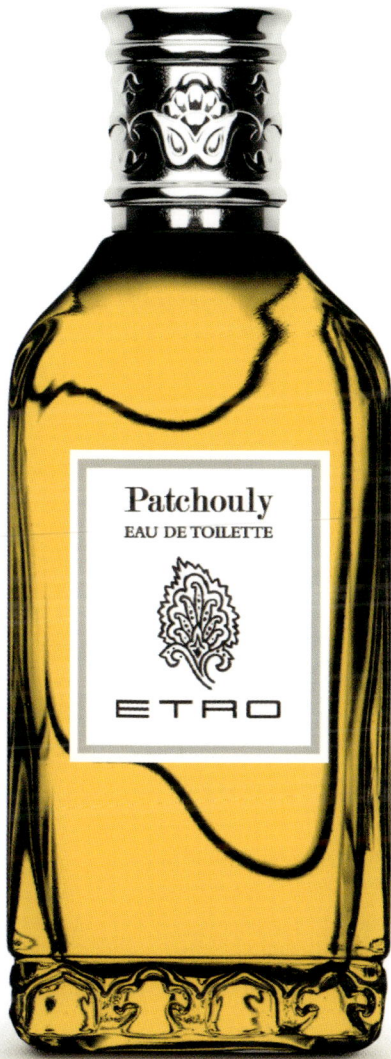

Iceberg

Brand: Iceberg
Gender: feminine
Year of launch: 1989
Status: relaunched in 2007
Analyzed version: original Eau de Toilette
Author: Sophie Labbé
Classification: aldehydic floral
Bottle design: Joel Desgrippes
Glassware Company: Bormioli Luigi

"Iceberg" has been able to build up a long line of admirers over four decades: an exceptional result that would on its own suffice to draw anyone into a perfumery to discover the strengths of this fragrance.

Wealth and sophistication are not the focal point of "Iceberg": considering the period it first came out in, this is an unusually composed fragrance, with the accent on a clean-cut structure and fresh, translucent sensations created by a bouquet of transparent flowers.

All these characteristics would not become trendy until two decades later. Bright and lively right from the opening thanks to the citrus notes of bergamot and lemon, teamed with the green, pungent notes of basil and galbanum, "Iceberg" is softened by a deliciously feminine rose, in an accord with other flowers that have shed much of their specific weight (lily of the valley, jasmine, lily, ylang ylang) and are illuminated by a dash of aldehydes. Light, clean and delicate. The musky bouquet of the base, softened by iris, vegetable musk and amber notes, offers a stable base for the flowers and lengthens duration, adding other green, dry, subtle face powder notes.

Although the base accord of "Iceberg" features a chypre vibration, it is insufficient to give the fragrance the statuesque humoral character of the chypres from the period. At the same time, its clarity does not take on board the ozonic/detergent edge that was making its way into perfumery during those years; so Iceberg has never been particularly aligned with the trends of the moment. It has style, however: a style all of its own that was ahead of its time, and that has remained unaltered over the years, except for a few little adjustments due to age.

"Iceberg" has a projection of medium intensity for an hour, after which it calms down, giving out green, powdery notes for another couple of hours.

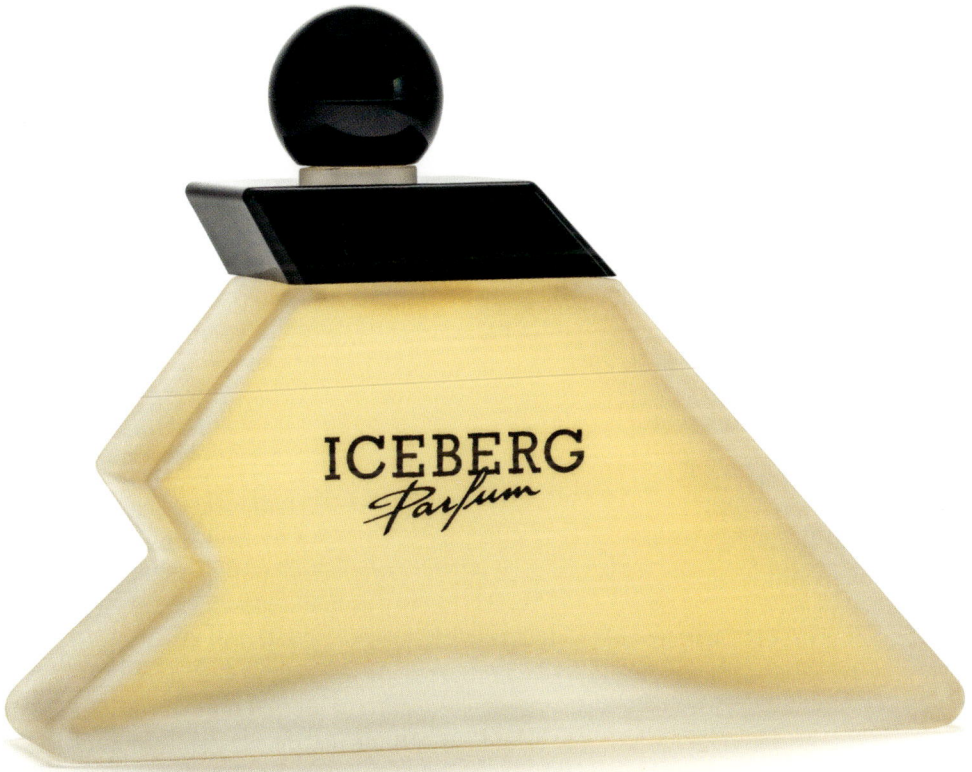

Romeo

Brand: Romeo Gigli
Gender: feminine
Year of launch: 1989
Status: discontinued
Analyzed version: original Eau de Toilette
Author: Sophie Labbé
Classification: green floral
Bottle design: Romeo Gigli and Serge Mansau

Perhaps it is because our temperate climate allows us to enjoy long spells of time outdoors, or because our gardens are full of aromatic plants with grassy scents (lavender, rosemary, sage, verbena, oregano, basil, myrtle, laurel, marjoram, thyme and all sorts of other marvellous varieties). Whatever the reason, the green facet has always been much loved by Italians, and "Romeo" by Romeo Gigli is one of the finest green floral fragrances ever produced in Italy. "Romeo" slides gracefully over the skin, with its citrus bouquet of lime, mandarin and bergamot that welcomes aboard a triumph of flowers now a thing of the past: rose and carnation give a compact, satisfying texture; cassia, freesia and neroli bring contribute their honeyed breath, while lily of the valley and jasmine give "Romeo" a lush, green accent, amplified by pot marigold and basil, a pairing so resinous, aromatic and astringent that it resembles the note of galbanum. A fruity undertone of mango acts as a magnificent counterpoint to the grassy nuance, making it even more evident, if possible, throughout the formula.

The backbone of "Romeo" remains the green floral bouquet, even when the sandalwood and iris base notes come through, bringing powdery tones, while benzoin and incense maintain the freshness right through to drydown. The effect on the skin is natural, vivid, open, evocative of the time of the year when plants begin their cycle once more, just before spring. Although flowers are still wrapped tightly up inside their corolla, the sap is already beginning to rise up within the stalks, filling the surrounding air with its fragrance and infusing it with the promise of new life. "Romeo" is one of the first fragrances by Sophie Labbé, offering a clear perception of her love for delicately processed flowers and spring sensations. Thanks to its outdoor ambience, "Romeo" is also perfectly suitable for men to enjoy, taking on spiced, aromatic sensations; the projection is moderate, lasting about two hours and stretching to four with the superbly delicate drydown.
The spectacular bottle, designed by Romeo Gigli, features a white chiffon drape being blown away by the wind.

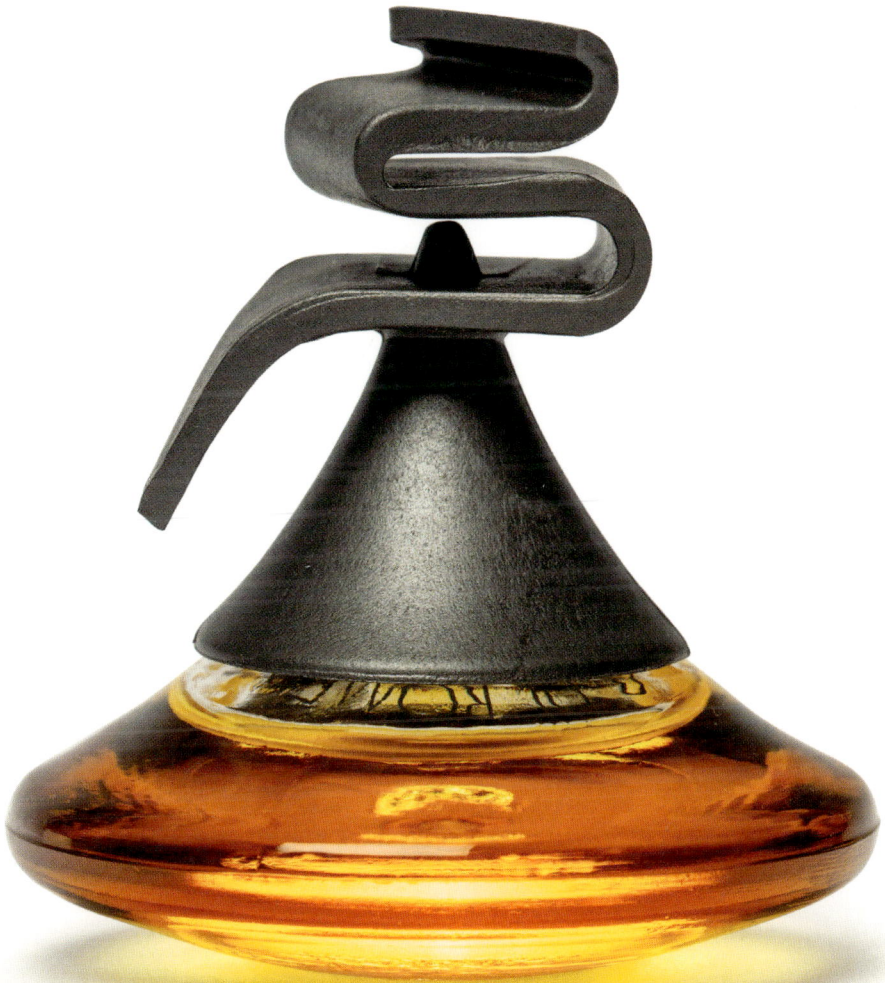

V/E

Brand: Gianni Versace
Gender: feminine
Year of launch: 1989
Status: discontinued
Analyzed version: original Eau de Toilette
Author: Jean-Pierre Béthouart (Firmenich)
Classification: fresh floral/floral chypre
Bottle design: Thierry Lecoule
Glassware company: Christallerie Baccarat

This little gem from Versace has such a variety of nuances and undertones that it's difficult to catalogue: citrus floral? fresh floral? aldehydic floral? rose soliflore? floral chypre? Capturing the essence of this fragrance is no easy task. Capturing the essence of a Real Women never is.

"V/E" opens with bergamot, lemon, mandarin and a note of light, vibrant rosewood with floral/aromatic nuances, accompanied by a delightful, spirited fresh floral accord of hyacinth, violet and rose. Aldehydes envelop the floral accord in a pearly, milky, translucent cloak.

As the minutes go by, the rose rises up from the floral bouquet and begins to sing with a full, vibrant voice featuring rough, subtly spiced undertones and capturing all the attention.

An hour from application, an iris note comes through and winds its way around the middle and base notes, binding to the rose above and the sandalwood and cedar notes below, and in particular to the oak moss, which takes "V/E" into the realm of the chypres with a husky, sensual voice.

Three perfectly performed movements, three complex personalities concentrated into a single bottle, where they alternate smoothly in a formula calibrated to the millimetre.

"V/E" is the heir of both "Diorella" (1972, a floral chypre with green nuances) and "Anaïs Anaïs" (1979, a fresh floral). "V/E" has a more amiable, fashionable personality than "Diorella", while it is more adult and emancipated than "Anaïs Anaïs", shaping up into a petite blonde with a rebellious temperament, a sort of Debbie Harry in a silver catsuit singing "Heart of Glass" on the disco floor.

"V/E" comes forth proudly for the first hour, creating a metre-wide bubble around the wearer, before toning down slightly, although it makes itself clearly heard for another two hours. By the fifth hour, once it has entered the drydown phase, "V/E" matures enough to leave the rebel attitude behind, finally settling on the skin where it starts to whisper with powdery tones.

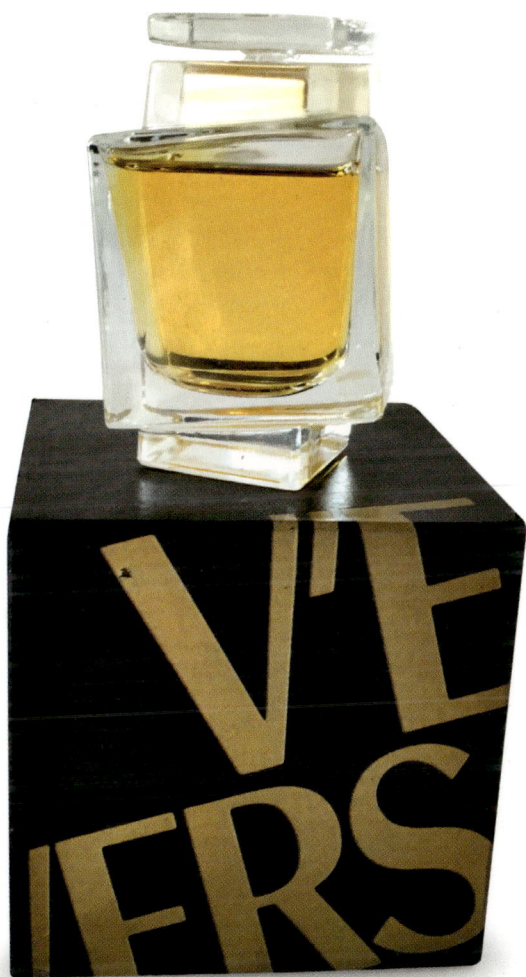

90

The Great Italian Perfumes of the 1990s

The social and cultural background

The 1990s began with the outbreak of the Gulf War, which brought an end to the rampant materialism of the 1980s. The years that followed would continue to be marked by conflict, as the Gulf War was followed by a bloody war in the former Yugoslavia, which redrew the borders of a significant portion of Europe, by the war in Chechnya and by the brutal genocide in Rwanda.

In Italy, with the "Tangentopoli" scandal, and the "Mani Pulite" investigation it prompted, the Italians became aware of the widespread system of corruption involving Italian politics and business.

For the whole decade, in many countries in the West, AIDS became a social scourge that killed hundreds of thousands of young people, without the possibility of an effective treatment.

Society's reaction to these shocking events was for people to take refuge in what they held dearest, prompting them to rediscover the value of solid relationships founded on friendship, trust and a sense of belonging; new aspirations came to the fore, focusing on greater purity and a return to nature and to integrity. New Age philosophy and alternative medicine spread decisively throughout the West.

Meanwhile, the spread of Internet shaped the new, Global Village, and TV, cellphones and the satellites in orbit around the Earth began to change the way we communicate, creating the impression of a shrinking world.

Techno music took hold in discos, and rave parties drew crowds of young people with a shared desire to be at one with Nature, with their fellow human beings and with the Divine; a longing for experiences able to transcend an everyday existence dominated by the violent images on TV.

The trends of the decade

By the 1990s, perfume was no longer considered a status symbol, and had become accessible across the board in the West. Many new brands were appearing on the market alongside cosmetic companies, designers and jewellery brands.

Marketing became the main instrument used to "construct" perfumes: consumers are segmented into categories (based on gender, age, nationality, socio-economic and cultural condition, lifestyle, spending capacity, etc.) on which the composition of perfumes was then based. This placed considerable restrictions of the creative freedom of perfume composers, turning them into mere "fragrance makers".

Promotional images became increasingly sophisticated and exciting, and perfume companies invested heavily for the chance to work with visionary directors of the calibre of Ridley Scott, David Lynch and Luc Besson, able to transmit a completely new, engaging visual aesthetic. Among the most memorable commercials of the decade were those for "Égoïste" (Chanel), with dozens of women looking out of the windows of the Carlton Hotel shouting "Égoïste!"; "Trésor" (Lancôme), featuring a se-pia-toned Isabella Rossellini; "Obsession" (Calvin Klein), starring a very young, naked, disquieting, irresistible Kate Moss; "CKOne" (Calvin Klein), with a multi-ethnic, multi-gender, multi-age tribe rigorously portrayed in black and white; "J'Adore" (Dior), with the molten gold lake that became an icon; "Coco" (Chanel), featuring a very young Vanessa Paradis as a splendid caged bird, and finally, Estella Warren in the guise of Little Red Riding Hood, in the "N°5" (Chanel) commercial directed by Luc Besson.

From the point of view of the fragrances, compared to the "larg-er than life" ones of the 1980s, the perfumes of the 1990s seemed to have just come through gastric band surgery: subtle, watery and purified, they were a reaction to the "exterior" trend of the previous decade, in search of greater interiority. This was the decade in which the desire for nature, unspoilt settings and connections with primeval energy burst through powerfully, and was masterfully interpreted by the world of perfumery.

The olfactory expression of these new values was entrusted to new materials obtained thanks to the advances made in Headspace technology, which allowed for the analysis and reproduction of all possible places, objects and situations.

In the mid-1990s, Firmenich laboratories discovered and patented the macrocyclic musks (including Habanolide, Muscenone, Exaltenone, Paradisone, Romandolide), a category of synthetic molecules with a musky scent resembling that of the marvellous nitromusks used between the 1930s and 1960s, but more stable and with no risk to health, which were to become fashionable with "Classique" (Jean Paul Gaultier, 1993), "Bulgari for Men" (1995), "Pleasures" (Estée Lauder, 1995).

In addition to the new "fresh" musky notes, woody and amber musky notes were patented, as well as made-up fruity notes and salty notes defined as "ozonic/marine".

The discovery of these new olfactory notes offered perfume composers a wealth of new options to express themselves, and this decade saw the dawn of the three most important categories of contemporary perfume composition: the fruity florals, the ozonic/marines and the gourmands.

The fruity florals teamed the floral notes with an endless variety of fruit notes, featuring sweet, sharp, exotic, ripe and red fruit nuances. To bring out the best in the new fruity notes, the floral accords were kept fresher and lighter than the classic florals, and many flowers with an excessively strong character were thus abandoned in favour of a softer, more subtle floral sensation. The trend took off with "Happy" (Clinique, 1992), Moschino "Cheap & Chic" (1995), "Baby Doll" (Yves Saint Laurent, 1996) and "Envy" (Gucci, 1997), and continued with the most famous: the legendary "J'Adore" (Dior, 1999).

On the opposing side, the marine/ozonics provided a response to the desire to get away from it all, for open, unspoilt spaces, with their salty notes evoking the fragrance of a stroll along the ocean front, breathing in the sea air. The trailblazer of this family was a men's fragrance, "New West" (Aramis, 1990), followed by "Escape" (Calvin Klein, 1991) and "Kenzo homme" (1990), but it was the launch of "L'Eau d'Issey" (Issey Miyake, 1992) and "Acqua di Giò" (Armani, 1996) that brought resounding success.

With "Cašmir" (Chopard, 1991) and "Angel" (Thierry Mugler, 1992), the market welcomed the successful family of oriental/amber fragrances with gourmand nuances, characterised by a prominent vanilla note, accompanied by other sugary, praline, candies, cocoa, coffee, almond, milky and caramel notes that remain popular to this day. "Cašmir" and "Angel" were followed by Lolita Lempicka (1997), "Hypnotic Poison" (Dior, 1998), "Emporio Armani" (1998) and many others.

For men, modern fougère fragrances held up well, with examples including "Cerruti 1881" (1990), "Polo Sport" (Ralph Lauren, 1993), "Dolce&Gabbana Uomo" (1994), "Hugo" (Hugo Boss, 1995). Men's fragrances also continued to explore the floral avenue ("Insensé" by Givenchy, 1993), as well as the oriental/amber route ("Égoïste" by Chanel, 1990; "Le Male" by Gaultier, 1995; "Allure homme" by Chanel, 1997 and "Rochas man", 1999).

In Italy

The perfumes by Italian designers held up well among the most successful fragrances; while not everyone can afford models from the catwalks of Milan, we can all wear the brand of our dreams in the form of a fragrance. A perfume costs less than a coat or an evening dress by the same designer, yet it's just as luxurious and creative.

And Italy remains marvellously creative, transmitting its essence though visionary fragrances that often open up entirely new veins of expression. The restrictions imposed by the regulations governing the use of materials compelled composers working for Italian brands to explore alternative avenues: "Gieffeffe", "Bulgari Black" and "Gucci Rush", for example, succeeded in bringing a modern, allergen-free twist to the structures typical of the great chypre, amber and floral fragrances of earlier decades, and the sublime creativity of the results was widely admired worldwide.

"Eau Parfumée au Thé Vert" (Bulgari) is another wonderfully creative fragrance, thanks to the dry, grassy edge of the innovative green tea note, destined to become a very popular olfactory trend in the years that followed thanks to the success of this particular *jus*.

The most markedly innovative developments, however, came from Byblos, which at the start of the decade opened up both the fruity floral and ozonic floral routes.

As the decade progressed, Italian fragrances gradually moved away from the exuberant, full-bodied chypre nuance of the previous decades towards the fresher, greener, more natural scents of "Eau Parfumée au Thé Vert", "Light Blue" and "Bulgari for Women". The olfactory structures were dominated by tart fruit notes, accompanied by delicate, almost ethereal floral notes, enveloped in clouds of soft musks.

For men's fragrances, fougères such as "Grigioperla" remained popular, often enriched with deep, woody notes (found in "Roma Uomo" by Laura Biagiotti and "Dolce&Gabbana pour homme") contributing sensuality and extreme sophistication.

This decade saw the launch of two perfumes destined to achieve tremendous success worldwide: "Acqua di Giò" (Giorgio Armani) and "Eau Parfumée au Thé Vert" (Bulgari) became a permanent fixture in the top ten all over the world, where they were to remain for at least two decades.

Italian perfume bottles stood out for their elaborate details, offering a visual reflection of the stylists they represented. Some of the most interesting bottles included the splendid "Vendetta" (Valentino), with its marvellous pleated glass; "1881" by Nino Cerruti, a parallelepiped in satin-finish glass with a relief design; "Blonde" (Versace), featuring a carved, satin-finish Medusa on the back, and "Blu" by Blumarine, with a sophisticated pattern reminiscent of a soft matelassé cushion. Also interesting are the plastic casings of "Asja" (Fendi) and "Proibito" (Soldano); "Mariella Burani" and "Byblos", with their sophisticated floral tops ("Byblos" was also one of the first, along with "Blu" by Blumarine, to bring the blue bottle back into fashion) and Blumarine, with its beautifully elaborate top. The most iconic of them all remains "Moschino Cheap&Chic", in red and black plastic in the shape of Popeye's Olive Oyl; the tongue-in-cheek style would make it an unmistakable design icon, able to get people talking about the brand on its own.

Perfume boutiques began opening up in a number of cities, with the Olfattorio Bar à Parfums stores in Turin among the pioneers, offering the most discerning customers olfactory gems away from the industrial mainstream, reserved for a select few experts. Among the most successful brands in this pioneering new niche market were French brands such as L'Artisan Parfumeur, Diptyque or Maître Parfumeur et Gantier, as well as Italian names of international renown such as Etro, Lorenzo Villoresi, Bruno Acampora, Laura Tonatto and classification-run new business such as the Farmacia del Castello (Genova), together with long-established brands such as Santa Maria Novella and SS. Annunziata, Borsari and Acqua di Parma (which had just been purchased by a handful of young entrepreneurs including Luca Di Montezemolo and Diego Della Valle with the aim of restoring its heritage).

Niche stores began to introduce an exclusive clientèle to an alternative perfumery, awakening such enthusiasm that customers were delighted to spread the word, proving to be the most formidable advertising resource.

Ocean Rain

Brand: Mario Valentino
Gender: masculine
Year of launch: 1990
Status: discontinued
Analyzed version: original Eau de Toilette
Author: Edmond Roudnitska
Classification: citrus chypre

"... if Edmond Roudnitska were still alive, how would he approach a contemporary men's fragrance, with the ozonic notes of Calone, white musks and all the rest?" Edmond Roudnitska has been the greatest Master Perfumer of them all, he composed masterpieces such as "Femme and Moustache" by Rochas, "Eau d'Hermès", "Diorella", "Diorama", "Diorissimo" and "Eau Sauvage" (Dior) and many more. Roudnitska is the composer everyone respects, indeed reveres, for both his creative talent and human qualities.

The answer to the question posed above is that Edmond Roudnitska, at the grand old age of 84, did author a modern men's fragrance featuring all the characteristic notes of contemporary male perfumery: Mario Valentino's "Ocean Rain".

The first spray lights up the air with the vigorous opening typical of Roudnitska's men's fragrances (lemon and bergamot, glazed with a whisper of Hedione), almost immediately joined by a classic fougère mix of lavender, artemisia, thyme and basil) over which a floral bouquet of rose and cyclamen breathes a soft, humid, moving, subtly melancholy sensation. Calone, in addition to the salty note also adds a touch of sugar, with a melon facet enlivening the top and heart notes. The lingering chypre base accord features leathery nuances shaped by cedarwood, musk, frankincense and amber; its indefinable opaque, chalky quality is as uncommon as it's interesting. Despite the fougère mid notes and the leathery base accord, it's almost impossible to classify "Ocean Rain" as an exclusively men's fragrance, because the perfumes it is reminiscent of are for the most part women's fragrances: "Femme" (Rochas) and "Diorella" (Dior), composed by Roudnitska himself.

The only men's fragrance it recalls is its contemporary "Fahrenheit" by Dior (by Jean Louis Sieuzac), which is also laden with floral notes.

It came out the same year as "New West" (Aramis), the first fragrance to contain those ozonic notes that were a brand-new element at the time.

The difference between the two could not be more evident, however: in "Ocean Rain", the task of Calone is merely to counterbalance the floral breeze, enliven the chypre base accord and bring a modern edge to a jus that without these ozonic notes would be a slightly dated, through splendid, classic.

"Ocean Rain" was the last fragrance to be composed by Edmond Roudnitska, a tribute to his idea of delicacy, like all his earlier creations. It has a very contained radiance, its strong character designed for the sole enjoyment of the wearer, with a longevity of about a few hours.

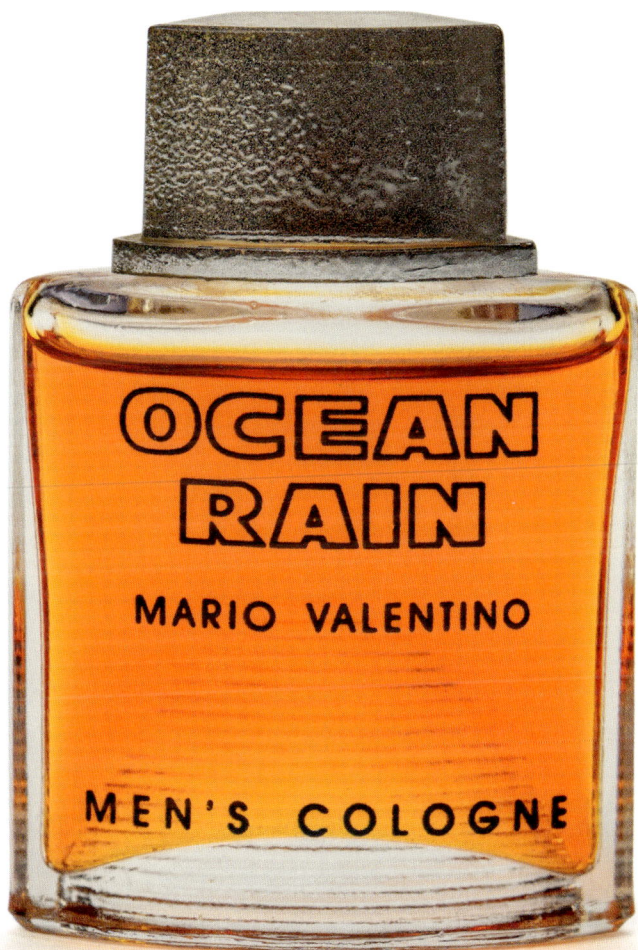

1881

Brand: Cerruti
Gender: masculine
Year of launch: 1990
Status: in production
Analyzed version: original Eau de Toilette
Author: Martin Gras (Dragoco)
Classification: aromatic fougère
Bottle design: Serge Mansau

"1881" was launched by Nino Cerruti to celebrate the year in which his family's textile business was founded, the first chapter in an entrepreneurial success story destined to last over a century. This splendid celebration took the form of an elegant, generous fragrance composition: stylish, yet laid-back and casual.

Like many other Italian fragrances, "1881" is a difficult one to pin down. It has a clean, refreshing "barber's shop" vibe, a typically fougère aromatic vibe, a gentle floral vibe and a vaguely chypre vibe. The most interesting aspect of this perfume is that all these vibes are diligently, thoroughly explored: none of them are left as an undertone, none of them are merely hinted at; they alternate over time, each one with its own development and duration. Such a dynamic composition is rarely found in a "masculine" fragrance, and is responsible for a success stretching across three decades, and for the endless number of clones it has generated.

"1881" has a terse, bright citrus opening, soon taking off down a dry, pungent road where it encounters tarragon, rosemary, juniper and lavender, as well as a potent green, almost resinous cypress note.

The aromatic notes are joined by rose, ylang ylang and a touch of forest berries, gently touching upon the aromatic accord. Coming through at this point are both the "barber's shop" and the fougère aspects, as well as the breath of flowers that vaguely recalls "Joop! Homme" (1989). As the barber's shop nuance gradually fades and the aromatic notes tone down, the flowers continue to interact, reached by a base accord that binds the smoky sweetness of the birch tar to the sensual, tender sandalwood nuances and the sweetness of the amber notes. The texture of the fragrance, resembling crisp, pure white linen throughout the first part, settles into a wonderfully soft, comfortable, sensual pashmina.

In contrast to the fashion of its time, which had a preference for amber fougères and ozonic/marine fragrances, "1881" is reminiscent of the grand classics, yet has that sassy, contemporary edge that continues to make it hugely popular today.

"1881" spreads with amiable confidence around the wearer, with the amber end notes whispering on the skin for a few hours.

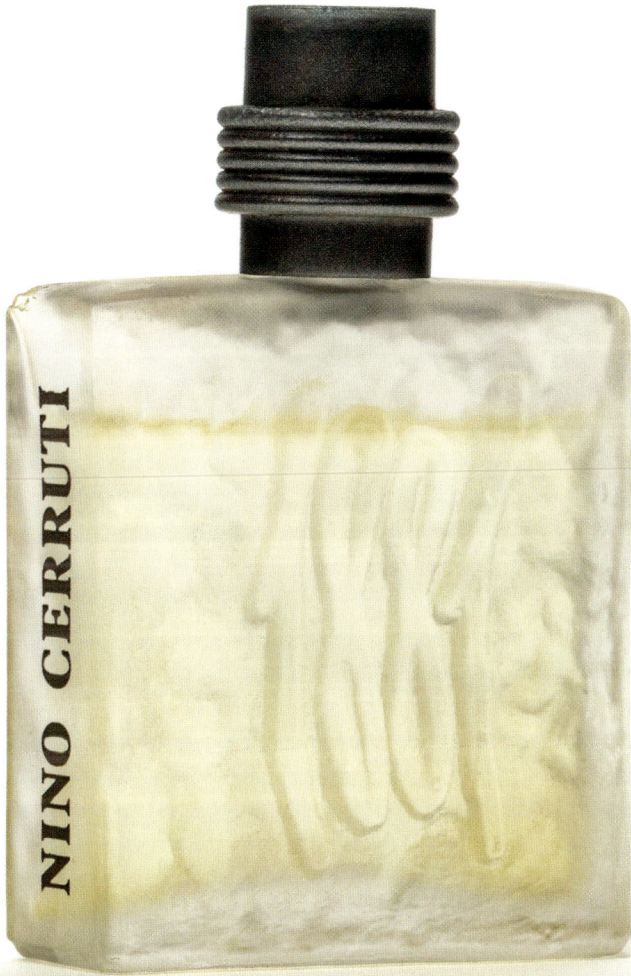

Byblos

Brand: Byblos
Gender: feminine
Year of launch: 1990
Status: discontinued
Analyzed version: original Eau de Toilette and Eau de Parfum
Author: Ilias Ermenidis (Firmenich)
Classification: ozonic fruity floral

Listen up! One of the most innovative fragrances of the last thirty years enters on stage!
"Byblos" opens with a juicy blast of citrus and fresh fruit (raspberry, blueberry, plum and nectarine peach) enhanced by a carefree floral breeze of mimosa, violet and heliotrope, with delicate powdery tones. Powdery notes are also evident in the base, with the iris and vetiver anchoring the fragrance to the skin without increasing its specific weight. Even if this had been all there was to "Byblos", it would have sufficed to make it worthy of note, because fruity florals of this calibre would start popping up only a few years later, with "Chiffon Sorbet" by Escada (1993). Fruity florals are the leading trend in today's market, but while they often appear confused, inconsistent or sickly sweet, "Byblos" was a burst of energy and *joie de vivre*, composed with rigour and balance.
And it had another surprise up its sleeve: the overall sweetness of the fruity floral bouquet is complemented by a discreetly salty note, creating a delightfully refreshing interplay that holds the attention firmly without either of the two sensations prevailing over the other. Salty notes would not become fashionable in perfumes for women until 1996, with the launch of "Cool Water Woman" (Davidoff), with its fruity bouquet complemented by marine notes (not to mention the blue bottle...).
So "Byblos" paved the way for both the fruity florals and the ozonic florals: a sort of World Champion in originality. Its exhilarating sunny, outgoing character proved popular with the public, and although it has not obtained international recognition, its audacity is obvious if examined a few decades on.
The packaging, too, was amazing, poised on the far edge between visionary design and vintage kitsch: a blue shaded bottle - decidedly unusual for the period - directly calling to mind the sea, with a contrasting copper top in the shape of a flower, resting on a circular platform.
In the Eau de Toilette, the note of black pepper adds a sharp, vivid touch that enhances the marine note, while in the Eau de Parfum the fruity accord is rounder and the fragrance is denser, with a liqueur-like texture.
The projection is good without being over the top, and persistence is perfectly satisfactory.
With its cutting-edge innovation, good taste and immediate appeal, "Byblos" was an expression of Italian perfumery at its very best.

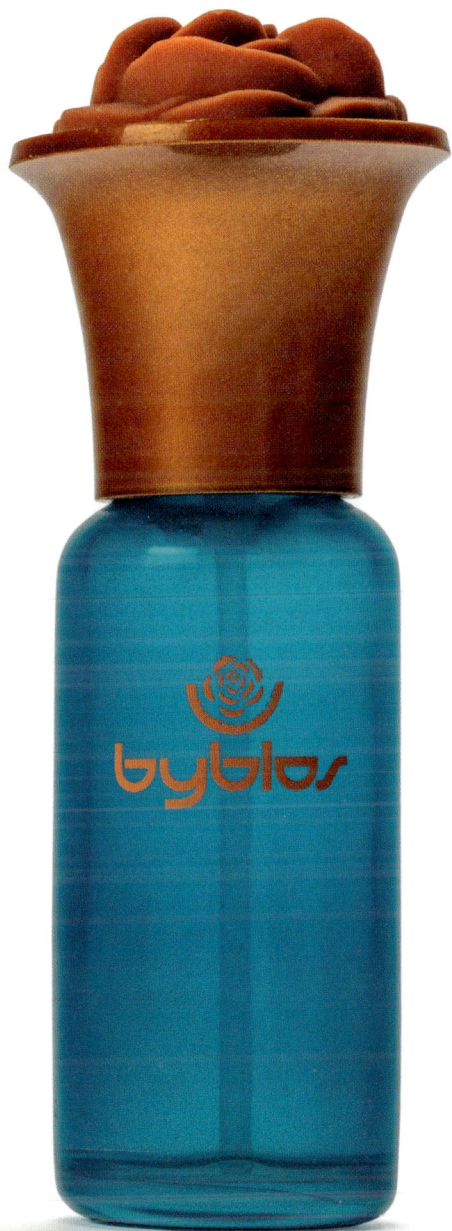

Moschino Pour Homme

Brand: Moschino
Gender: masculine
Year of launch: 1990
Status: discontinued
Analyzed version: original Eau de Toilette
Author: Francoise Caron (Roure)
Classification: leather chypre

The first fragrance for men by Moschino has the exact amount of genius and unruliness you might expect from this extraordinary punk-inspired designer. Audacious to the point of being extreme, yet at the same time incredibly sophisticated, "Moschino Pour Homme" was incomprehensibly out of fashion at the time it was launched, surrounded as it was by fragrances with a clean, ozonic "push". The reason was that "Moschino Pour Homme" was composed following the personal taste of Franco Moschino, who used it himself every day for years, making it his signature fragrance. Thirty years later, many ozonic successes of the 1990's have been completely forgot, while "Moschino Pour Homme" is still loved and sought after; it would surely make a fortune for any niche brand that made the effort to catch up its unusual, edgy character (and let's hope someone does, because it's been discontinued for too long). "Moschino Pour Homme" bursts forth from the bottle with an aromatic fougère top of bergamot, lavender, rosemary and mace, soon reached by a spicy, moody floral pair (rose and carnation). While the opening of "Moschino Pour Homme" may seem that of a classic fougère of its time, its sensual ambery, base takes just a few minutes to rise up, with resinous notes of labdanum and ambergris, vegetable musk, styrax officinalis, tonka bean and a powerful leathery edge.

"Moschino Pour Homme" conveys both the statuesque sophistication of "Bel Ami" (Hermès) and "Aramis", and the extravagant genius of "Yatagan" (Caron), pumping up the leather tone until it becomes animalic and dirty as in "Ten" (Knize). Yet, "Moschino Pour Homme" is different from all four, more contemporary extreme and unbridled. "Moschino Pour Homme" is the second-last of the heirs to the glorious dynasty of the leather chypres (which would come to an end with "Bulgari Black"), and its regal position is right in the front row, alongside its more vibrant, complex forebears.

Why this gem of inestimable value has been discontinued is completely at odds with any kind of commercial logic, given the fan base it was able to count on. I have my own theory. Because it was Franco Moschino's personal fragrance, the people who worked with him may have decided to take it off the market for the same reasons the shirt numbers of the footballing greats are not reused: out of a mixture of love and respect.

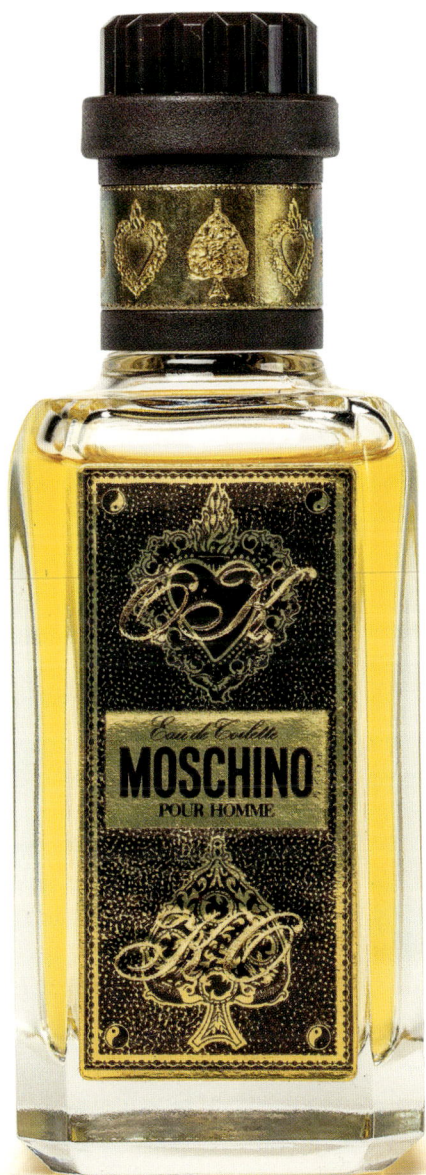

Vendetta Uomo

Brand: Valentino
Gender: masculine
Year of launch: 1991
Status: discontinued
Analyzed version: original Eau de Toilette
Author: Edouard Fléchier
Classification: woody fougère
Bottle design: Serge Mansau

"Vendetta" was composed by Edouard Fléchier, a master perfumer with the ability to create smooth, full, generous fragrances. His rich compositions are satisfying and rounded, with formulas that often focus on splendid materials and powerful concepts, such as the resounding tuberose of "Poison" by Dior (1985), or the fruity floral "C'est la Vie" by Christian Lacroix (1990), bursting with cheerful, happy thoughts, or "Lys Mediterranée" and "Une Rose" by Frédéric Malle (2000 and 2003), beacons bringing out the best in lily and rose respectively, thanks to their peerless three-dimensional quality. With its middle accord featuring verbena, neroli, laurel and cloves, "Vendetta" is one of his finest creations. This accord spreads from the heart throughout the fragrance, with an austere elegance all the other nuances revolve around.
The lavender and geranium at the heart of the fragrance form a fougère core; jasmine, patchouli and oak moss bring a confident chypre facet, labdanum, benzoin and incense envelop it in resinous and amber notes, while the leather note that comes through an hour after spraying, lasting throughout drydown, contributes a dry, incisive edge. All these currents flow around the heart accord, overlapping and gradually replacing one another, swinging back and forth between warm and cold, bright and gloomy, smooth and sharp undertones that are so intriguing it is difficult to pin the fragrance down.
This marvel by Valentino has a compact texture that spreads out discreetly, giving off an aura of extreme class; this makes it easy to wear on any occasion: if I were a man, I'd definitely wear it on a date. The fragrance has a duration of a few hours.
The transparent, disc-shaped bottle, adorned only by an original ring-shaped top, perfectly shows off the golden nuance of the perfume, offering a visual reflection of its luxurious, distinguished content.

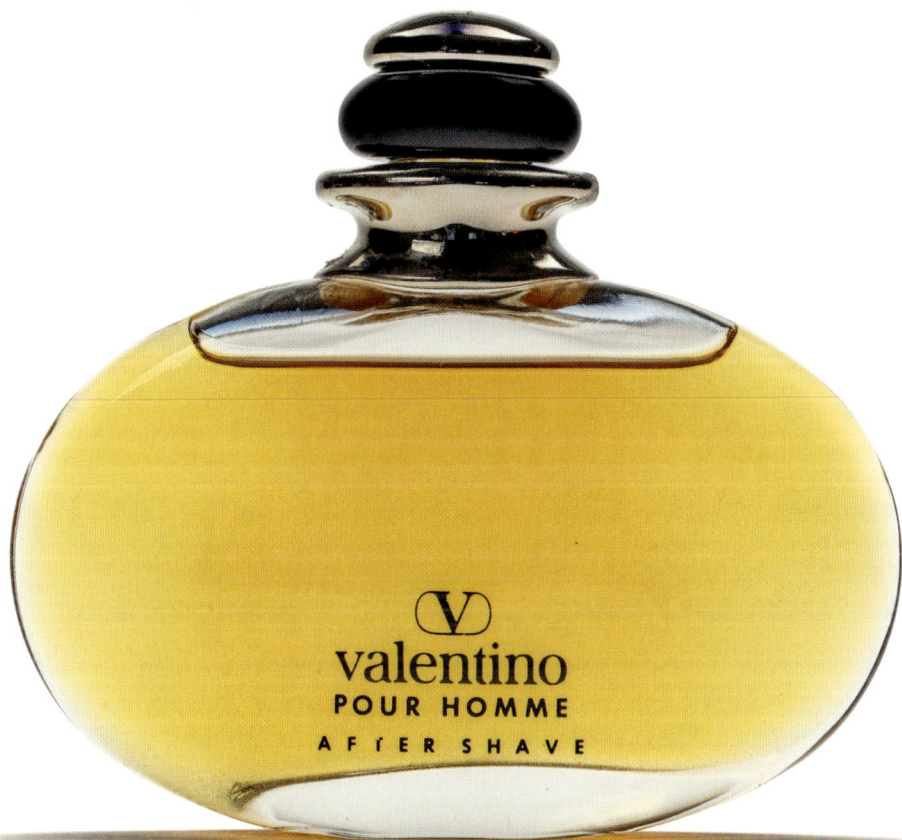

L'Arte

Brand: Gucci
Gender: feminine
Year of launch: 1991
Status: discontinued
Analyzed version: original Eau de Toilette
Classification: floral chypre
Bottle design: Serge Mansau

"L'Arte" by Gucci, brings Her Majesty the Rose onto the stage.

A velvety, temperamental rose that shifts between affable and austere, enveloped in an illuminated formula that shines the spotlight firmly on her.

Her Majesty is accompanied by aldehydes, coriander and green tones in the top/heart notes; other flowers (jasmine, tuberose, geranium and lily of the valley) come through at the heart of the fragrance, while the base accord is formed by patchouli, vetiver, amber and leathery notes and oak moss.

And right in the centre, there She is, sparkling like a diamond.

The flowers and the green notes accompany her as faithful servants are held under Her firm, imperious hand. The woody notes form the throne She sits upon, offering her support and strength. The amber notes soften the effect, rendering Her almost gentle: but only for a moment, because as soon as the chypre accord comes through, Her Majesty's dry, haughty allure returns. Yet surprisingly, the leather notes and the benzoin make her tremble with desire, awakening a wave of sensuality She can hardly restrain.

"L'Arte" is an exceptionally beautiful fragrance: complex, three-dimensional and enriched with materials of extraordinary quality.

Although I haven't been able to trace the perfume composer, I suspect it may have been someone of the calibre of Maurice Roucel or Sophia Grojsman, whose creativity has taken the rose to heights of unparalleled vibrancy: Roucel with "Tocade" (Rochas, 1995), Grojsman with "Vanderbilt" (1982), "Paris" (Yves Saint Laurent, 1983), "Trésor" (Lancôme, 1990).

Today, a fragrance such as L'Arte could come only from a niche brand, or feature in the "exclusive" line of one of the major brands; and it would be so successful that it would never occur to anyone to discontinue production.

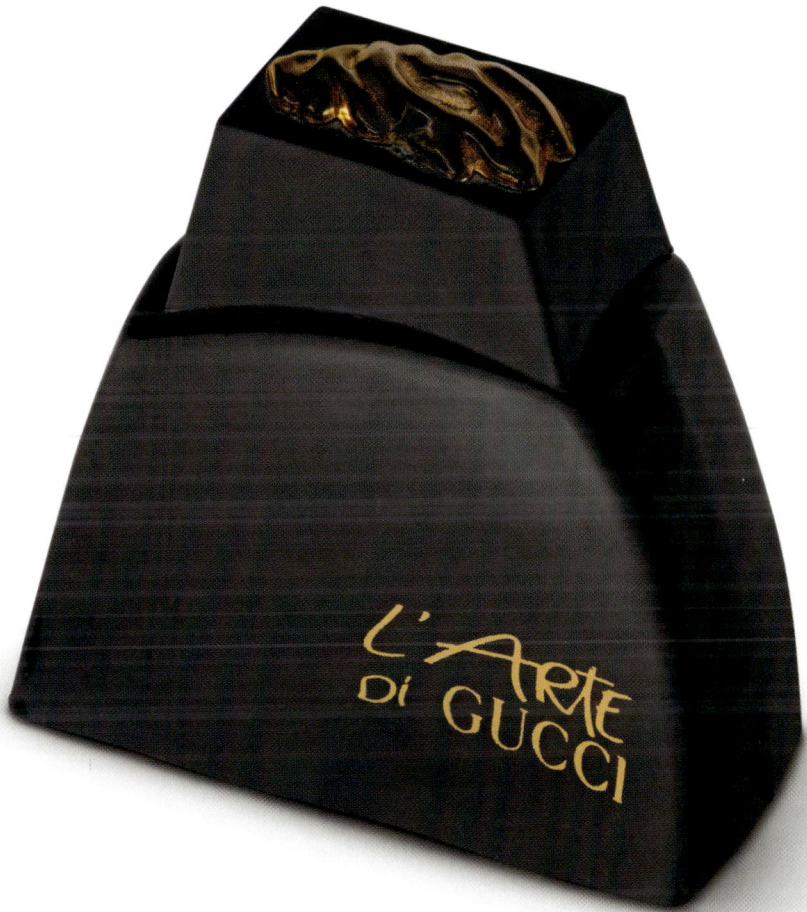

Asja

Brand: Fendi
Gender: feminine
Year of launch: 1991
Status: discontinued
Analyzed version: original Eau de Parfum
Author: Martin Heindereich (Quest)
Classification: floral oriental
Bottle design: Atelier Dinand

"Asja" may be described as an oriental perfume, embellished with a gentle floral heart and a handful of warm spices. Such a description would makes it sound like a floriental similar to many others, but in fact "Asja" does not resemble any of them. An oriental with a classic structure (wood, spices and vanilla), "Asja" gives off a naturally lush, exotic scent, thanks to the minimal amount of ripe peach and apricot, accompanied by flowers with a lusciously green facet (jasmine and ylang ylang). The spiced sensation is created by cinnamon and cloves, gently placed within an exceptionally smooth, velvety heart and base.

"Asja" is demure, serene, with an appealing finesse and a snowy white skin, able to rise above the infernal chaos of everyday life; a sort of younger sister of "Bois des Isles" (Chanel, 1926). It has good projection and perfect duration. The glass bottle hidden by the oval box, reminiscent of Chinese lacquers, was as beautiful as it was impractical; it also gave the impression of a weightiness and austerity that in no way reflected the pleasant fragrance inside. Nonetheless, it was so original and precious that it's hard to criticise: shape and function are not always perfectly compatible, and in the early 1990s, the former decidedly still prevailed over the latter.

When sampling all Fendi's earliest fragrances together (Fendi, "Asja" and "Theorema"), the uniformity and consistency of the style is really impressive. Although they differ significantly from one another – we're talking about a woody chypre, a floriental and a spiced oriental – they share the same velvety texture, the same warm, golden glow, the same spiced, liqueur-like texture, and above all, powerful base accords that share a clearly recognisable "Fendi hallmark". We're accustomed to considering olfactory consistency a given in the fragrances produced by companies with a parfumeur maison (Guerlain, Chanel, Hermès, etc.); finding that same consistency in perfumes created by different composers in different decades means that the composition of the master perfumers (Bernard Ellena, Martin Heindereich and Christine Nagel) was guided by a clear, distinctive style, a strong vision able to make those fragrances an authentic olfactory manifesto of the brand. *Chapeau*!

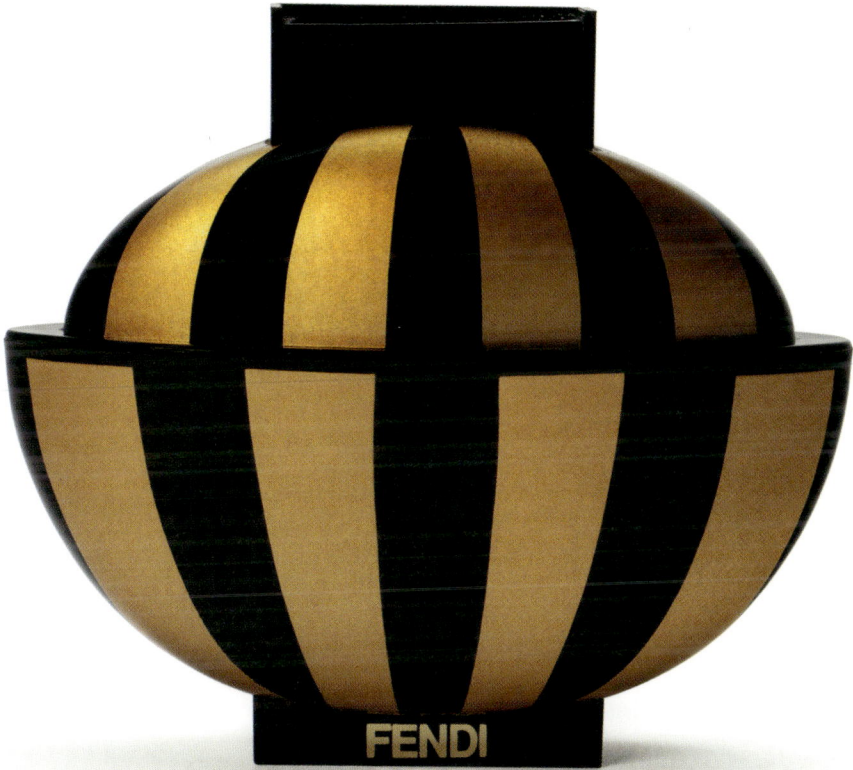

Vendetta

Brand: Valentino
Gender: feminine
Year of launch: 1991
Status: discontinued
Analyzed version: original Eau de Toilette
Author: IFF
Classification: rich floral
Bottle design: Serge Mansau

For "Vendetta", the great Serge Mansau designed one of the most striking, sophisticated bottles ever seen, immediately identifiable with the Valentino concept of *Haute Couture*. The shape of a stylish evening dress in pleated silk, floating in the breeze is a sublime, magnificent piece of work, absolutely deserving of the fragrance inside – a triumph of Baroque, with an almost overpowering opulence. "Vendetta" is essentially a floral, but with an incredible array of accords and undertones: a citrus opening, a green accord that moves through the top and heart, an aromatic accord, bright, slightly soapy aldehydes, white flowers (tuberose and jasmine), notes of ripe fruit, a woody bouquet, endless resins, musky notes – and perhaps civet, too.

There really is all sorts in "Vendetta", offering a kaleidoscope of floral, fruity, woody, green, soapy, resinous, musky sensations that alternate and link into a perfectly orchestrated – if slightly bombastic – whole, before settling down into a *Grand Soirée* finale, bejewelled and dressed to kill for a première at La Scala.

Compared to some of its more timeless contemporaries, "Vendetta" had a very recognisably 1990s style, and today it appears rather dated. Nonetheless, it remains a fragrance of incredible complexity, very much worth discovering. It has excellent projection, with a fairly extensive sillage and a duration of several hours.

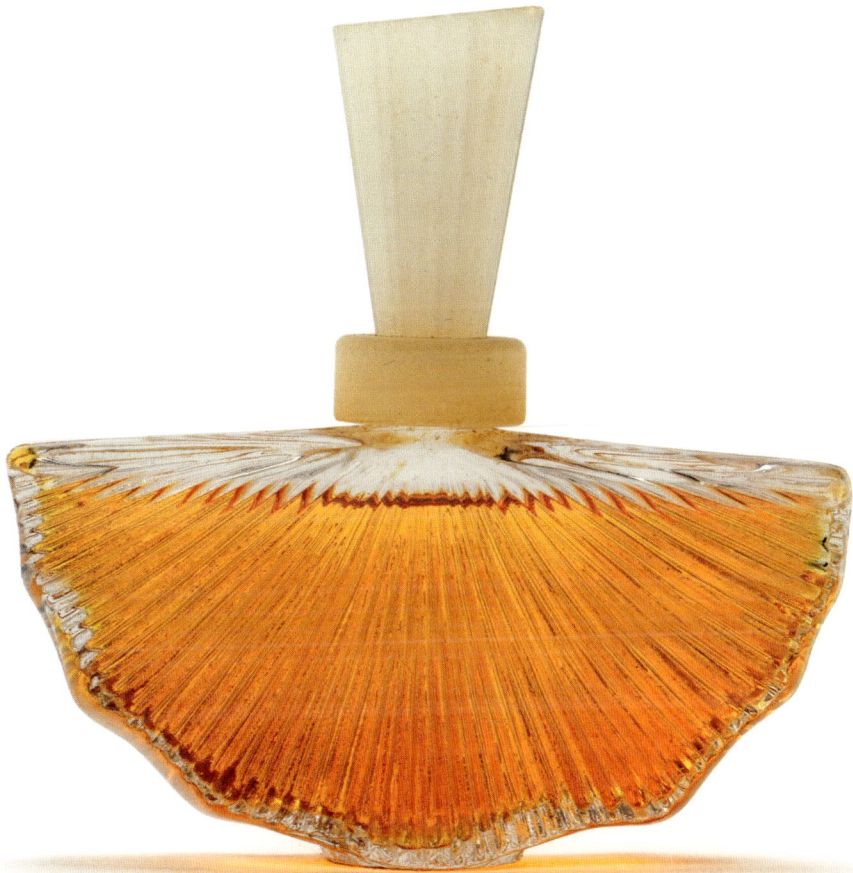

Krazy Krizia

Brand: Krizia
Gender: feminine
Year of launch: 1992
Status: discontinued
Analyzed version: original Eau de Toilette
Author: Dominique Ropion (Dragoco)
Classification: fruity oriental
Bottle design: Atelier Dinand
Glassware Company: Bormioli Luigi

The second fragrance launched by Krizia was almost more appealing than the first: in those years, Italian design could do nothing wrong. It must be said, though, that the composer of "Krazy" is none other than Dominique Ropion, considered one of the most talented, visionary perfumers ever known, an undisputed authority on the skilful use of materials and the nose behind masterpieces such as "Amarige" and "Ysatis" by Givenchy (1984 and 1991), "Trésor" by Lancôme (1990), "Safari" by Ralph Lauren (1990), "Kenzo Jungle L'Elephant" (1996) and another half dozen extraordinary fragrances for Frédéric Malle.

The early 1990s was the golden age of amber fragrances, which thanks to trailblazers like "Cašmir" (Chopard) and "Angel" (Mugler) began to take on new gourmand nuances of vanilla, condensed milk and caramel. On the same wavelength in those years was "Krazy Krizia", with its ambery formula suffused with a motherly gentleness, bathed in an enchantingly dense, languidly sensual autumn glow. This is an embrace from Sophia Loren in a black corset: beautiful, generous and scandalously inviting yet gentle and motherly at the same time. The top accord features a bouquet of citrus notes, accompanied by sassy green notes of basil and galbanum; this green sensation extends into the heart of the fragrance, with lily of the valley, jasmine, carnation and rose, while the aldehyde c-12 envelops the whole bouquet in a velvety sensation like the skin of a peach. The vegetable facet acts as a counterpoint to a powerful base accord that places the accent firmly on the sticky notes of labdanum, tonka bean, benzoin, vanilla, musk, civet, patchouli, cedar and sandalwood.

Where sweet meets green it is undoubtedly the former that prevails, but the green note effectively performs its duty of keeping the sugar from going overboard.

"Krazy Krizia" is a close relative of the fragrances mentioned above, yet it differs significantly from them, with a more mature, sophisticated personality than "Cašmir" and a softer, subtler texture than "Angel".

"Krazy Krizia" has excellent duration and textbook projection. Enthusiasm must be reined in when spraying it, however; three sprays are one two many, the explosive olfactory sensations of the 1980s being just around the corner.

Krizia was to work successfully with Ropion again in 1995, with "Accenti" and "Fiori di Krizia".

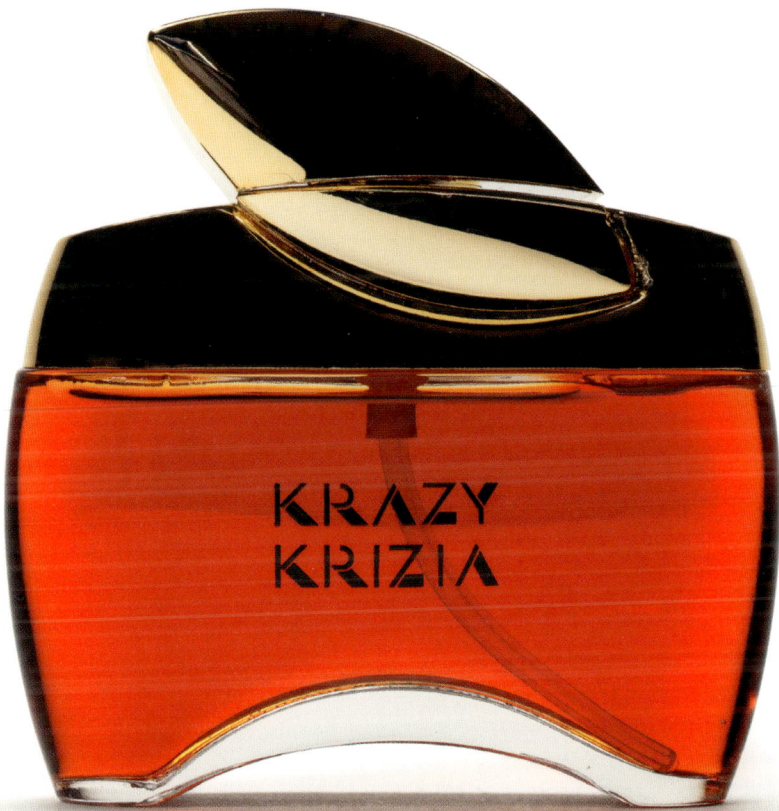

Venezia

Brand: Laura Biagiotti
Gender: feminine
Year of launch: 1992
Status: relaunched in 2011
Analyzed version: original Eau de Toilette
Classification: gourmand amber
Bottle design: Peter Schmidt

In the Middle Ages, Venice played a key role in trade between the West and the East, with spices, silk and other valuable goods travelling through the city's port on their way towards the rest of Europe. Gold, fine fabrics, monumental architecture, beautiful women, culture... all this is perceptible in the fragrance by Laura Biagiotti, thanks to its fabulously Baroque formula, with middle notes reminiscent of "Cašmir" (Chopard, which preceded it by a year) and a base accord resembling "Samsara" (Guerlain, 1989) combining to form a structure that is more elegant and complex than the former, and is more generous in nature than the latter.

"Venezia" opens with a fruity/floral top/ middle accord of peach, plum, neroli, blackcurrant, jasmine and ylang ylang, with its green floral tones embraced by a deliciously tasty, thick, smooth fruit compote enhanced with a stick of cinnamon.

The heart of the fragrance is almost immediately reached by the heavier notes of the base accord, originally a marvellously creamy mix of sandalwood, vanilla and Tolu balsam it is impossible to obtain today due to the prohibitive costs of the vanilla and sandalwood, now a protected species as a result of the intensive exploitation it was subjected to over the preceding decades.

"Venezia" is composed for the most part of natural materials of heart-stopping beauty, skilfully combined into a perfectly smooth whole: every note of "Venezia" is soft, luxurious and opulent, like a crimson brocade cloth glistening with golden reflections.

Its sweetness is never excessive, and tones down after the first half hour, as the fruity notes gradually fade. What remains on the skin after an hour is a languid, woody, supremely elegant whisper of fragrance that lasts several hours.

"Venezia" has excellent projection for the first half hour, with a breath-taking sillage the wearer must take account of in order to dose it wisely.

Unavailable for a long period of time due to the need to render the fragrance compliant with IFRA regulations, "Venezia" has been back on the shelves for a few years now: Michel Almairac and Lucas Sieuzac have trimmed the fragrance down somewhat, and Venezia is today less Baroque than the original, enveloped in musky notes that give it a more contemporary slant, so it can easily be enjoyed even by those born after 1990.

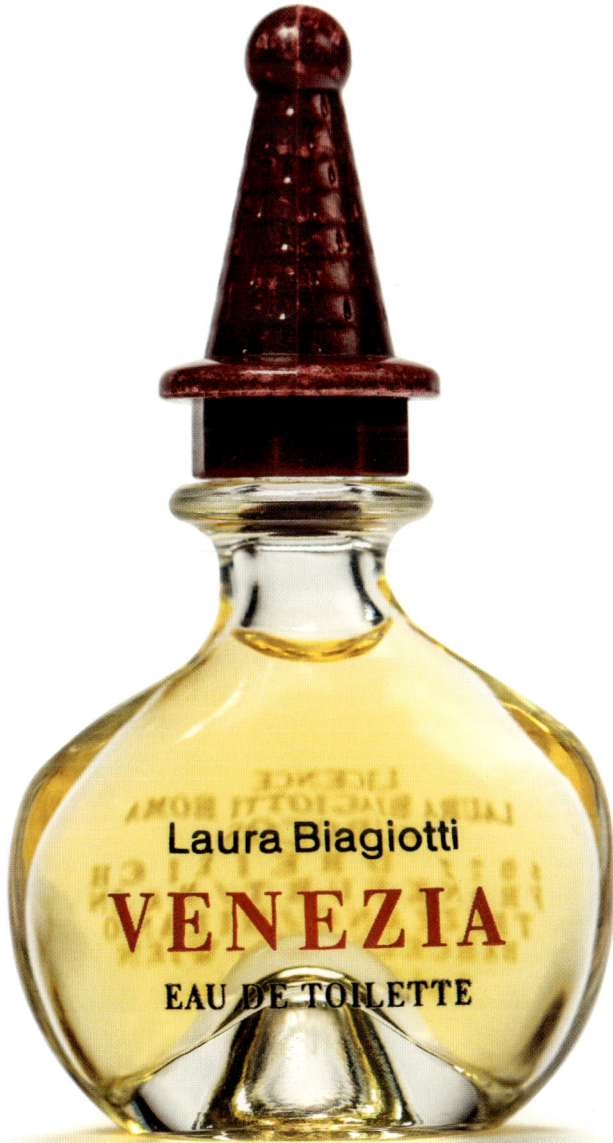

Mariella Burani

Brand: Mariella Burani
Gender: feminine
Year of launch: 1992
Status: discontinued
Analyzed version: vintage Eau de Toilette
Classification: floral oriental
Bottle design: Atelier Dinand

Pinning "Mariella Burani" down into a single olfactory category was no easy task: it has such a wealth of nuances and undertones that any official classification runs the risk of defining just a part of this complex, marvellously generous, feminine fragrance: dreamy and romantic, yet solidly rooted in much of the history of modern perfumery.

"Mariella Burani" is composed of a wide variety of mostly natural materials, starting from the rich bouquet of sun-drenched citrus notes (lemon, bergamot, sweet orange and mandarin), following through with a hint of spices, a rich floral bouquet of rose, geranium, lily of the valley and ylang ylang with an aldehydic slant cutting through it, a delicious hint of peach, coconut and vanilla, a powder-pink touch of iris and violet, an amber nuance of labdanum, Tolu balsam and benzoin, a magnificently woody base accord of cedar, sandalwood and vetiver, oak moss and an animalic note of castoreum.

More than a mere fragrance, Mariella Burani is an olfactory journey through perfumery at its finest and most vibrant, with sophisticated accents reminiscent of "Chanel N°5" (the top and heart notes), half a dozen of the classic orientals (heart and base notes) and the most enchanting chypres ever composed (base notes), along with an intriguing "sun cream" sensation that was a brand-new feature at the time. "Mariella Burani" undoubtedly owes its sublime formal balance to the experience of a renowned, exceptionally talented perfume composer: fragrances like this do not emerge from nowhere. Unfortunately, I haven't been able to discover the composer's name.

"Mariella Burani" creates a perfect sillage (clearly perceptible at a distance of half a metre), with a duration of several hours. The fragrance is an exhaustive expression of all the nuances that characterise Italian perfumery: the pursuit of immediate appeal, a generous scent with a velvety texture, all enhanced by a sense of humour that is all too rare: far too many fragrances take themselves too seriously, without sufficient reason to do so.

Unfortunately, "Mariella Burani" has been discontinued for some time, and is difficult to come by; but I assure you it would be worth tracking down, and worth every penny.

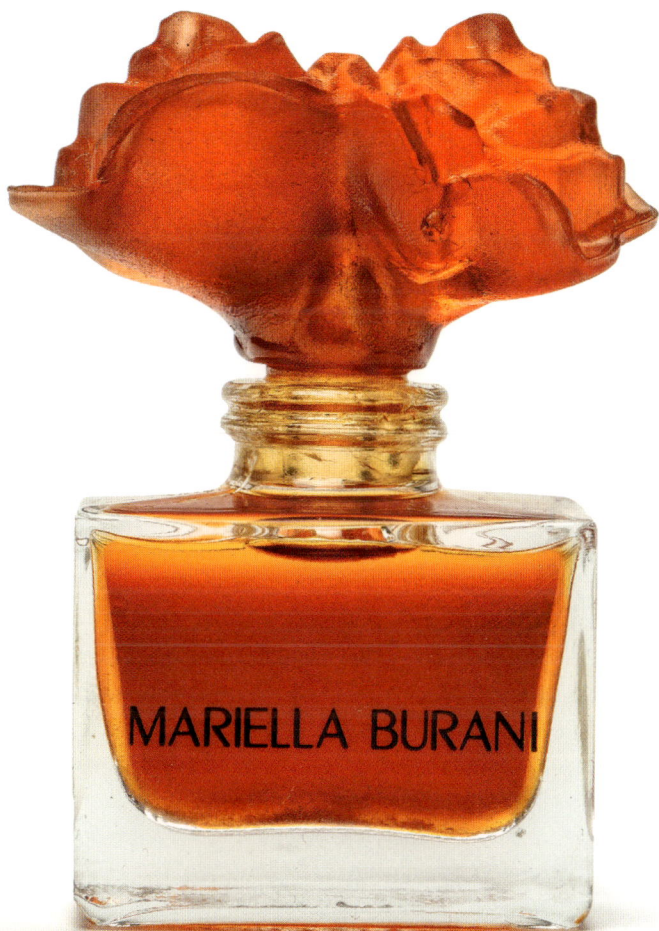

Giò

Brand: Armani
Gender: feminine
Year of launch: 1992
Status: discontinued
Analyzed version: original Eau de Toilette
Author: Françoise Caron
Classification: rich floral
Bottle design: Giorgio Armani in collaboration with Michel Blanc

"Giò" is a typical example of a rich floral composed in the grand manner, with a formula featuring magnificent floral materials, in which rose, jasmine, neroli, ylang ylang, gardenia, freesia, hyacinth, carnation and violet twirl around a marvellous tuberose. Yet there's nothing in "Giò" that's evocative of that retro, "old lady" opulence you might expect from such an abundance of flowers, nothing that conjures up images of dresses with a long train or diamond-studded tiaras. "Giò" has an innate, minimalist elegance, with the accent firmly on substance rather than impression. Giò is a woman in a simple, crisp, white shirt, with her hair tied back and no visible make-up, her only embellishment a slender, beautifully stylish bracelet. She has a sophisticated, slightly introspective, contemplative air that's both tremendously appealing and just out of reach. When you meet a woman like "Giò", how beautiful she is matters not; she always ends up making you feel like the ugly duckling before a graceful swan.

A bright, summery mandarin note ushers in the fragrance's floral bouquet, dominated by white flowers and a soft, frothy tuberose. This floral nectar gradually releases all its marvellous green and pinkish nuances, with the tuberose acting as the conductor's baton that brings the two forth alternately. Half an hour after application, a subtle hint of honey envelops the flowers in a cloak of velvet, bringing a gentler, more mature, serene, slightly syrupy glow to them. Sensational. Almost insuperable. Two hours after application, when the typically 1990s base accord of amber, benzoin and sandalwood comes through, it becomes easy to tell "Giò"'s age. This takes nothing away from her appeal; quite the reverse, because when you realise how old she is, it simply makes you wonder how such a mature woman has lost nothing of her powerful magnetism.

"Giò" is one of the finest creations by Francoise Caron, the author of absolute masterpieces such as "L'Eau d'Orange Verte" by Hermès (1979) and "Ça Sent Beau" by Kenzo (1988).

The fragrance develops for about six hours, settling perfectly onto the skin with a moderate sillage best maintained as such, without weighing it down by spraying it too liberally.

This is one of the true treasures of Italian perfumery, now unfortunately discontinued and hard to get hold of.

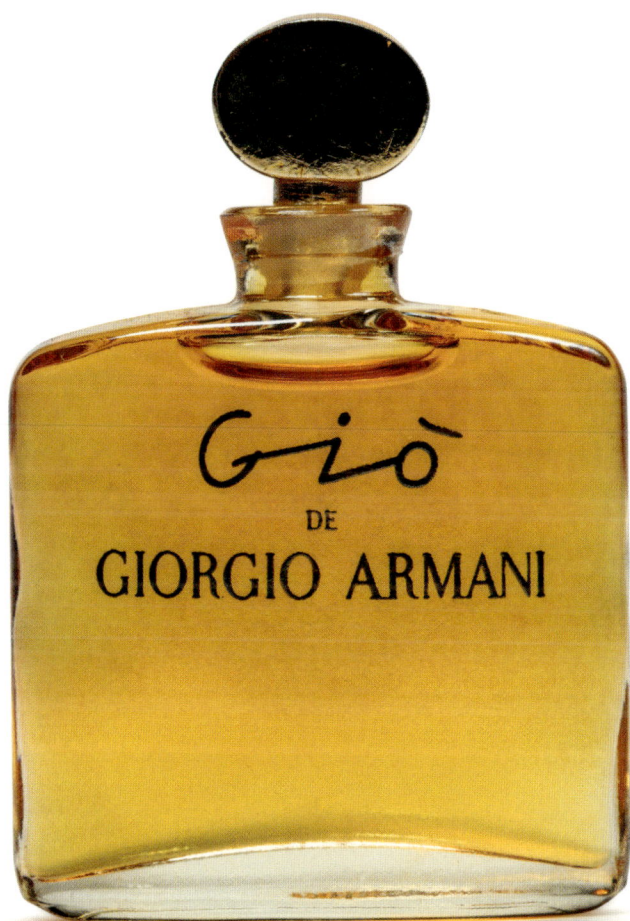

Dolce & Gabbana

Brand: Dolce & Gabbana
Gender: feminine
Year of launch: 1992
Status: relaunched in 2012
Analyzed version: original Eau de Toilette
Author: Jean Claude Mary (IFF)
Classification: oriental

The personality of the 1990s fragrances by Dolce & Gabbana closely resembled that of the couture creations by the two stylists: the marvelous "Dolce e Gabbana pour homme", together with its feminine counterpart, are among their finest.

The feminine version opens with an exhilarating citrus accord with the accent on the green/dry note of the petitgrain polished and refined by an aldehydic touch, and moves on into a floral bouquet of carnation, freesia and lily of the valley triumphantly bringing forth a magnificently sunny, feminine neroli; the heart accord would later be taken up and amplified in Sicily, with a higher dose of aldehydes and white flowers. The splendid central accord has the open, direct personality of a confident, self-assured woman with a sensual, affable tone of voice. As the flowers gradually fade, the aldehydes take on base notes (warm, sensual amber, sandalwood, sweet vanilla and tonka bean), creating a musky trail radiating a seductive, intimate sensation.

Dolce & Gabbana boasts good projection without raising its voice, offering an invitation to move closer, to smell the scent directly on the skin, creating an intimate contact.

The duration is perfect.

Dolce & Gabbana belongs to the oriental family; this is more evident in the Eau de Toilette, which is more floral, especially soft and inviting, while the Eau de Parfum, although from the same family, has a more markedly aldehydic tone. The current reformulation has replaced the sandalwood – no longer available – with a bouquet of creamy white musks.

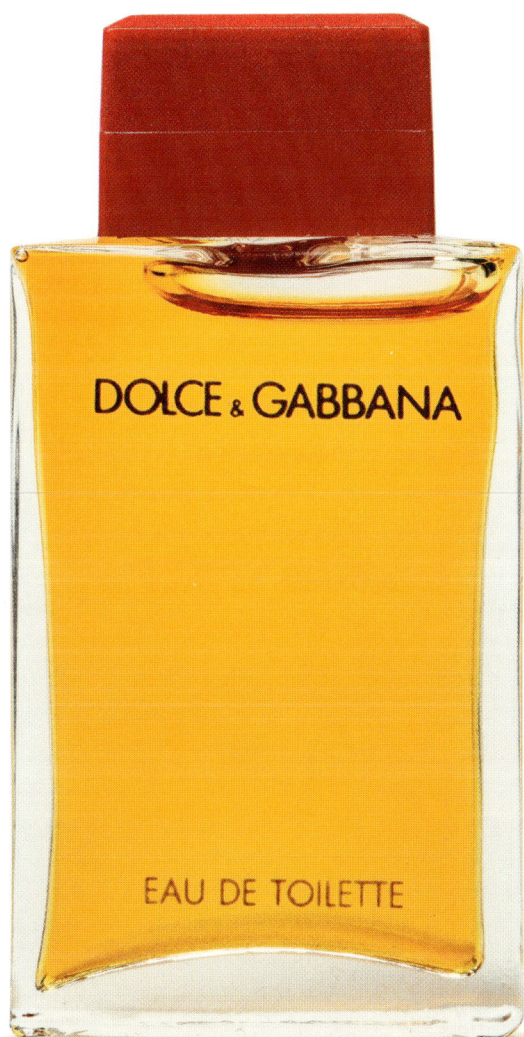

Donna

Brand: Trussardi
Gender: feminine:
Year of launch: 1992
Status: discontinued
Analyzed version: original Eau de Toilette
Author: Jean Guichard
Classification: aldehydic floral
Glassware Company: Bormioli Luigi

"Trussardi Donna" is an aldehydic floral situated outside of the vortex of time, in a parallel dimension inhabited by heavenly creatures with snowy-white wings, tuneful voices and splendid, natural notes used with a happy intent. "Trussardi Donna" develops around a floral accord with green facets of jasmine, tuberose, carnation, ylang ylang, lily of the valley and a full, rounded rose, brightened with a minimal amount of aldehydes. The delicate, feminine opening of the first few minutes gradually acquires more bite from the heart notes onwards, when the flowers are enveloped by an audacious, "typically Trussardi" leathery note conferring stability and impressive character to the whole. The ambery base notes of labdanum, benzoin, patchouli, cedar wood, musk and vanilla emerge slowly and deliberately, when the flowers are already beginning to fade away on the skin, bringing the fragrance to a delicate close that mirrors the opening.

It's hard to put an age to "Trussardi Donna", although it's safe to say she's over thirty. She's dressed in jeans and a white t-shirt, she's lightly tanned and without a trace of make-up, her straight hair blowing in the breeze as she makes her way through the world at a reserved, light pace respectful of those around her and the earth supporting her footsteps (creatures like this undoubtedly have a pair of snowy-white wings tucked away somewhere that only a select few have permission to take a close look at)... "Trussardi Donna" has a discreet projection throughout all three phases (top, heart and base), and lasts a few hours in total.

The fragrance was created by Jean Guichard, former director of the prestigious Givaudan Perfumery School, with a lenghty carrer and many successful perfumes including "Obsession" (Calvin Klein, 1985), "Parfum de Peau" (Montana, 1986), "Loulou" and "Eden" by Cacharel (1987 and 94). Perceptible in "Trussardi Donna" is his love for the rose, a material he has been particularly fond of since his childhood in Grasse, and which is found in many aldehydic floral of the past – and indeed a few of the present today.

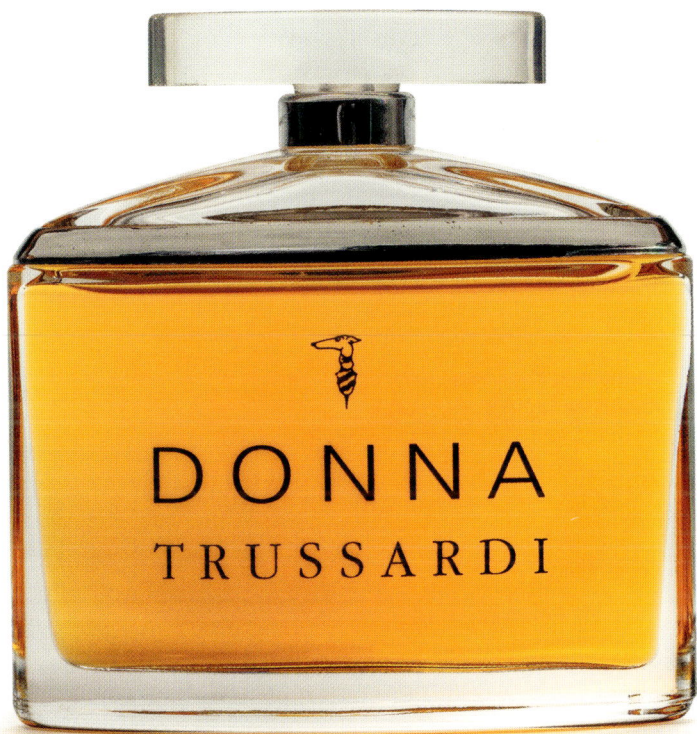

Eau Parfumée au Thé Vert

Brand: Bulgari
Gender: unisex
Year of launch: 1992
Status: in production
Analyzed version: original Eau de Cologne
Author: Jean Claude Ellena
Classification: aromatic citrus
Bottle design: Thierry de Bachmakoff/Paolo Bulgari

"Eau Parfumée au Thé Vert" is one of those rare fragrances able to shift the axis perfumery revolves around – not by flexing its muscles in a display of brute force, but thanks to a delicate, sincere voice ready to tell a brand-new story. When fragrances like this enter the scene, something changes forever.
A few years prior to its appearance, Givaudan headspaced the prestigious Mariage Frères tea boutique in Paris, to capture its subtle, distinctive aroma. Skilled chemists were able to artificially reconstruct it into a "tea base" Jean Claude Ellena found immediately appealing, hoping someone would show enough audacity to ask for it in a fragrance. It was Bulgari.
"Eau Parfumée au Thé Vert" revolves entirely around this green, clean, invigorating tea sensation, lit up by a rich bouquet of white musks. The green tea is bolstered by top notes of bergamot, coriander, pepper and cardamom, a Hedione/rose/violet heart and a woody/musky base. It envelops the wearer in a herb-scented cloud, creating a purifying, relaxing, tonifying sensation.
The whole fragrance is kept low-key, delicate and transparent, yet it has an amazingly powerful radiance that many outspoken perfumes do not even come close to. It has a longevity of up to two hours; no longer can be asked of an Eau de Cologne!
The international success of "Eau Parfumée au Thé Vert" confirmed Jean Claude Ellena in his path towards a new compositional style, characterised by purity and essentiality, and above all by that rare quality Edmond Roudnitska had named "delicacy". Delicacy is the ability to tell a story not with the booming, structured voice of an actor on the stage, but with the confidential, authentic tone of the storyteller, whose emotions make it vibrate and even break it, when they become too intense to bear. The followign Ellena's works will get progressively brighter, more dynamic and subtly diffusive, full of desaturated notes, almost deprived of their specific weight, surfacing the composition like watercolours.
Their marvellously subtle nuances are exactly what gives Ellena's fragrances their powerful emotional impact. In a world always ready to yell, and to hurl insults, a moving whisper is something to be treasured.

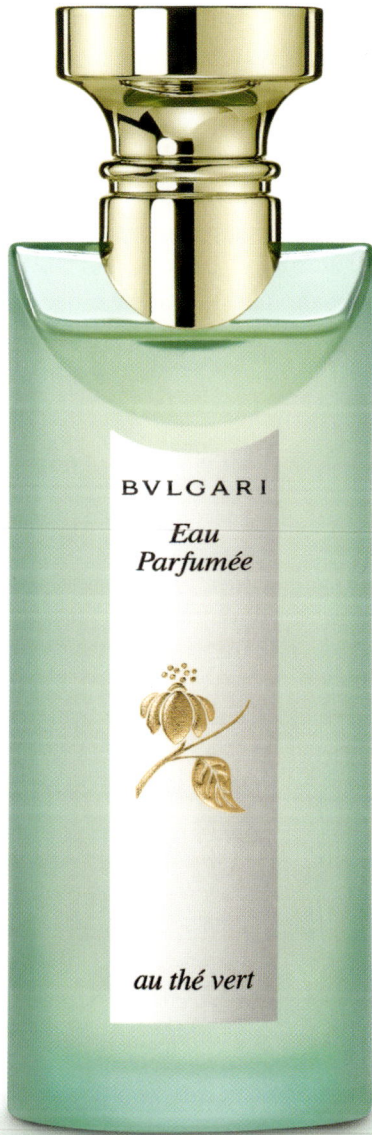

Tribù

Brand: Benetton
Type: for women/unisex
First produced: 1993
Status: discontinued
Version analysed: original Eau de Toilette
Author: Bernard Ellena (Symrise)
Classification: Green chypre

In contrast with its elder sibling "Colors", which emerges from among the fragrances of its period as the only transgender product - whether it is transitioning from female to male or vice versa is unclear -, "Tribù" is a fragrance that is proudly unisex in the sense that, instead of switching fluidly from masculine to feminine and viceversa, it prefers to explore the expressive possibilities common to both genders, with original and convincing results.

Here the floral, gourmand note of many women's fragrances is set against the greener, woody note typical of many men's fragrances. The two heart notes of this strange, extremely interesting creature are then enveloped by a powerful scent of oak moss, placing "Tribù" in the chypre lineage of both genders. More complex and intellectual than most, "Tribù" is unquestionably the fruit of a wealth of experience, courage and visionary power, so it is no coincidence that its creator is Bernard Ellena - also author of "Colors" -, who had the genius to reshuffle the cards, creating a composition above and beyond convention, the originality of which is still striking today.

"Tribù" opens dry and decisive, the tart green note of cassis (blackcurrant) enlivens the floral violet/rose/geranium/ylang ylang accord, propelling it towards unrivalled heights of stylization. There is no distinct perception of flowers, but rather a solid, compact floral sensation; even the woods of the base note (vetiver, sandalwood, cedar) are fused and melded into one another, creating a dense, opaque sensation, dry and intensely green. "Tribù" could be the olfactory version of a Shadow Theatre, where the story is not told by flowers and petals but by cardboard cut-outs, whose archetypal black stylized silhouettes move behind a screen that is totally white.

Curiously enough, although "Tribù" is often cited among the first perfumes to recall the scent of tea - a kind of green jasmine tea - the formula contains neither jasmine nor tea.

Its subtle and elusive personality makes it extremely recognisable: there is nothing out there that even remotely resembles it. "Tribù" does not have a particularly strong impact and does not leave a sillage, but its fragrance lasts for up to four hours. In keeping with the fragrance it contains, the "Tribù" bottle is also a strange object with a surprising design: a sort of angel/totem/space rocket designed by Tamotsu Yagi, on permanent display at the Museum Of Modern Art in San Francisco. Once again, the stylistic consistency between brand, container and content is an indication of a strong brand vision, which brings indisputable added value to any product. If you come across it, don't think twice. Go for it.

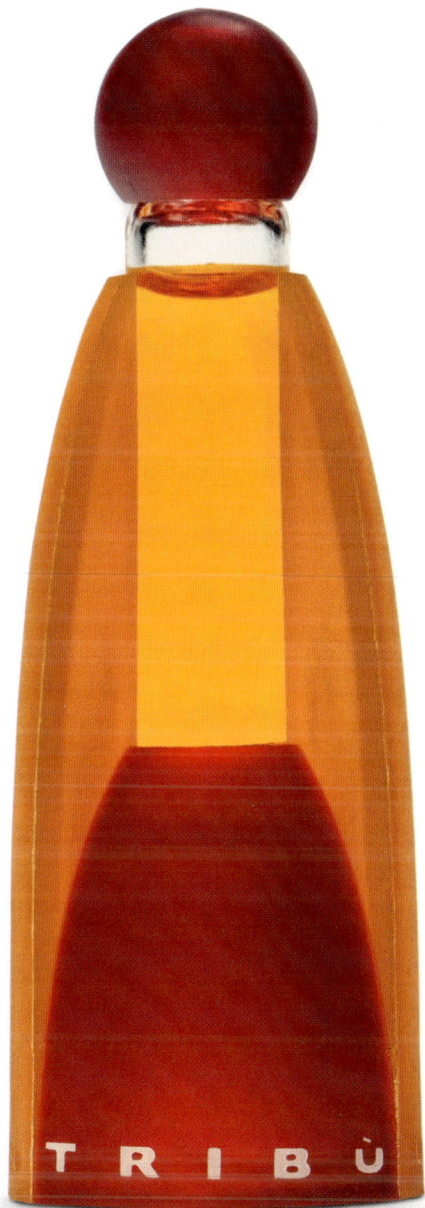

Roma Uomo

Brand: Laura Biagiotti
Type: for men
First produced: 1994
Status: in production
Version analysed: original Eau de Toilette
Author: Annick Ménardo (Symrise)
Classification: amber fougère
Glassware Company: Bormioli Luigi

Creatively speaking, there are many interesting, original, avant-garde and even visionary compositions. In terms of how pleasant they are to wear, however, many of the more "extreme" perfumes don't even pass the test. Other perfumes, on the other hand, opt for formal beauty as an end in itself, and if they stick to the beaten tracks – often perfecting them – it is only because they tend less towards the revolutionary intellectual, and more towards the relaxed and seductive gentleman. "Roma Uomo" is one of these. Indeed, it is at the top of its class. Rich in warm, sumptuous, elegant accords, "Roma Uomo" picks up the amber fougère theme developed thirty years earlier by "Brut" (Fabergé, 1964) and perfected by "Minotaure" (Paloma Picasso, 1992), and fashions it with a taste that is Italian through and through: the sparkling opening of citrus fruits gives way, in a matter of minutes, to a fougère of sublime elegance (laurel, basil and geranium), joined almost immediately by a warm, mellow amber accord, enhanced by sandalwood, myrrh and benzoin. A slight hint of vanilla melds into the woods and the resins, adding sensuality and maturity; the texture is as satisfying as a damask silk dressing gown in warm autumn hues. Many amber fougères were launched after the clamorous success of "Minotaure" and "Roma Uomo", with results that were even more modern and original. Nevertheless, "Roma Uomo" remains a textbook example of "Italian style" men's perfumery: formally impeccable, elegant, rich in interesting nuances, full of humour and witty conversation. Men like that never grow old. If anything, they improve as years go by.

"Roma Uomo" is ideal for both formal occasions and romantic evenings out, and it expresses itself to the full in autumn and winter. Its tenor voice resounds, spreading proudly and lasting surprisingly.

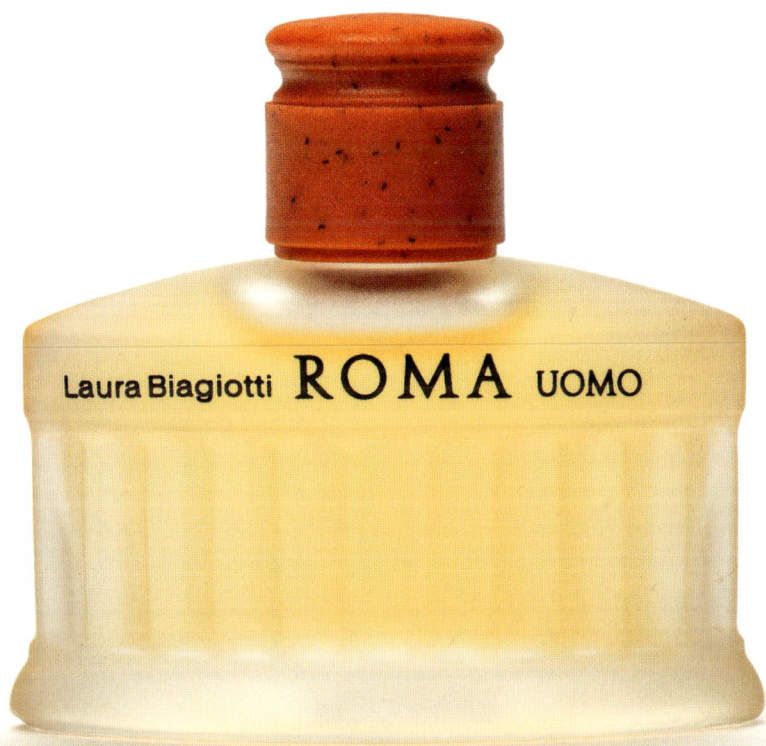

Messe de Minuit

Brand: Etro
Gender: unisex
Concentration: eau de Cologne
Year of launch: 1994
Status: relaunched in 2002
Analyzed version: original cologne
Author: Jaques Flori
Classification: aromatic woody

"Messe de Minuit" has a formidable evocative power. More than an actual fragrance, it's a vivid olfactory Polaroid taken inside an Orthodox church during a night of full moon. The church is bathed in the dim light of candles trembling in the cold breeze blowing in from the door, while the full moon lights up the white marble floor with a silvery glow. In the half-light, churchgoers are kneeling on the freshly polished pews, heads bowed. The priest begins to intone the holy litany, shaking the thurible and enveloping the central nave in a thick, aromatic cloud of incense. Some worshippers in the front pews fall into a trance, and start to mumble strange words in an unknown language. Sends shivers down your spine, doesn't it? To achieve such a complex storytelling result, Etro entrusted the creation of the fragrance to the refined talent of Jacques Flori from Robertet, a world leader in natural raw materials.

Flori constructed "Messe de Minuit" around a mystical, cold, subtle, central note of frankincense, complemented with dark-nuanced resins such as labdanum and myrrh. The vivid, fresh top of lemon, cedar and bergamot is counterpointed by a hypnotic woody-resinous base accord with dry, earthy patchouli and smoky vetiver.

"Messe de Minuit" is a mesmerizing scent, nocturnal as and cold as marble. On an olfactory scene that was slowly and wearily heading in the direction of globalised monotony, the audacious "Messe de Minuit" was probably the biggest shock ever to contemporary noses. Its growing success made it one of the beacon fragrances of artistic perfumery at the beginning of the 2000s. Is this a fragrance with an Italian soul? Absolutely: its message comes across loud and clear, with a breathtaking vibrancy and abundance of detail.

Although it is an Eau de Cologne, ù"Messe de Minuit" spreads confidently with a fair sillage, lasting for several thrilling hours. However, it's highly emotional nature doesn't belong to everyday life: for example I find it perfect for winter nights, when Nature is at rest, and a full moon lights up an inky black sky. If on a night like this you should ùfeel the urge to venture out into the forest to howl with the wolves and dance naked among the trees, you'll find nothing more suitable to wear. "Messe de Minuit"'s current version is slightly less gothic, with fuller citrus notes contributing a brighter, more extrovert tone.

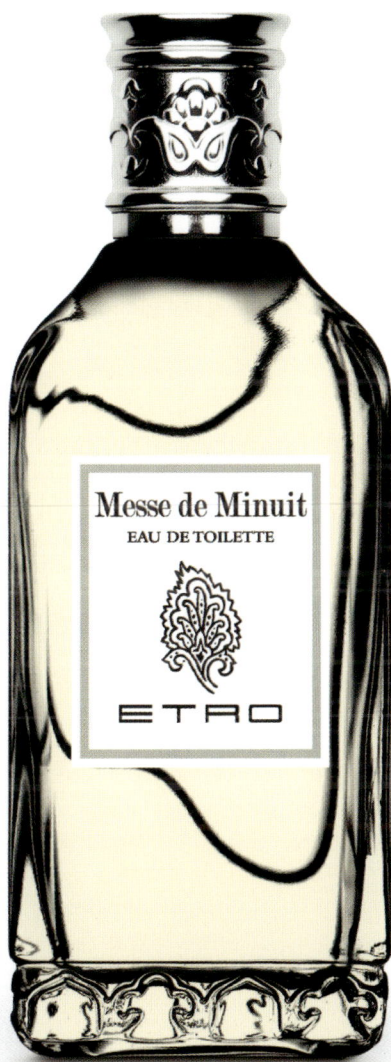

Messe de Minuit

EAU DE TOILETTE

ETRO

Acqua di Giò

Brand: Giorgio Armani
Gender: feminine
Year of launch: 1995
Status: in production
Analyzed version: original Eau de Toilette
Author: Edouard Flèchier
Classification: fruity floral
Bottle design: Giorgio Armani

With all the sparkle of a tonic water enriched with flowers, the women's version of "Acqua di Giò" is one of the most graceful works ever composed on a musky base. The three facets of this perfume – the flowers, the fruit and the ozonic notes – remain perfectly balanced for the entire longevity of the fragrance, in a deliciously fresh, carefree interplay of sweet, sharp and salty nuances that recall to mind holidays by the sea and lemon ice lollies enjoyed between dips. The musky/ozonic accord builds a bright, clean base, radiating out from the fruits (lemon, orange, mandarin, lime and peach), immediately followed by the flowers (rose, freesia, violet, hyacinth and jasmine), offering a general impression of confident simplicity, as if the formula were short and linear (which in fact it isn't at all).

"Acqua di Giò" is the ideal companion on all those occasions in which you need to relax, chill out and just enjoy the moment; its fresh scent spreads subtly and with impressive duration.

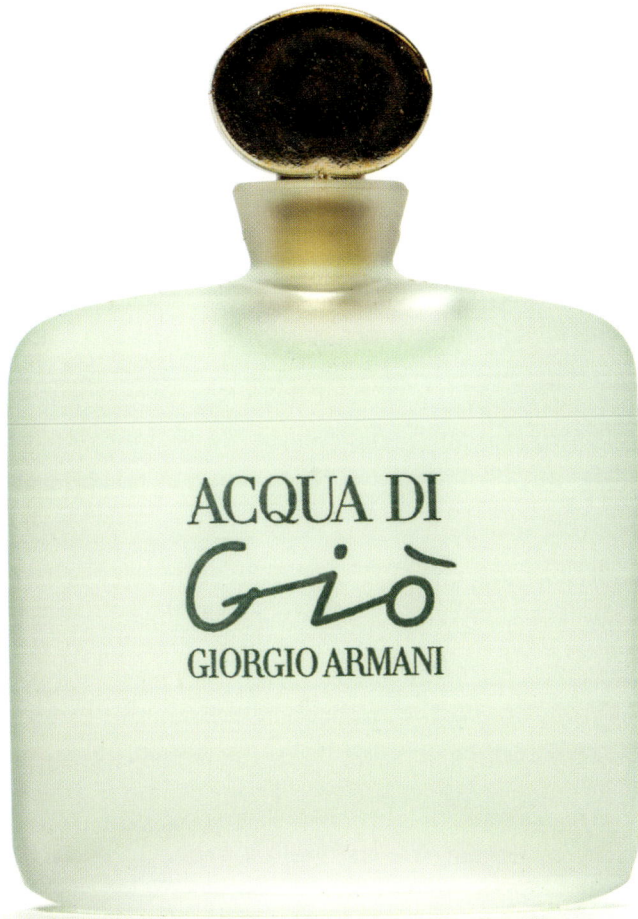

Cheap & Chic

Brand: Moschino
Gender: feminine
Year of launch: 1995
Status: in production
Analyzed version: original Eau de Toilette
Author: IFF
Classification: fruity floral
Bottle design: Atelier Dinand
Glassware Company: Bormioli Luigi

The odd name of this perfume teams the two concepts of *chic* (something luxurious and sophisticated) and *cheap* (inexpensive) into a strange oxymoron that initially seems puzzling. When I read it for the first time, the first thing that sprang to mind was a marketing ploy. I was wrong, of course: Moschino had a very clear idea of the message to be transmitted, and did so masterfully, with an uncommon – and thus particularly precious – sense of light-hearted irony. The first thing that captures the attention about Moschino "Cheap & Chic" is the bottle designed by Bormioli Luigi. It's not just your usual glass bottle that attempts to boost the appeal of the liquid inside with sophisticated details or visual finesse. The bottle – which I imagine doesn't come cheap – is in red and black plastic in the shape of Popeye's girlfriend Olive Oyl. Not Monica Bellucci, Carla Bruni, or any other icon of female beauty. Olive Oyl. Who isn't even a real woman, but a cartoon character, and indeed one that represents a bland femininity, devoid of character, unable to choose between a brute that carries her off over his shoulder to make her his and a Sailor destined to spend long periods away from her: a sort of ambassador for the sad reality of everyday life rather than the glossy existence we read about in magazines. In this plastic-covered bottle, the liquid is not visible. Perhaps this means that it's not the main thing? Yes, that's right. The fragrance itself is a pleasant mix of aldehydes, flowers and white musks, with a delicate scent, softened by a subtle hint of fruit. Its apparent simplicity is perfectly consistent with the rest, because Moschino "Cheap & Chic" is to be considered a concept rather than a perfume: a concept transmitted in a surprisingly coherent fashion by the combination of the name, the bottle and the fragrance. When it arrived on the shelves, Moschino "Cheap & Chic" announced an incontrovertible truth that at the time was becoming obvious to everyone: "Luxury is Dead". In other words: "Take perfume for what it is: a cheap treat. Because if it's real Luxury you're looking for, you're no longer going to find it in a perfume. Not even this one". This was a stroke of absolute genius. And such genius is rarely understood by the critics. "Cheap & Chic" was one of the first-ever fruity florals, and the public fell in love with it precisely for its pleasant, comfortable, clean, feminine, superbly discreet essence. This is what has made it so successful for over twenty years. Even if luxury may be dead, a well-made perfume remains very much alive and popular.

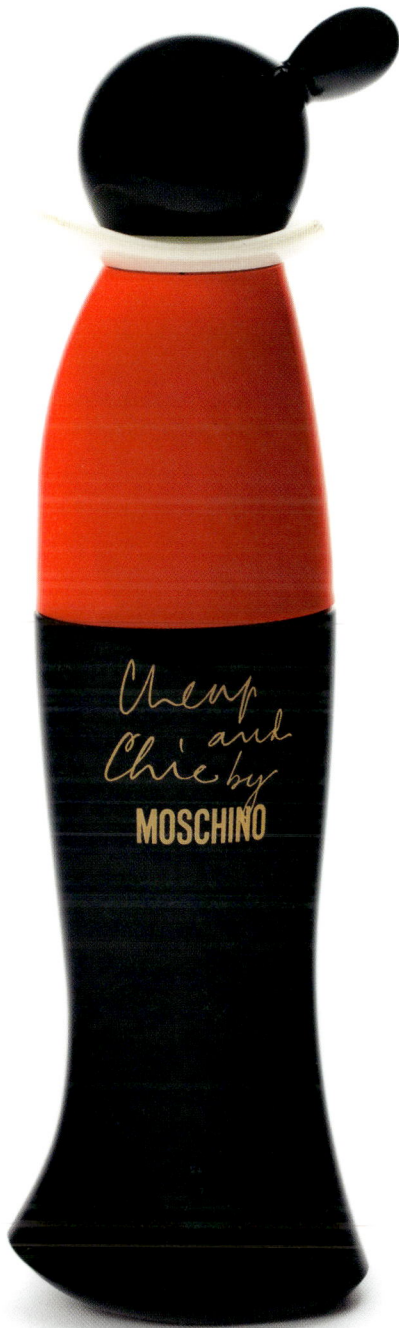

Gieffeffe

Brand: Gianfranco Ferré
Gender: feminine
Year of launch: 1995
Status: in production
Analyzed version: original Eau de Toilette
Author: Michèle Saramito (Robertet)
Classification: green chypre
Bottle design: Gianfranco Ferré

Starting from the name – not the full name, "Gianfranco Ferré", but just the initials, "Gieffeffe" – and continuing with the round bottle with a peculiar lid-free spray cap, and lastly, the light, airy jus, everything about this fragrance suggests a minimalistic, fluid character; two features not much sought-after in the 1990s which, a decade later would turn essential for the success of any fragrance.

The bitter citrus opening of "Gieffeffe" binds with the rose/jasmine accord (softened here by the osmanthus, which adds a fruity undertone) in a particularly green/vibrant manner. The cold, rather pungent notes of nutmeg and cardamom give a boost to the effervescent effect. The base perfectly supports the green feeling developed by the top/heart, but lacks the chypre austere temperament of the past chypres: patchouli remains in the background, and is fractionated (not the whole essential oil, but the driest, crispest fraction of the distillation); oak moss is replaced by a molecular alternative, and more contemporary clean, aquatic molecules are added. "Gieffeffe" is indeed a must for anyone wishing to understand two events that set down roots precisely in this period: the advent of musky colognes and the transformation of the traditional chypres into their modern-day heirs.

The new concept of Cologne presented here for the first time (citrus bouquets paired with airy, purified floral notes, enveloped in soft clouds of white, clean musks), would later be masterly explored by Alberto Morillas in the "Cologne" by Mugler (2001), setting one of the strongest trends in modern perfumery. "Gieffeffe" also ushered in the revolution in the chypre structure, which gets progressively desaturated, partly to satisfy the tastes of a public interested in fresher fragrances and simpler structures, and partly as a result of the restrictions gradually imposed by IFRA on the use of raw materials.

In some cases the regulations diminished the amounts of naturals that could be used and in other cases allowed their use only if deprived of possible allergens (unfortunately, it is precisely the allergens that make a significant contribution to the olfactory profile of a raw material). "Gieffeffe" was one of the first "new" chypres based with some of the notes pared down and a huge musk bouquet (like a musky cologne), but it is still recognisable as a chypre.

"Gieffeffe" has a subtle projection, enveloping the wearer in a green aura that lasts a couple of hours.

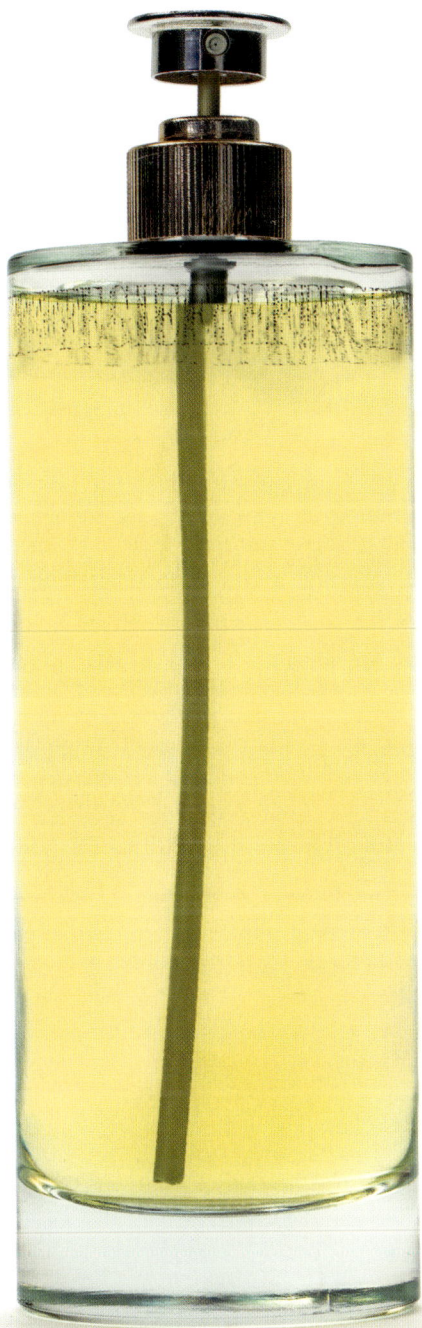

Blonde

Brand: Gianni Versace
Gender: feminine
Year of launch: 1995
Status: relaunched in 2010
Analyzed version: original Eau de Parfum
Author: Nathalie Feisthauer
Classification: rich floral
Bottle design: Serge Mansau

"Blonde" by Gianni Versace is a quintessentially Italian perfume: communicative, casual and with a broad smile, it's the perfect olfactory ambassador of a cheerful, tongue-in-cheek style, in love with life and its pleasures.

"Blonde" is composed of an abundance of white flowers (magnolia, orange blossom and tuberose) bursting into a song of the *dolce vita*, holiday lifestyle, amid chiffon skirts in gorgeous shades of colour, pergolas heavy with flowers and relaxing chatter over a chilled glass of Prosecco. The resemblance to "Giorgio Beverly Hills" (Charles of the Ritz, 1981) and especially "Fracas" (Piguet, 1948) appears obvious, as for all fragrances focused on a tuberose/orange blossom accord: these two notes are impossible to combine without a nod to "Fracas". However, while "Fracas" has a *grande soirée* projection and density, "Blonde" is exhilarating and extrovert, curling down onto a delightful musky note that gives it a modern, versatile edge.

Blonde is one of those few fragrances able to brighten the mood and raise a smile, yet it's not a frilly, superficial fragrance, but a balanced perfume with its very own mature, sophisticated elegance. "Blonde" is the friend we'd all like to have: lively, fun, fashionable, able to get herself noticed when necessary, but also an emotional, sympathetic listener, able to look us straight in the eye and whisper: *"Don't worry, baby, everything's going to be okay. I'm here for you"*.

"Blonde" spreads out exuberantly for the first ten minutes, then settles down into an exhilarating floral/amber/musky breeze that lasts around three hours. Unfortunately, it's now discontinued, but if you're able to track down one of the few bottles still around, don't hesitate – and wave goodbye to the benzodiazepines.

Engraved on the back of this prestigious bottle is a satin-finish Medusa, the symbol of the Versace brand. "Blonde" would be worth having even for this marvel alone.

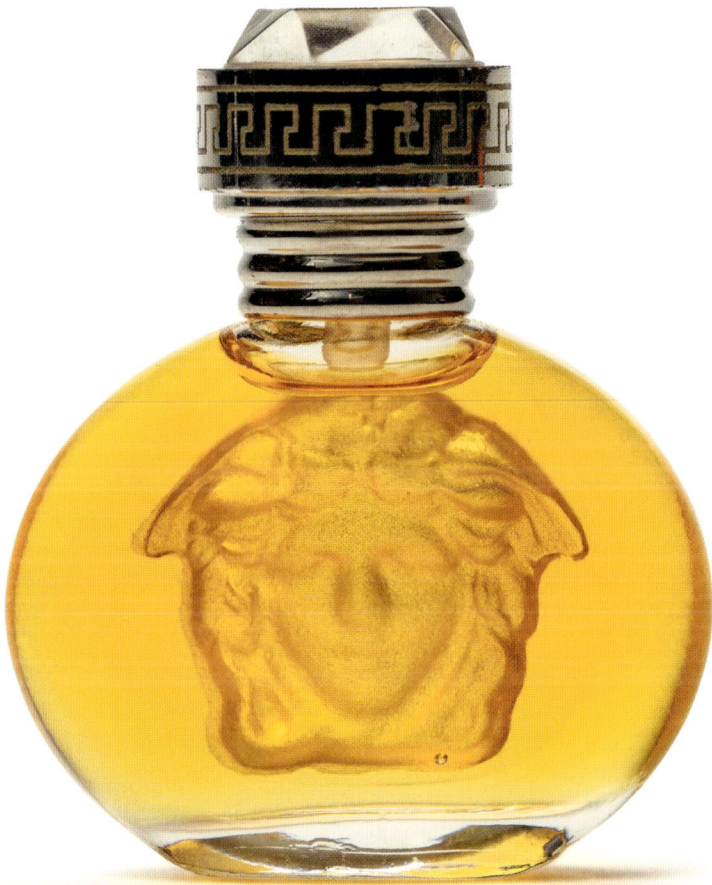

Acqua di Giò

Brand: Giorgio Armani
Gender: masculine
Year of launch: 1996
Status: in production
Analyzed version: original Eau de Toilette
Author: Alberto Morillas
Classification: aquatic/aromatic citrus
Bottle design: Giorgio Armani

"Acqua di Giò" made such an explosive impact on the men's fragrance market that for a long time you could perceive its presence wherever you went. Twenty five years later, its success still goes strong in many markets, where "Acqua di Giò" is among the top five men's fragrances.

When it was launched, at the height of the ozonic/marine trend (the similarity to "Cool Water" is clearly perceptible), two main factors made "Acqua di Giò" stand out. The first was the absence of any embellishments and nuances: in this fragrance, there's nothing more than the elements strictly necessary to convey a disarming impression of discretion and cleanliness, two sensations that market was crying out for, in a period dominated by a subtle sense of social disquiet. The citrus opening is enriched with a note of Hedione (a molecular jasmine that brings a soft, delicate floral sensation) and an interesting, dry aromatic note of rosemary binding the top with the woody base. A mix of white musks, Dihydromyrcenol and Calone are at the heart of a splendidly clean, dazzling, sculptural jus, a sort of silver monolith standing starkly out against a snow-covered hill. "Acqua di Giò" has an impressive longevity, without any particular evolution, settling down onto a dry base of musky wood of simple clarity. This is the second reason for its success: "Acqua di Giò" spreads out confidently, creating a highly recognisable sillage that lasts for eight hours without ever fading. Men apply their fragrances in the morning before they leave the house, their fragrances need to remain fresh and persistent, keeping them fresh and presentable for hours both in the office, at the gym and for aperitif time. "Acqua di Giò" ticks this box like very few other men's fragrances: it can be casual or sophisticated, as required; it's supremely pleasant in the summer, and suitable for all seasons, without ever going unnoticed or being overpowering.

"Acqua di Giò" is one of those seemingly simple conjuring trick that make you think: "That can't be so difficult, can it? Anyone could do it". Yet all you have to do is try one of the thousands of copycat fragrances to appreciate the outstanding talent and vision necessary to create something so unique, perfectly distinctive, linear and sharply focused for its entire eight-hour duration. Standing ovation.

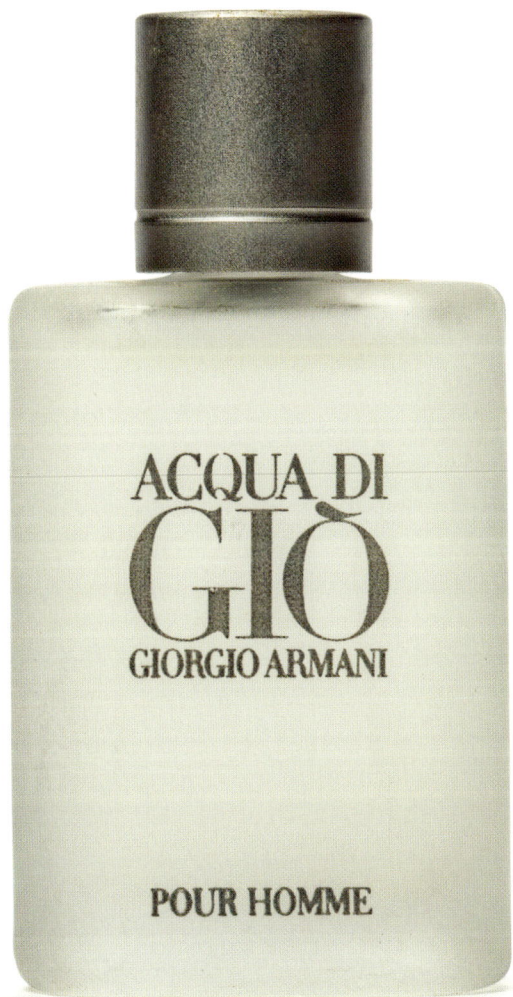

Gucci Envy

Brand: Gucci
Gender: feminine
Year of launch: 1996
Status: discontinued
Analyzed version: original Eau de Toilette
Author: Maurice Roucel
Classification: green floral

Within the floral family, the green facet began to develop with "Vent Vert" (Germaine Cellier for Balmain, 1946), a legendary perfume focused on an overdose of galbanum, a dry, green resin that conjures up a sensation of open spaces and green fields. "Diorissimo" (Edmond Roudnitska for Christian Dior, 1956), the most famous and widely acclaimed lily of the valley soliflore ever composed, came ten years after "Vent Vert". This green edge was taken up again after another ten years, in 1966, by "Fidji" (Guy Laroche), which was followed by "Chanel N°19" (1971) and "Amazone" (Hermès, 1974). From the start of the 1990s onwards, this green edge saw a return to favour, thanks to the success obtained by a handful of new green florals enriched with fresh fruity notes and white musks: "Cabotine" (Grès), "5th Avenue" (Elizabeth Arden), "Parfum d'Eté" (Kenzo), "Pleasures" (Estée Lauder), "Tommy Girl" (Tommy Hilfiger) and "Gucci Envy", whose audacious, distinctive character elevated it above the others. The floral notes of "Gucci Envy" (hyacinth, magnolia, lily of the valley, jasmine and violet) come together to shape a perfume there is nothing naive and dreamy about: this is an assertive, forthright fragrance that demands immediate attention. Its natural habitat is not wide-open, natural spaces blooming with spring flowers, but glossy magazines and neon lights. Because "Gucci Envy" is all about Fashion, with a capital F: that glamorous, parallel universe beyond our reach, inhabited by delicate, translucent, emotionally detached creatures that grace the catwalk with confident steps, moving in a perfectly straight line as hordes of sweaty photographers fire off their flashes in an attempt to capture their most intimate essence.

There's no other perfume in the world able to paint a sharper, more convincing portrait of the Fashion universe. And since it's by Gucci - one of the brands that created Fashion and continues to convey it at the very highest level - "Gucci Envy" is just the perfect fragrance for the perfect brand, and this rare occurrence needs to be highlighted. "Gucci Envy", composed by the great Maurice Roucel, the nose behind a host of outstanding feminine fragrances with a perfect balance of pride and floral notes; slides over the skin, enveloping it in a vibrant floral allure that remains perceptible for a couple of hours, followed by a drydown of approximately a further two hours.

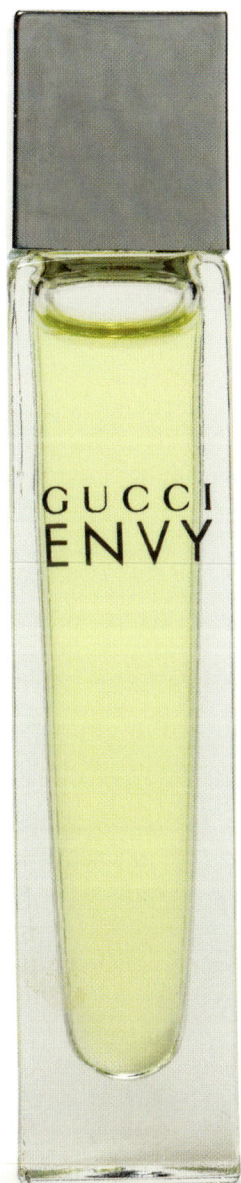

The Dreamer

Brand: Gianni Versace
Gender: masculine
Year of launch: 1996
Status: in production
Analyzed version: original Eau de Toilette
Author: Jean Pierre Béthouart
Classification: ambery fougère
Bottle design: Gianni Versace

"The Dreamer" proved one of the richest men's fragrances on the 1990s scene: it has that fine, luminous, aquatic quality typical of its contemporaries, together with an unmistakable fougère reference, all of it resting on an oriental base enhanced by an unusual note of fresh tobacco.

The complex, multifaceted formula, with a rich variety of undertones, required an experienced composer of the calibre of Pierre Béthouart (who also created "Boucheron, 1988 and "Parfum Sacré" by Caron, 1990) to preserve its dry, restrained character and avoid getting lost amid a myriad of inconclusive trickles. Béthouart was also the author of another Versace fragrance, "Blue Jeans", launched two years earlier, and of which "The Dreamer" is a more adult, mature, "complete" version.

"The Dreamer" has a clear, refreshing opening, with a mandarin note accompanied by aromatic juniper, sage and lavender in an aquatic accord of crystalline purity. The top notes spread their bright presence out until they encounter the floral accord of rose, carnation and geranium, whose green undertones bind with the aromatic top notes, bringing a green tinge to the heart, and conjuring up an image of open spaces stretching out beyond the horizon. Tobacco, vetiver, cedarwood, iris, vanilla and tonka bean form a classic, elegant, oriental base with a slightly powdery edge, which rises into the aromatic top notes, pushing them upwards almost to the opening of the fragrance. The grassy, aromatic facet of the tobacco note strikes a further connection between the top and the base, keeping the green/fresh aromatic sensation clearly perceptible throughout the entire development of the fragrance, giving "The Dreamer" a measure of simple, intimate, suspended linearity, the dreamy quality the name suggests. When a fragrance truly reflects its name in this way, it denotes a strong vision on the part of the brand, which the talent and experience of the composer were able to breathe pulsating life into.

Thanks to the fougère structure, "The Dreamer" by Versace also echoes the timeless class of vintage men's fragrances from the Fifties. The Dreamer is both tasteful and restrained, and this – together with its moderate projection and eight-hour duration – makes it suitable for almost any occasion; only the intense heat of the summer penalises it somewhat. Gianni Versace designed the marvellous bottle featuring the relief Medusa head pattern and the distinctive spray cap integrated into the top.

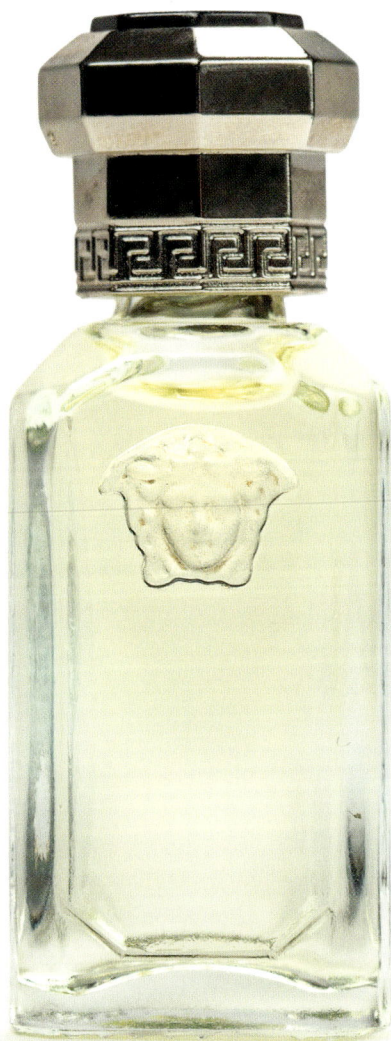

By Woman

Brand: Dolce & Gabbana
Gender: feminine
Year of launch: 1997
Status: discontinued
Analyzed version: original Eau de Toilette
Author: IFF
Classification: oriental

Animalier prints have been a feature of the Dolce & Gabbana visual universe since day one, and the prints on the perfume bottles are right in line with this style hallmark of the brand. The bottle of "By Woman" is a compact metal cylinder that distinguishes itself from the similar "Rive Gauche" (Yves Saint Laurent) bottle thanks to the animalier decoration promising an adult, dangerously sexy fragrance. The sensual bouquet lives up to this promise, although it is more subtle and discreet than the striking bottle suggests.

A squeeze of bright, sweet citrus fruit brought straight from Sicily blows a gentle, sunny breeze across a few modest, almost retiring flowers (lily of the valley, cyclamen and lily). Perceptible from the heart notes onwards is a clean, gentle breath of aldehydes, which blows down into the base of the fragrance, dominated by an audacious accord of coffee, vanilla and sandalwood, enveloped in a musky bouquet. The perfume gradually tones down towards a sort of skin scent, with delightfully crisp, powdery tones.

This is when the sensuality of the fragrance comes into its own: neither aggressive nor provocative, indeed particularly calm and intimate, evocative of a pleasantly sincere, inviting, familiar skin. This rather original, amazingly sophisticated oriental has little in common with the banal, loud, larger-than-life orientals beloved of the *femme fatale*, and is classified in this family exclusively because of the vanilla note, which remains soft and takes a back seat here.

Despite its modest spread, "By Woman" boasts a surprisingly long duration of over six hours, indicative of a construction carried out to perfection in order to keep the accent on delicacy. Now discontinued (perhaps due to its unusual essence, out of line with the trends of the time and thus poorly understood), "By Woman" is very difficult to come by, and requires an expert eye, because most of the bottles in circulation are fake.

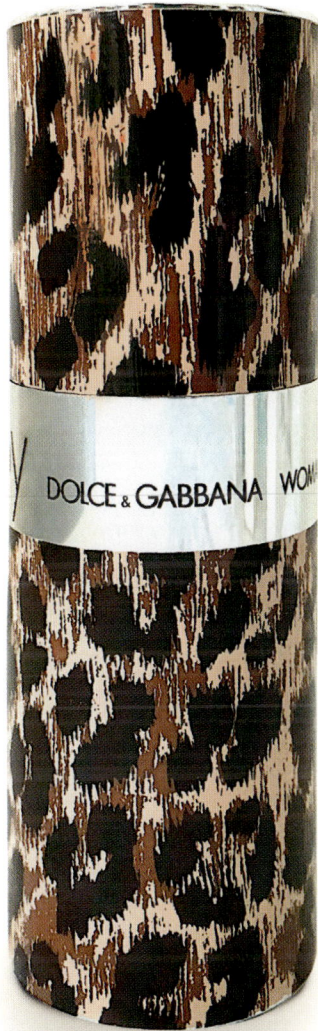

By Man

Brand: Dolce & Gabbana
Gender: masculine
Year of launch: 1997
Status: discontinued
Analyzed version: original Eau de Toilette
Author: IFF
Classification: oriental

Unfortunately, "By Man" has also been discontinued long enough for most warehouses to have run out of stock. It's a pity, because this was a brilliantly, unusually crafted men's fragrance: a sort of strange oriental with an aromatic heart of lavender, spiced with nutmeg and black pepper, two facets drawn together in a magnetic embrace. Woody and amber notes, musks and a touch of vanilla gather the spices and the lavender together, plunging them into a sensual, warm, enveloping amber accord with a vaguely crisp hazelnut nuance. A leathery accent brings depth to "By Man", rendering it alluringly dark, with a low, husky voice that whispers close to the skin. The duration is extraordinary.

The amber notes and leathery touch place it firmly in the 1990s, yet "By Man" has none of the bold, "manly", spirit that characterises the fragrances of the time. Quite the reverse: it has an intimate, slow, persuasive, milonga-like sensuality. What makes it so appealing to us today is probably exactly what explains its lack of success at the time.

The zebra-print bottle is the perfect complement to the leopard-print bottle of its female partner fragrance, and when placed side by side, the coherent overall style approach becomes evident, boosting the appeal further.

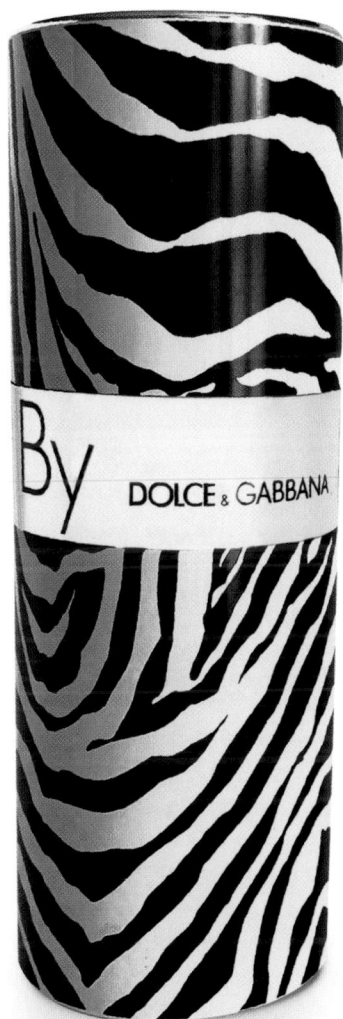

Moschino Uomo?

Brand: Moschino
Gender: masculine
Year of launch: 1998
Status: in production
Analyzed version: original Eau de Toilette
Author: Olivier Cresp
Classification: ambery fougère

As for other fragrances created by the brand, running through "Moschino Uomo?" is a subtle, interesting tension between opposing poles.

It's undoubtedly a fougère, yet it has the "melting" sensuality of an ambery; it's masculine, for sure, yet with an intuitive, magnetic sensitivity that's incontrovertibly feminine. It's clean, freshly shaven and appropriately dressed, yet there's a glint of subversive genius twinkling in its eye.

"Uomo?" rises up from the skin with a broad smile, thanks to the aromatic herbs (artemisia and sage) and the spices (coriander and cinnamon) of the top/heart to which a soft breeze of rose and rosewood and a vibrant note of kumquat give a gentle edge. The humid freshness of the Hedione and the peach aldehyde linger over the opening, settling like dew on the notes and making them transparent, like a stained-glass window against the light. The vanilla/ambery base emerges slowly, binding with the rose to form a peculiar floral fougère with a woody/musky undertone that gradually takes over. Even if laden with musky notes, the dominant sensation is not "fresh and clean", as in most of the musky/marine fragrances from the period, because clary sage contributes a "dirty", "human" edge, together with a strange, undefinable dry, warm, almost salty note reminiscent of oak moss (which at that time was hardly ever used any more) and Ambroxan (which did not yet exist). Musky, yes; clean? Not quite...

In "Moschino Uomo?", the expressive tension between opposites (male/female; classic/contemporary; clean/animalic; light/shade) keeps running high for the first two hours, before the musky notes - heavier and slower to evaporate - rise to the fore and last endlessly. Despite its complex structure, "Uomo?" remains easy-going, open and instantly appealing from the first note to the last, with a lively projection that can also be enjoyed by women, in any setting and with no fear of overdoing. The most recent version of "Moschino Uomo?" showes a less evident tension within; the "dirty" edge is subtler, and the whole fragrance has a cleaner, bubblier register, more musky in the contemporary sense.

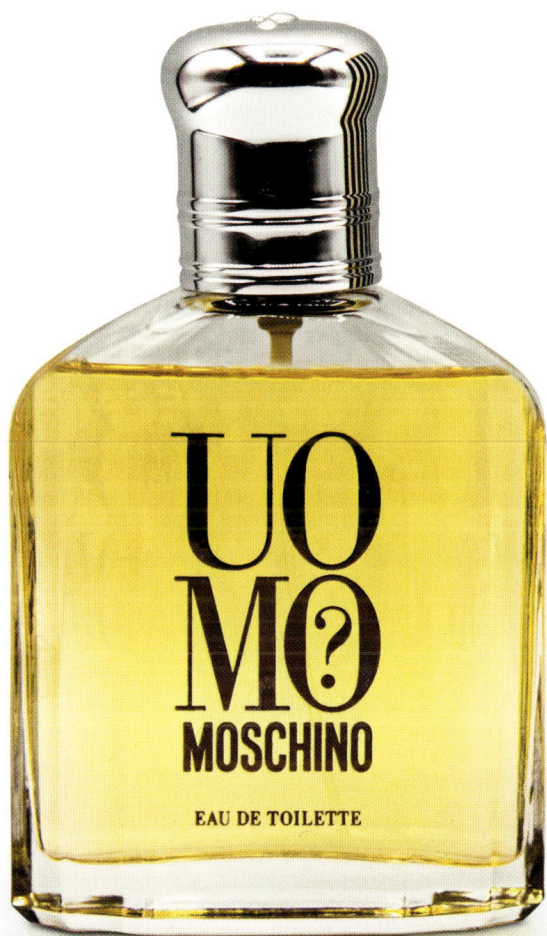

Salvatore Ferragamo pour femme

Brand: Salvatore Ferragamo
Gender: feminine
Year of launch: 1998
Status: in production
Analyzed version: original Eau de Toilette
Author: Jacques Cavallier
Classification: fruity floral
Bottle design: Thierry Baschmakoff

The first Ferragamo fragrance, "Gilio", dates back to 1960, and was followed by "F." (a new version of which appeared in 2006) and "Monsieur F.", which appeared at the start of the 1970s. For its third fragrance, the *maison* took the market by surprise, by opting for the trendiest family of the decade, the fruity florals. The fruity floral theme was executed with the mature, rigorous approach that is the brand's hallmark, with no hint of *tuttifrutti* frivolity, entrusting its composition to a master of style and restraint, Jacques Cavallier, who during his honoured career spanning over 30 years has composed outstanding fragrances for all the leading brands: Dior ("Midnight Poison"), Yves Saint Laurent "M7" and "Nu"), Jean Paul Gaultier ("Classique"), Issey Miyake ("L'Eau d'Issey"), Cartier ("Pasha"), Rochas ("Absolu"), Bulgari ("Blv" and "Bulgari pour homme"), Ermenegildo Zegna ("Essenza di Zegna"), Lancôme ("Poême"), Giorgio Armani ("Armani Mania"), Calvin Klein ("Truth").

For Ferragamo, Cavallier composed a fragrance introduced by a spiced accord of black pepper and nutmeg, which add dynamism to an ultra-feminine heart accord of carnation, rose, peony and lily of the valley. When the spices begin to tone down, a deliciously sweet note of blackberry and almonds starts to emerge, and although this presence is clearly perceptible, it does not smother the flowers, simply lighting them up with deliciously intriguing nuances. A bitter, vegetable trail of iris and wood, together with an aquatic nuance, form a polite counterpoint to the gourmand floral heart. All this makes for a mature – and thus highly versatile – fruity floral, perfectly consistent with the rigorous, tasteful style typical of Ferragamo, one of the few brands that remains Italian through and through. The fragrance has a discreet projection and a perfectly satisfying duration.

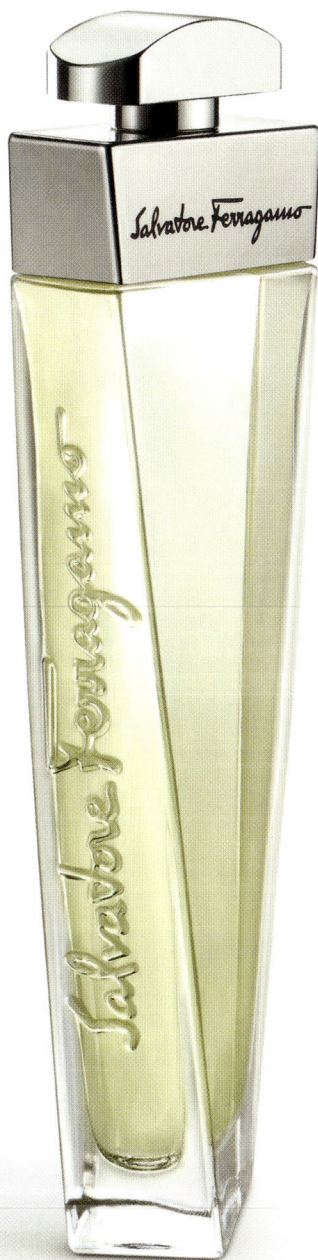

Theorema

Brand: Fendi
Gender: feminine
Year of launch: 1998
Status: discontinued in 2005
Analyzed version: original Eau de Toilette and Eau de Parfum
Author: Christine Nagel
Classification: spicy oriental
Bottle design: Catherine Krunas

"Theorema" was the perfume that brought its composer, Christine Nagel, into the spotlight of the fine perfumery universe, thanks to its serene, measured composition: authoritative without being overpowering, illuminated from top to base by a glistening, golden glow with an intensely autumnal allure.
"Theorema" is everything an oriental should be: warm, audacious, sensual, generous, exotic, distinctive; and fortunately, it has none of the showy, blaring tone that accompanies many modern orientals, replete with excessively cloying notes, loud, aggressive personalities and neon lights... On the contrary, it is imbued with a bright, sparkling sensitivity, with a joy of being alive...
Already evident from the opening are the elements the fragrance is built around (fruit, spices and amber notes), and indeed it does not develop significantly from this deftly constructed beginning. All that evolves is the tone, which gradually becomes more intimate.
The spices the formula revolves around (cardamom, cinnamon, pepper, nutmeg and cumin) appear bathed in a warm, citrus glow, in an accord at times reminiscent of "Eau d'Hermès" (1951), but developed in a surprisingly warm, soft manner. Citrus fruit and spices accompany a floral breath of rose, ylang ylang and osmanthus, a wonderfully precious flower with ripe apricot nuances, added purposefully to strengthen the soft sweetness of the top and heart notes. The base accord combines macassar (obtained from the same plant ylang ylang is extracted from) with sandalwood, guaiac wood and patchouli, amber notes and benzoin into a generous amber liquor that melts at the back of the palate, making the taste buds literally explode with pleasure.
"Theorema" has a lively spread for the first half hour, before toning down into a soft, gentle whisper that lasts for several hours. It has aged without a wrinkle, and is perfectly in line with current tastes: it would be considered a priceless gem had it been produced under a niche label such as Lutens or Frederic Malle, not least because of its natural notes of rare beauty. Its misfortune is that it was launched by a traditional brand: the average consumer was not able to recognise its greatness, while it never occurred to the more sophisticated perfume connoisseur to give it a try while it was still in production. This was a shame, because many were heartbroken when it was discontinued. If you ever have the chance to purchase a bottle, do so without hesitation.

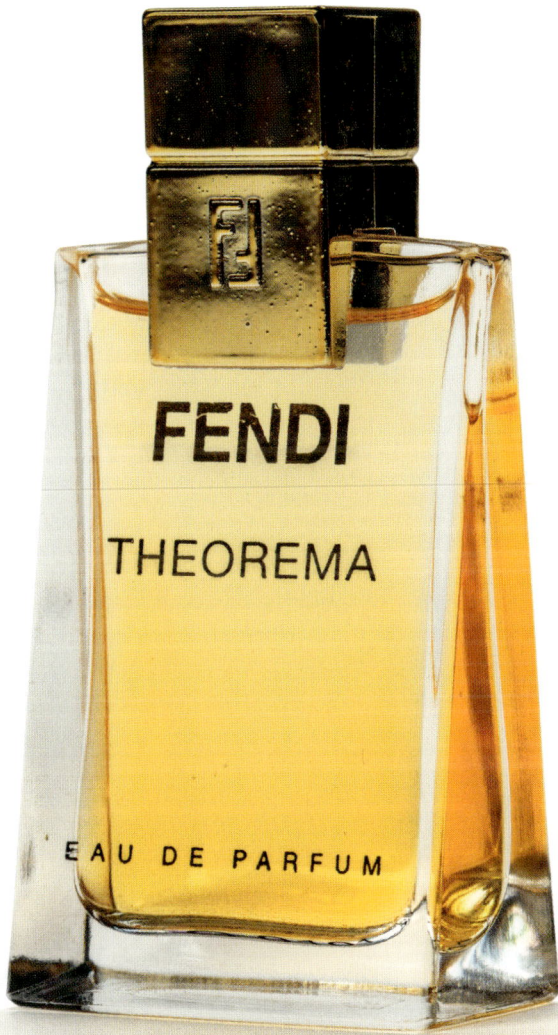

Black

Brand: Bulgari
Gender: unisex
Year of launch: 1998
Status: discontinued
Analyzed version: original Eau de Toilette
Author: Annick Ménardo
Classification: leather chypre/sweet amber
Bottle design: Thierry de Baschmakoff

When it was launched over twenty years ago, there was nothing even remotely similar to Bulgari "Black". Its notes of tea, rubber and vanilla shaped an alien creature, with such blurred lines it was difficult to classify: was it a chypre? An amber? A leather fragrance? On close inspection, "Black" is poised right in the middle between a sweet amber and a leather chypre, a new unisex, hybrid species that works oddly and magnificently. Unisex fragrances are usually linked to marine notes, fresh citrus, or white musks, while "Black" revolves around warm, smoky, woody notes with no top accord as such: the bouquet slides out of the bottle in one piece. Lapsang suchong (a dry, slightly smoky tea note) curls its way around the rose, sandalwood, cedar, amber and musky notes, along with vanilla, leather and vegetable musk bringing out one element after the other, with the vanilla, leather and sandalwood remaining constantly to the fore.

The amber accord of resins, sandalwood and vanilla places it within the lineage of "Ambre Antique" (Coty, 1910), "Habanita" (1921), "Shalimar" (Guerlain, 1925) and "Must" (Cartier, 1991), while at the same time, the chypre core awith a leather facet takes it in the direction of "Cuir de Russie" (Chanel, 1924), "Bandit" (Piguet, 1944) and "Cabochard" (Grès, 1959). "Black" succeeds in turning all his weighty heritage into an absolutely contemporary, thanks to the perfect balance it strikes between exquisitely constructed, "strong" accords, and to the innovative lapsang suchong note, which binds all the elements together with a fil rouge perceptible from beginning to end. "Black" envelops the wearer with its confident presence for the whole of the first hour, before toning down and remaining delicate on the skin for a further four hours. This modern masterpiece was created by Annick Ménardo, who between 1997 and 2006 composed "Hypnotic Poison" Eau de Toilette (Dior), "Lolita Lempicka" and "Lolita Lempicka au Masculin", "Bois d'Argent" (Dior) and "Bois d'Armenie" (Guerlain). Many of her works skim over the flowers and the top notes to focus on dense, opaque, textured heart/base accords giving her creations an opaque vibrancy and a tactile quality that are supremely satisfying. Bulgari "Black" is one of her finest compositions. The fabulous round bottle, encircled by a rubber disc, offers both a visual and tactile foretaste of the fragrance inside; and despite its striking design, it's surprisingly simple to use.

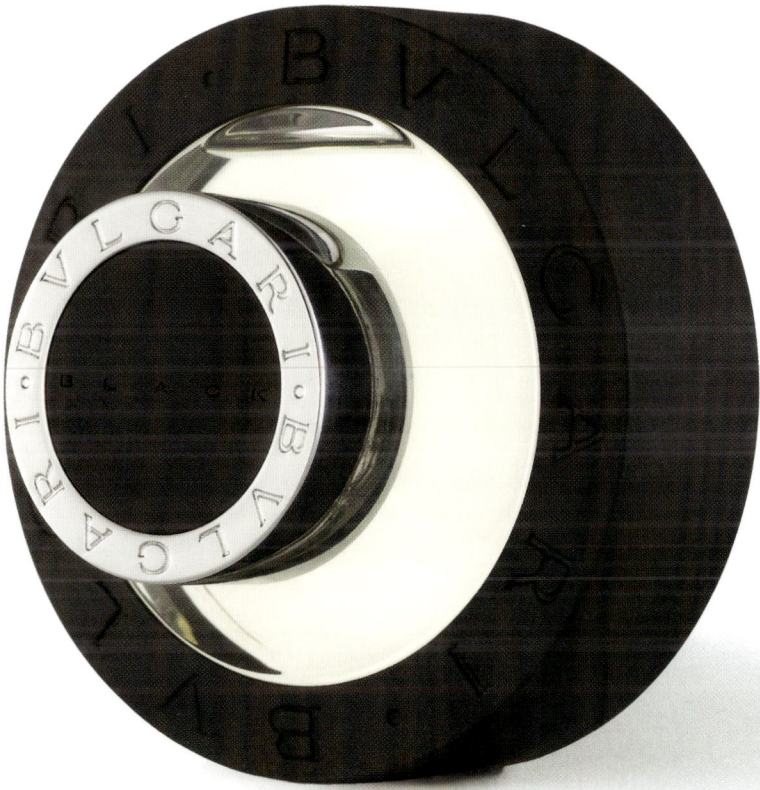

Very Valentino

Brand: Valentino
Gender: masculine
Year of launch: 1999
Status: discontinued
Analyzed version: original Eau de Toilette
Author: Harry Fremont
Classification: ambery fougère
Bottle design: Pierre Dinand

The modern ambery fougères descend from the world-famous "Brut" by Fabergé (1964), whose humid, sweet, warm forest floor notes of geranium, lavender, vetiver, oak moss, coumarin and tonka bean drew millions of dads into the world of fragrances, perpetuating in the generations to come - especially in Italy – a love for this classic, elegant, reassuring olfactory structure, forever associating it with an idea of manliness. After three generations lingering in the wings, this family confidently seized back its leading role on the perfumery stage in the 1990s, with the launch of "Zino Davidoff" (1986) and "Le Male" (Gaultier, 1995), followed by an impressive trio of fragrances *pour homme*: "Allure homme" (1998), "Yohji homme" (1999) and "Very Valentino pour homme".

"Very Valentino" has the classic fougère structure composed of aromatic herbs (lavender, sage, thyme and anise), given a warmer, livelier touch here by a pinch of spices (coriander and nutmeg). The sweet amber and sandalwood notes of the base accord are lit up by a wonderfully deep tobacco note that rises up into the heart, bonding with the herbs and spices to form a warm, sensual mix, with the density and maturity of a prestigious Port wine aged in ancient wood barrels.

"Very Valentino" has a natural feel, a thick, satisfying texture and an intimate, comfortable, nocturnal character.

This splendid fragrance is the work of the prolific Harry Fremont of Firmenich, and when it was launched was much more audacious and interesting than how it is perceived today, twenty years – and thousands of copies - later.

"Very Valentino" has a duration of about four hours, with more than moderate projection, making it easy to wear even on working occasions. Thanks to its amber sweetness, it also appeals to women.

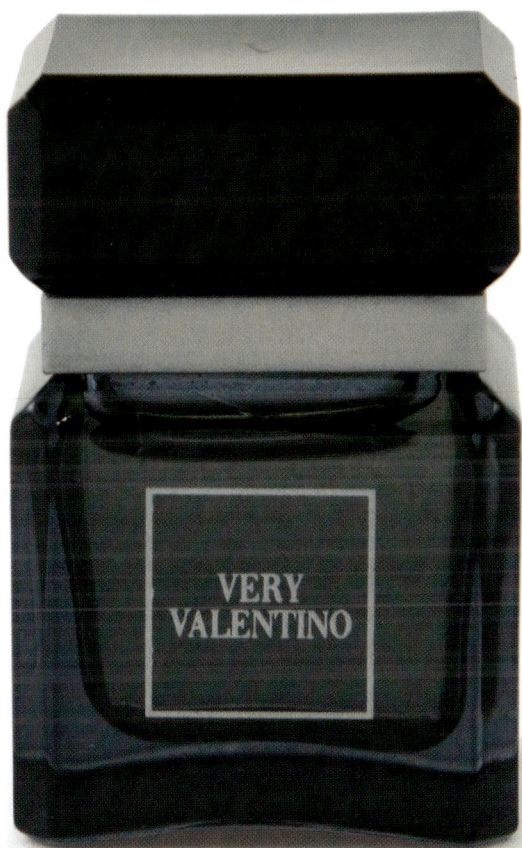

Gucci Rush

Brand: Gucci
Gender: feminine
Year of launch: 1999
Status: discontinued
Analyzed version: original Eau de Toilette
Author: Michel Almairac
Classification: aldehydic floral
Bottle design: Tom Ford

"Gucci Rush" has a truly unique quality: electricity. A cool, electric current runs right through the fragrance, sparkling like a glitter ball in a disco struck by neon lights. "Gucci Rush" bursts forth from the bottle with a floral outfit in bloom, enveloped in a peach aldehyde cloak. You might expect gardenia, freesia, jasmine, rose and lily of the valley to form a classic-style accord, able to whisper softly and smoothly over everything in its path; instead, the flowers in "Gucci Rush" create a cool, pearlescent effect with no resemblance to dewy fields in spring, but to the hydroponic hothouse inside a spaceship orbiting the Moon. Strange and interesting.

The base of vanilla, patchouli and vetiver, nestled within a bright bouquet of white musks, makes for an even drier fragrance, contributing a lively, metallic, pulsating edge, perhaps not entirely human, building a sort of ultra-sophisticated, latest-generation cyborg with brilliant white silicone skin.

"Gucci Rush" has a shrill, resounding, clarinet-esque voice it's impossible not to notice on the skin. Its projection is potent enough to fill a whole room, remaining linear and stable for at least four hours, after which it comes gradually closer to the skin, where it settles down after another five hours.

"Gucci Rush" is a perfume that polarises opinions like few others ever composed: while many detest it, at least as many adore its eccentric, absolutely over-the-top character. In a word, this fragrance is unique. And this should come as no surprise, given the winning combination of the brand that commissioned it and the composer who created it: none other than Michel Almairac, one of the perfume world's most innovative composers, who has created absolute masterpieces for Dior, Chloé, Burberry and Calvin Klein. "Gucci Rush" is a milestone in his career: the story goes that it took Tom Ford – creative director for Gucci at the time – less than three seconds to choose this perfume over the others proposed. His intuition proved correct: "Gucci Rush" was perhaps the first perfumery masterpiece of the new millennium, able to bring a surprisingly contemporary edge to the style canons of the floral aldehydics.

"Rush" by Gucci has a clarinet-like vibrant and shrill voice; impossible to go unnoticed while wearing it. Its scent spreads till saturating a whole room, staying linear and steady for at least four hours; then it flows ever nearer to the skin, completely appeasing after another five hours.

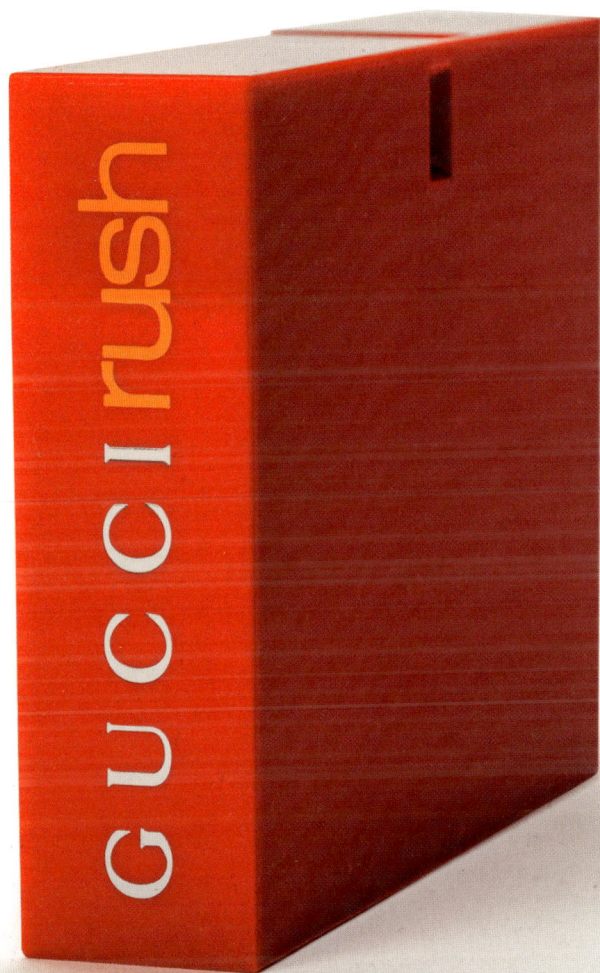

20
00

The Great Italian Perfumes of the 2000s

The social and cultural background

The new Millennium began with the riots on the streets during the G8 summit in Genoa and the attack on the Twin Towers in New York (2001), followed by the start of the US offensives in Afghanistan (2001) and Iraq (2003). For the first time, audiences all over the world had the opportunity to witness these events in real time on TV, thanks to the efforts of hundreds of reporters who often risked their lives to allow those audiences to get "in on the news".

Terrorist attacks in Madrid and London sowed panic and death, creating a climate of fear and social uncertainty all over Europe; added to this was the major economic crisis in America, which had a negative knock-on effect throughout the world, forcing many countries to adopt extraordinary measures that impoverished the population.

At the end of December 2004, a tsunami razed to the ground entire communities looking onto the Indian Ocean, killing 200,000 people.

Frightened by terrorism and worried about the economic crisis and the future of the Planet, many people began to feel an urgent need to take a closer look at their role in society and to make a personal, active contribution to it. The spread of internet offered access to information and opportunities to engage with others and to create groups of activists focused on environmental and social issues, and allowed us to learn more about the work of organisations such as Greenpeace, Legambiente, Medici Senza Frontiere and Save The Children.

Increasingly sophisticated and affordable mobile phones, digital video cameras and MP3 readers became a part of everyday life for most people, making the distances separating them shorter; the world became increasingly interconnected, and thanks to forums, blogs and the first social networks (My Space and Netlog), people were able to meet up virtually and remain connected 24/7 to the communities of interest to them.

On TV, Big Brother paved the way for other Reality Shows, a form of entertainment able to attract huge audiences by satisfying the voyeuristic instinct that is a part of all human beings. The Fantasy genre was popular in cinemas, with films and sagas (such as *The Lord of the Rings* and *Harry Potter*) able to evoke an other-worldly, reassuring universe in which Good wins through every time.

Dan Brown, with his *Da Vinci Code*, tuned into and amplified the yearning for a deeper spirituality, stripped of material interests, obtaining resounding success.

Trends in perfumery

In the 2000s, there were perfumes for all targets and all pockets. The decade constantly witnessed one launch after another, with many fragrances inspired by – or openly copied from – the most successful perfumes.

Gas chromatography made it possible to break down the top sellers into their main accords, mixing them with one another to create products that were new, yet contained familiar elements, in the same way as certain singers introduce sound loops from other tracks into their songs.

These repetitive olfactory structures nudged many consumers – in search of an individual, exclusive scent – towards the artistic fragrances, consecrating niche perfumery once and for all. Internet began hosting websites and forums where perfume aficionados all over the world could come together and engage in a dialogue regarding the aesthetics of perfumery, sharing information, opinions, reviews and precious perfume bottles. These soon became fertile terrain for cultivating a passion for a less standardised approach to perfumery, and often played a direct role in the development of the artistic, "niche" sector that was emerging during those years.

In the search for new fragrances able to surprise bored consumers once more, a number of long-established brands such as Lancôme and Givenchy launched "vintage" lines, with historical perfumes re-edited adding more innovative raw materials. Other brands preferred the exclusivity of the limited edition, focused on a specific raw material (the rose, for example), harvested in a particularly favorable production year. Other brands, including Chanel, Armani, Prada, Dior and Hermès, went a step further. Having grasped that the public's interest in artistic perfumery opened up new business opportunities, they launched alternative, highly creative lines, reserved for connoisseurs and available only in a number of brand-name boutiques. These lines, situated mid-way between the mass fragrance market and artisanal perfumery, offered more vibrant, audacious fragrances, composed using particularly expensive materials, and immediately found favour with consumers.

The macrocyclic musks discovered in the preceding decade made their way into dozens of fragrances for both men and women, plunging the formulas into a delicate, subtle, translucent light that from this moment on was to become synonymous with modernity and an essential element in every fragrance. This ushered in the fashion for the "fresh and clean", "white musk" perfumes, including "Miracle" (Lancôme, 2000), "Flower" (Kenzo, 2000), "Cologne" (Mugler, 2000), "Narciso Rodriguez" (2004).

In some cases, the women's fragrances became unashamedly floral and ultra-sensual, such as "Insolence" (Guerlain, 2005), "Chloé" (2007), "Lady Million" (Paco Rabanne, 2010), or on the contrary, airy and transparent, such as "Ralph" (Ralph Lauren, 2000), "Flower" (Kenzo, 2000), "Narciso Rodriguez" (2004), "Infusion d'Iris" (Prada, 2007) and the new take on "N°5", "N°5 Eau Première" (Chanel, 2008).

The gourmand formulas remained popular, with perfumes featuring increasingly creamy, sweet, fruity nuances, such as "L'Instant" (Guerlain, 2003), "Hypnose" (Lancôme, 2005), "The One" (D&G, 2006) and "Prada Candy" (2010).

"M7", the seventh men's fragrance by Yves Saint Laurent, brought to the West a material traditionally used in oriental perfumery: oud. Oud is a resin secreted by an Asian species of tree (*Aquilaria*

Malaccensis) to defend it from an infection caused by a fungus that feeds on its wood. Oud has an olfactory profile situated mid-way between woody and animalic notes, and in "M7" it is accompanied by vetiver and other woods that create unrivalled effects of depth, elegance and sensuality. "M7" did not find favour with the public, and was withdrawn from the market after a few years; nonetheless, it inspired a large number of composers, who in the years that followed would take the oud note and use it in different ways (along with flowers, spices and other resins), making it familiar also to Western noses through dozens of fragrances for both men and women.

In Italy

The triumph of the Made in Italy concept worldwide persuaded many multinational groups to purchase the most successful Italian companies, and by the end of the decade, the most famous Italian brands were no longer Italian-owned.

Thanks to the large investments made by the multinationals, hitherto unthinkable, Italian brands were able to grow and develop further, and were finally able to compete on equal terms with French and American brands, in all the countries the multinationals sold their products in. Russia, China, India and the Arab countries were the new markets for the luxury and recognisability of the Made in Italy label.

Despite the limits imposed by the global market in which their new owners operated, a number of Italian brands continued to transmit that "Italian touch" that allowed them to obtain extraordinary success, keeping them at the top of sales rankings in many countries for over a decade.

Among these, "Light Blue" (Dolce & Gabbana) in 2001 and "Light Blue pour homme" in 2007 feature tonifying marine notes alongside fruity notes, on a mirror-polished base dominated by white musks; also in 2007, Prada launched "Infusion d'Iris", the first citrus perfume with a powdery edge, whose success would pave the way for others.

Back in vogue for both men's and women's fragrances were distinctive, full-bodied notes, with incense, spices and amber offering structure and character. On the other side, the Italians continued to love the fresh scent of the green facet, which brought success to "Versense" (Versace), "Bellissima" (Blumarine) and other female fragrances with a lush, green heart.

Gourmand perfumes continued to be successful also in Italy, with "Pink Sugar" (Aquolina, 2003) among the best-selling fragrances.

Released under a brand outside the luxury sector, "Pink Sugar" was a concentrate of reassuring sugary and vanilla notes that would soon be imitated both in Italy and abroad, turning it into a cult fragrance among fans of sweet notes.

Prada and Giorgio Armani launched confidential lines of artistic perfumery, which captured the attention of even the "serial" fragrance consumers.

During this decade, artistic perfumery nibbled away at a significant slice of the big brands' turnover. Leading independent perfumers included Profumi di Pantelleria, Carthusia, Eau d'Italie, Profumi del Forte, BOIS, Il Profvmo and Lorenzo Villoresi, whose "Teint de Neige", a floral, powdery woman's fragrance based on Florentine iris, was able to build up an extremely faithful fan base in Italy and abroad, in the space of just a few years. Its unmistakably powdery, elegant sillage was the secret of its success, getting a dreamy, vaguely retro allure back into fashion.

The most surprising perfume to appear during the decade was also Italian: "Black Afgano" by Nasomatto, teaming a potent, innovative oud note with resins and woods, both natural and synthetic. The power and the sillage of "Black Afgano" did not go unnoticed, and it became a signature fragrance for elegant young fashionistas seeking to show off their penchant for trends outside the mainstream, even when it came to perfume.

A number of companies dealing in the import and export of artistic fragrances – which for years had been contributing to the spread of niche perfumery in Italy – decided to step into the arena themselves with their own brands, such as Calé Fragranze d'Autore, Laboratorio Olfattivo and Nobile1942.

Dozens of "niche perfumeries" began making their appearance in all the big cities. This was an entirely Italian phenomenon, because in other countries, artistic fragrances were to be found along with traditional fragrances, both in large department stores and in neighbourhood shops. Italians, on the other hand, felt the need for these "special fragrances" to have their own distinct channel, placing them in boutiques reserved for a limited number of selected brands, following the distribution model applied in the wine industry, where the prestigious labels on sale in a well-stocked wine bar are not found on department store shelves.

In addition, since many "niche" perfumeries are the result of a passion for perfume as a means of artistic expression, their efforts to inform consumers and promote fragrances has helped shape more solid, mature tastes than in other countries.

Teint de Neige

Brand: Lorenzo Villoresi
Gender: feminine
Year of launch: 2000
Status: in production
Analyzed version: original Eau de Toilette
Author: Lorenzo Villoresi
Family: floral oriental

When it first appeared, "Teint de Neige" was such an original, distinctive fragrance that it drove many ladies to stop strangers in the street and ask them what perfume they were wearing. Its romantically retro vein did not go unnoticed in the industry either, which took the structure of "Teint de Neige" and inserted it into many perfumes composed in the years that followed; so while Teint de Neige remains unmistakable and extremely pleasant, it no longer has the amazing impact it used to have 20 years ago.

The main theme of "Teint de Neige" is formed by an ultra-traditional accord of rose, jasmine and ylang ylang, with a touch of aldehydes. Thanks to a generous measure of heliotrope, tonka bean and musks, what might have been a floral, feminine fragrance like so many others is transformed, almost immediately after application, into a tender, comforting, *very* powdery cotton wool cloud, a soft embrace to sink into when the world outside becomes too hostile and when an extra dose of hugs is required.

This is exactly what "Teint de Neige" is: an Italian *mamma* ready to welcome you in her warm, loving, reassuring arms. Perceptible in this intimate, heart-to-heart embrace is the fragrance of the talc *mamma* used after stepping out of the shower, the scent of her favourite face cream, her delicate rose fragrance; and a subtle hint of Panarellina (a soft cake with almonds and vanilla typical of Genoa) reassures you that she's already prepared your afternoon snack. Heaven, right?

Despite the powdery gourmand overall impression, neither the vanilla nor the retro sensation takes the upper hand, making this an elegant fragrance that can be enjoyed at any age.

"Teint de Neige" has such a faithful fan club composed of ladies of all nationalities that Lorenzo Villoresi would risk his very life if he ever dared discontinue it. And rightly so: with a spread that has no equal, this fragrance is able to create a hallmark scent that can identify the wearer in the middle of a crowd. So all it needs are two sprays, because with its record-breaking persistence, there really is no need to overdo it "Teint de Neige" is the fragrance that introduced the public to the talent of Lorenzo Villoresi, a pioneer of artistic perfumery and the only Italian composer ever to have won the prestigious "Prix Coty" (the Oscar prize of the perfume world), in 2006.

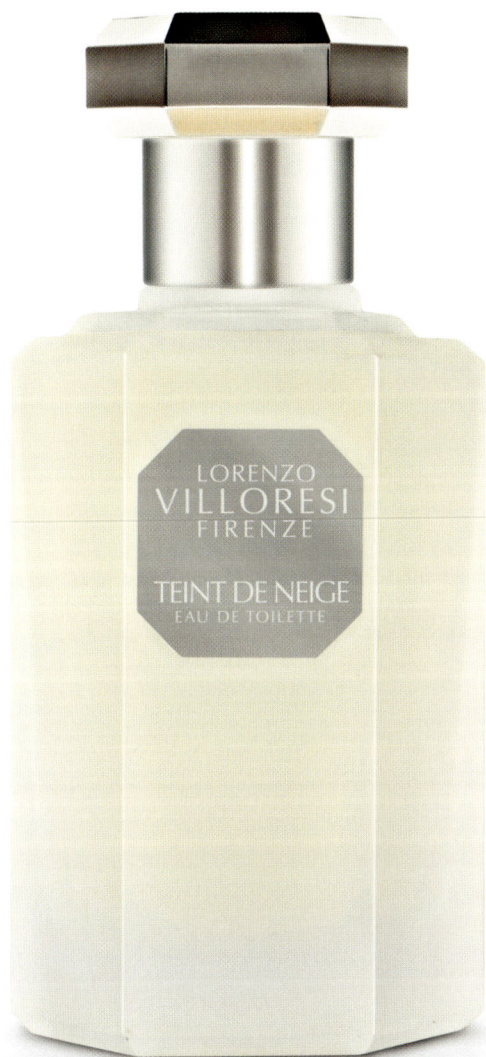

LORENZO
VILLORESI
FIRENZE

TEINT DE NEIGE
EAU DE TOILETTE

Ligea-La Sirena

Brand: Carthusia-Profumi di Capri
Gender: feminine
Year of launch: 2000
Status: in production
Analyzed version: original Eau de Toilette
Family: amber
Glassware Companies: Vetrerie: Bormioli Luigi (modern bottle);
Verreries Brosse (vintage bottle)

If this Siren were to rise up from the waves wearing a perfume, it would be a vintage Guerlain for sure! "Ligea-La Sirena" has a beautifully soft, classy old-school amber allure, with a sunny, optimistic edge. It's as if "Mitsouko" and "Shalimar" (Guerlain, 1912 and 1926) had bought a holiday home on the Amalfi Coast and finally discovered the joys of Limoncello.

Carthusia was one of the first alternative perfumery brands to surface in Italy in response to the massification of the perfumery market at the time. Among the fragrances in this line – all of them generous and graceful – "Ligea" is neither the most appealing nor the most interesting: "Io Capri", for example, is much more complex and sophisticated. Yet when "Ligea" was launched, it immediately received such an enthusiastic welcome that it made Carthusia – hitherto familiar only to a small number of connoisseurs – a benchmark label for those seeking that rich olfactory personality and distinction typical of Italian fragrances and no longer to be found in traditional perfumery.

"Ligea" is brimming with Mediterranean character in every note, from the sweet citrus fruit, through the rose and jasmine, closing with an amber accord dominated by the vanilla and opoponax (the Somalian myrrh, velvet-like, dry and sweet) unashamedly – indeed proudly – rooted in tradition.

"Ligea" does not seek special effects or fireworks, but that soft, serene, human sense of warmth and that relaxed mood that makes you feel you're on holiday every day of the year.

The wealth of materials that form the base guarantees truly impressive spread, especially for the first two hours, with a persistence lasting six full hours.

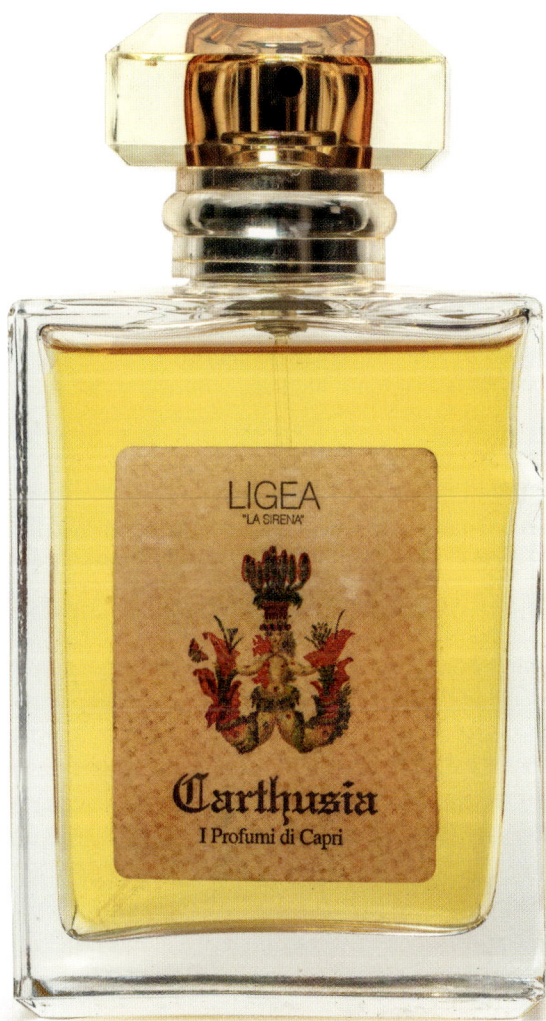

Scent Intense

Brand: Costume National
Gender: unisex
Year of launch: 2002
Status: in production
Analyzed version: original Eau de Parfum
Author: Laurent Bruyère
Family: amber
Bottle design: Ennio Capasa

Take a fashion brand with a distinctively sophisticated, avant-garde style (Costume National by Ennio Capasa); team it with an extraordinarily talented composer (the late lamented Laurent Bruyère), able to see synthetic molecules not as "cheap" replacers for natural and expensive materials, but as the ideal means to obtain innovative, extremely soft, dense tactile effects. If you're lucky, this sort of combination will generate something like "Scent Intense": interesting, unusual and futuristic, yet at the same time comforting, sophisticated and above all, instantly appealing.

The story of "Scent Intense" unfolds in two acts. The opening is characterised by a powerful note of slightly smoky black tea, enlivened by a counterpoint of hibiscus with delicately spiced, floral nuances. The second act, long and languidly orchestrated to bring out the notes at a purposefully slow pace, is composed of a soft, thick, opaque amber base, which instead of reflecting the light absorbs it like a black velvet curtain. Rising up from the amber base are undertones of leather and birch tar, over which the c-12 aldehyde blows an amazingly gentle peach note, adding a further velvety layer to the whole.

With a brief, concise formula, devoid of any glossy frivolity, "Scent Intense" is one of those rare fragrances best perceived at a distance: when smelled close to the skin, an elusive, restrained, enigmatic trace is barely perceptible, while the temperament of the fragrance can be fully appreciated only in the air around the wearer. Although it captures the attention, "Scent Intense" is a fragrance designed for the pleasure of the wearer, not to impress others: a statement of taste and character that requires a minimum of self-awareness for best results.

The projection of "Scent Intense" is perfect: half a metre of Gothic, nocturnal and subtly mystical aura, yet at the same time inviting, comforting, intimate and hypnotic, with a duration of over six full hours. "Scent Intense" does not have a clearly defined gender; although it has a subtle, gentle opening that places it close to the feminine sphere, the majesty of the amber base makes it equally appealing to men. In any case, it should be experienced on the skin for at least three hours, because the projection on paper is misleadingly two-dimensional. Among the other fragrances launched by Costume National, Juliette Karagueuzoglou's splendid "21" deserves a mention, it is an unusual oriental as white as a cup of milk, on whose opening the disembodied spirit of "Scent Intense" may be felt.

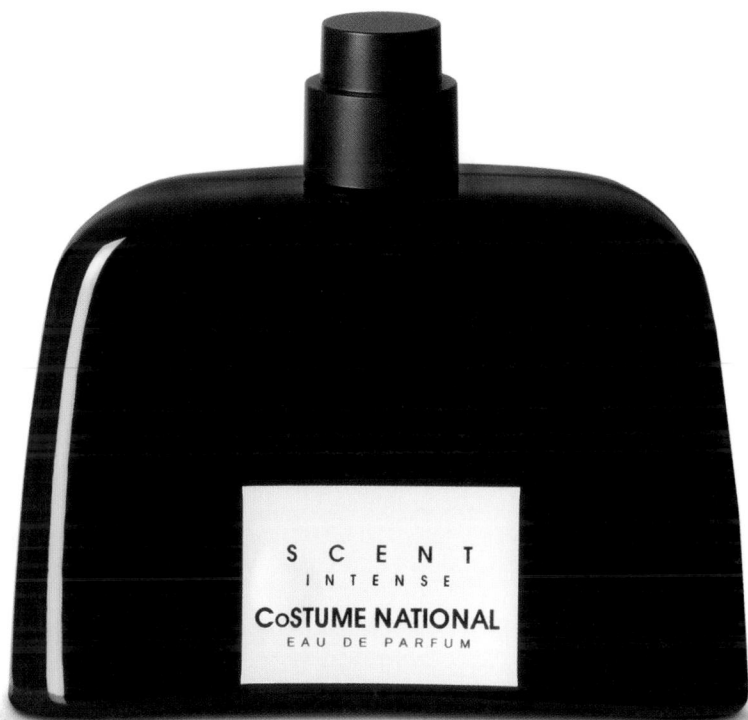

Essenza di Zegna

Brand: Ermenegildo Zegna
Gender: masculine
Year of launch: 2003
Status: discontinued
Analyzed version: original Eau de Toilette
Author: Jacques Cavallier in collaboration with Alberto Morillas
Classification: woody citrus
Bottle design: Doug Lloyd

The duo that created "Essenza di Zegna" – Jacques Cavallier and Alberto Morillas, two Giants in perfumery – is a sure-fire guarantee of a sophisticated composition, a musky freshness, with a contemporary allure. In "Essenza di Zegna", these characteristics are perfectly proportioned.

Reaching up into the splendid opening of bergamot, mandarin and cardamom is a dry, purified myrrh, forming an embrace as clear as an early summer day, in which the intense turquoise of the sky draws you right up inside the heavens, making you wish you had a pair of snowy-white wings. Beautifully delicate aquatic (not marine) notes bring an even gentler tone to the opening, adding a subtly melancholy shadow. The amber/woody base, supported by a crystal-clear vetiver, emerges slowly, bonding to the myrrh and fully coming through half an hour after application, as the citrus notes begin to fade from the scene.

The overall effect is clean and linear, almost minimalist, and the sensation is of a brief, concise formula. At the same time, "Essenza di Zegna" is more creative than other men's fragrances from the same period, thanks to the teamwork of Cavallier and Morillas and their consummate skills in creating citrus structures, evident here at their very best. Cavallier's works are a textbook example of formal perfection, teamed with a huge talent for innovation ("L'Eau d'Issey", "l'Eau Parfumée au Thé Blanc" by Bulgari), while those of Morillas offer extremely clean, modern sensations, with the accent on cotton wool impressions, reminiscent of rising clouds of vapour ("Mugler Cologne" and the whole "Omnia" series by Bulgari).

The projection of "Essenza di Zegna" is extremely discreet, best experienced directly on the skin. The duration is of little more than three hours, due to a structure in which the top and middle notes prevail over the base. Stock up while it's still available: I expect stocks to run out soon.

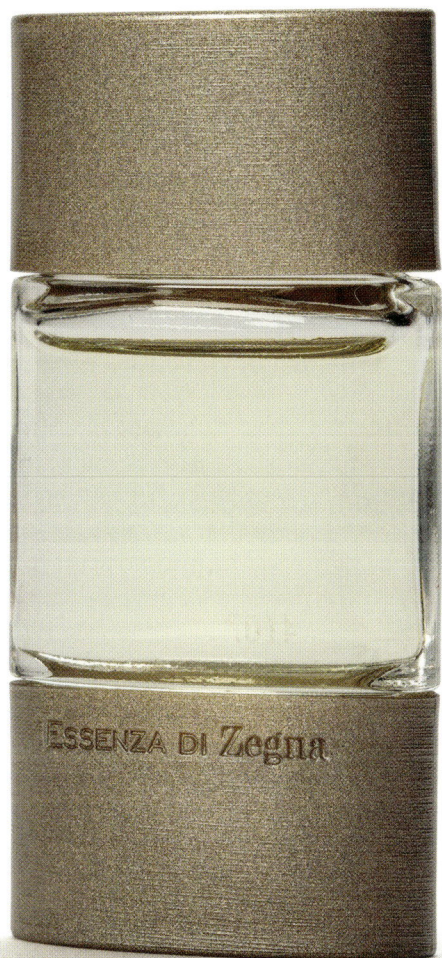

Essenza di Zegna

Gucci pour Homme

Brand: Gucci
Gender: masculine
Year of launch: 2003
Status: discontinued
Analyzed version: original Eau de Toilette
Author: Michel Almairac
Classification: aromatic woody

When it was launched, "Gucci pour homme" was not welcomed with the success it deserved. Recognition as one of the finest men's fragrances in its category came only a few years later, when the fragrance was on the verge of disappearing.

"Gucci pour homme" was created by Michel Almairac, the Maître Parfumeur of Grasse who composed masterpieces such as "Zino Davidoff" (1986), "Fahrenheit" (Dior, 1988), "Joop! Homme" (1989), "Jil Sander N°4" (1990), "Gucci Rush" (1992) and "Casmir" (Chopard, 1992), as well as numerous "niche" perfumes for "Bond N°9", "Le Labo", "Les Parfums de Rosine" and "L'Artisan Parfumeur".

"Gucci pour Homme" is a bouquet of woody, aromatic and resinous notes, seamed tightly together by a thread of incense, spreading a warm, raw, meditative, extremely sophisticated overall sensation. Rising above the sublimely woody middle accord of vetiver, sandalwood and vegetable musk is a magnificent, centuries-old cedar, accented by smoky and leathery notes and sliced from top to bottom by a blade of cold, extra-dry frankincense.

Many of Almairac's fragrances are built around a strong idea, and developed with a linear approach, and "Gucci pour homme" is no exception, with a monumental presence that starts to project an extraordinarily alluring, subtly mystical sillage of frankincense, benzoin and vegetable musk the moment it settles on the skin, and lasting for a good number of hours.

Gucci Pour homme was one of the best men's fragrances ever produced in living memory: distinctive, rich in natural raw materials and perfect in every respect. Far beyond any imitation. Should you find any bottle around, don't hesitate for a minute.

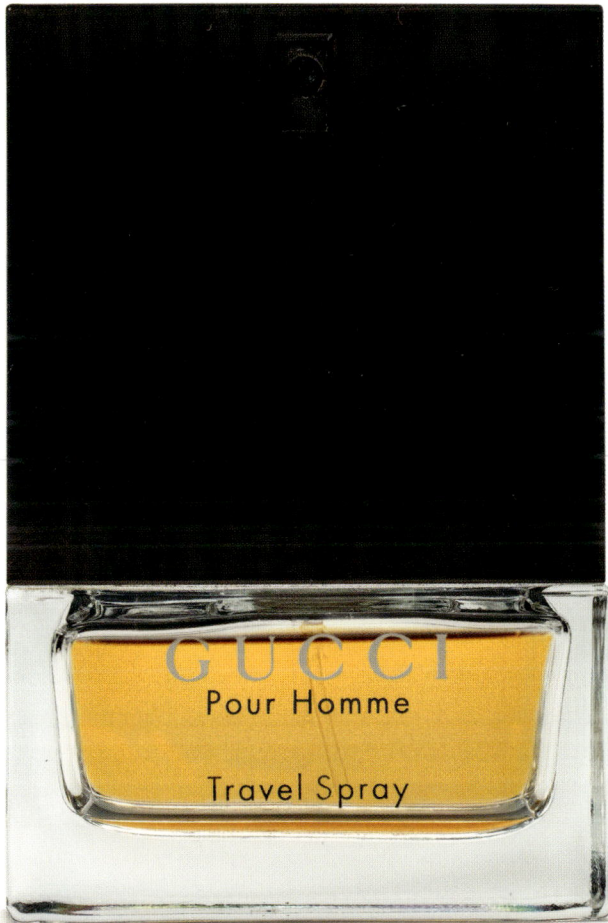

Sicily

Brand: Dolce & Gabbana
Gender: feminine:
Year of launch: 2003
Status: irelaunched in 2019
Analyzed version: original Eau de Toilette
Author: Nathalie Lorson
Classification: aldehydic floral
Glassware companies: Bormioli Luigi

Vulgar, fluorescent, plastic-coated, over-the-top. Tender, reassuring, clean, maternal. You'd think two different fragrances were being described here, wouldn't you? Yet in the world of perfumery, opposites often manage to find a spot next to each other, engaging in mutual enrichment thanks to the generous nuances they're made up of. The only other place in the world where opposites are able to coexist with such intrepid generosity is in the heart of a Woman.

"Sicily" opens with a sparkling burst of Sicilian citrus, while the heart beats with a traditional accord of jasmine, rose and orange blossom, the base is a tender blend of sandalwood, musky notes and heliotrope, a note from vintage perfumery at risk of disappearing because it has fallen out of fashion, despite its beauty and versatility. A significant amount of aldehydes blows a breath of white porcelain over the whole, like the clean scent of a soap bar lingering on milky-white skin. The result is a bright, floral, classic-style fragrance, with a measure of sweetness and such a large amount of aldehydes to recall "Chanel N°22" (1922), with a modern touch brought by the trail of white musks. Its intimate, retro essence, evident enough to be perceptible yet subtle enough to prevent it from becoming dated, makes "Sicily" a contemporary tribute to a century of perfumery for women. And by women, I don't mean those plastic, slightly disturbing creatures in vogue at the time, or giddy girls in search of the recipe for eternal youth. There are other types of fragrances for those. "Sicily" is for real flesh-and-blood, tears-and-laughter women: for those who have run up against situations that have cost them dearly; for women who have always followed their heart and always got it wrong; for women who always find the strength to carry on with a smile on their face – even if nobody knows how they do it.

Ultimately, "Sicily" is a perfume without a complex construction or particularly distinctive notes; it's simply a universal story of women, speaking through every individual wearer with a different voice. It has a truly impressive projection for the whole of the first half hour, after which it settles down onto the skin in a lingering accord of powdery tones that lasts for hours on end.

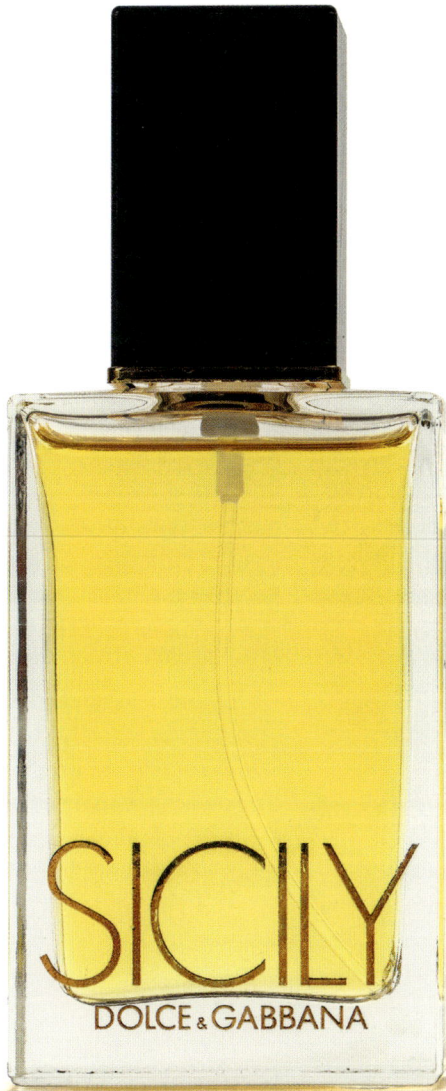

Bois d'Encens

Brand: Armani Privé
Gender: unisex
Year of launch: 2004
Status: in production
Analyzed version: original Eau de Parfum
Author: Michel Almairac
Classification: spicy woody

"Bois d'Encens" was one of the first fragrances in the Armani Privé collection, the artistic perfumery line created by the Armani brand in 2004. The Armani Privé line, similarly to exclusive lines of other brands (including Prada, Chanel, Dior and Hermès) is sophisticated, original and creative, featuring precious materials – every scent is an original interpretation of a single, splendid note– and with an extremely selective distribution. "Bois d'Encens" is one of the finest fragrances in the collection, a spicy/woody perfume enhanced with a note of frankincense that is much more spiritual than ceremonial, its subtle sugary nuance sets it apart from any other incense-based fragrance from the period (especially from the "3: Incense" series by Comme des Garçons, whose fragrances evoke an intensely religious experience).

The opening of "Bois d'Encens" is spicy citrus, with the black pepper in the foreground offering a cold, powdery sensation, immediately picked up by the incense note. Blowing through the heart accord is a green, floral breeze whose components are perfectly sewn together. The woods (primarily vetiver and cedar) come up almost immediately from the base, binding together flowers and spices into a calm, elegant, demure whole.

"Bois d'Encens" stands with one foot in spirituality and the other in luxury design, with natural and synthetic notes deftly mixed to evoke Armani's sophisticated, modern style, widely praised – and just as widely copied – all over the world.

No surprise that Bois d'Encens was the star of 2006's FiFi Awards, as the Best Fragrance Nouveau Niche and the Best Packaging Prestige (the black bottle, complemented with the sophisticated stopper is absolutely stunning). "Bois d'Encens" is a private pleasure with a moderate spread and a duration of a couple of hours.

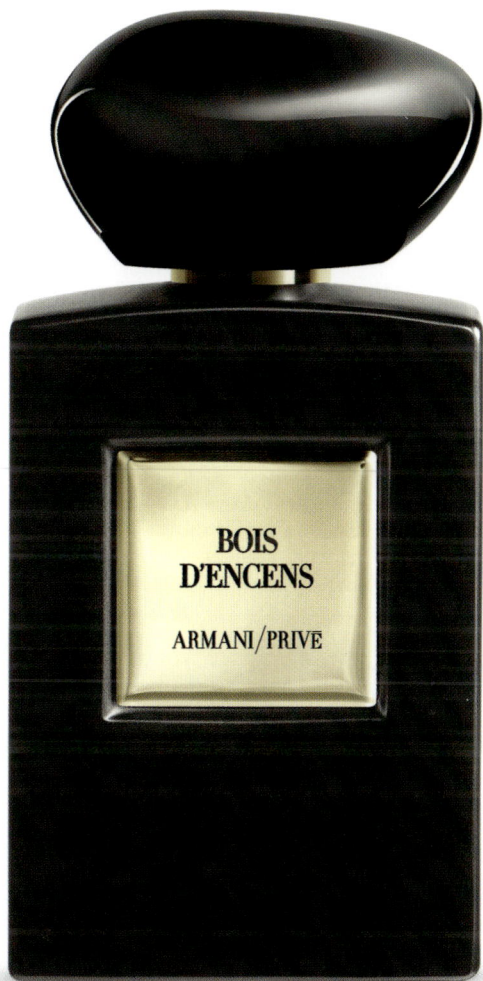

Max Mara

Brand: Max Mara
Gender: feminine
Year of launch: 2004
Analyzed version: original Eau de Parfum
Author: Daphne Bugey
Classification: musky floral
Bottle design: Thierry Baschmakoff

The first detail that catches the eye in "Max Mara" (the first perfume launched by the brand) is the bottle, a truncated parallelepiped rounded at the front, whose stopper is the bottle's continuation. This simple yet sophisticated design is perfectly in line with the values of a *maison* that shuns excess, placing the accent on a clean-cut elegance and sophisticated fabrics. The fragrance, meanwhile, has a surprisingly vibrant ginger and citrus opening, with black pepper offering a counterpoint that creates a cool/warm, transparent/opaque interplay able to keep interest high and ensure "Max Mara" is never banal. Once the turbulent opening strikes a spicy compromise – the effect lasts for several minutes – a dry, floral heart comes through, with a green facet of magnolia, lily and orchid. The flowers are soon reached by a bouquet of musks and a generous dose of sugary notes, which bring a pleasant, affable edge to a floral formula that might otherwise be too "reserved", almost austere. Elegant, skilfully composed and solid – exactly what transpires from the bottle – "Max Mara" has a moderate projection, remaining fairly close to the wearer's skin and a duration of several hours.

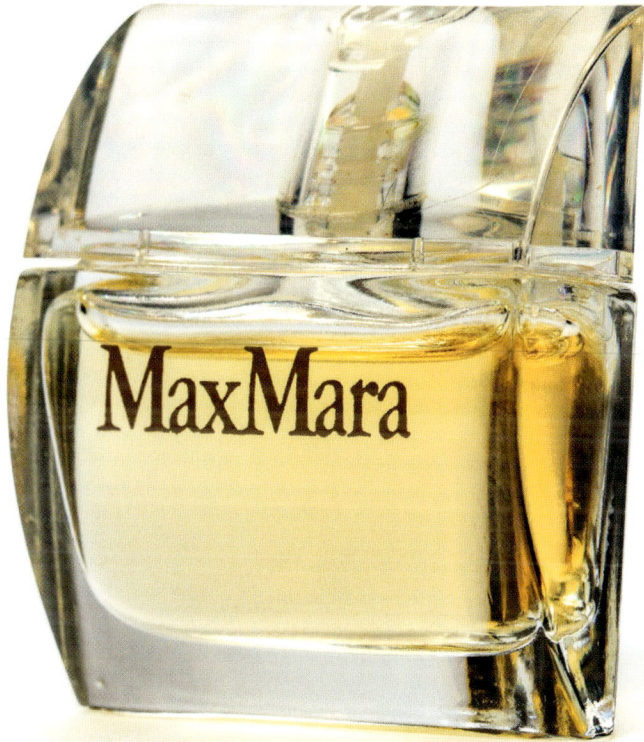

Armani Code

Brand: Armani
Gender: masculine
Year of launch: 2004
Status: relauched in 2006
Analyzed version: original Eau de Toilette
Author: Antoine Lie
Classification: oriental fougère

"Armani Code" (or "Black Code", the name with which it was released) is a textbook lesson on how to take a familiar structure - essentially a semi-oriental fougère like many others - and turn it into an Italian product through and through: elegant, velvety-smooth and sensual, one of those fragrances that draws you to the wearer with a smile and a desire to strike up a conversation. And perhaps even end up with an invitation to dinner by what just might be the man of your dreams. The citrus opening is soon reached by a powdery facet, creating a clean, subtly "barber's shop" sensation that lasts for a few minutes. As soon as the opening begins to fade out, star anise and olive blossom make their appearance in a warm, spicy, aromatic heart accord, bonding marvelously with the base of guaiac wood, tonka bean, tobacco and leather. "Armani Code" heads quickly towards a warm, nocturnal, sensual drydown, transmitting an air of elegance and self-confidence without ever falling into the macho-man trap: this fragrance is a triumph of warmth, restraint and good taste, with no style excesses or needless displays of power. "Armani Code"'s ideal habitat are formal evenings and romantic soirées, although with its delicate projection it can also be ventured for a business occasion. It has excellent persistence, lasting around six hours.

Z Zegna

Brand: Ermenegildo Zegna
Gender: masculine
Year of launch: 2005
Status: in production
Analyzed version: original Eau de Toilette
Author: Antoine Lie in collaboration with Pierre Negrin and Olivier Gillotin
Classification: woody ozonic
Bottle design: Ducati

"Z Zegna" is one of the most appealing members of the family of ozonic/musky men's fragrances, with a clean, vigorous core, which came into vogue in the wake of the success of forebears such as "Cool Water", "Acqua di Giò" and "Light Blue". Many of the descendants of these three legendary fragrances have unfortunately remained anchored to a rather basic model of virility, concerned above all with being perceived as clean, decent and inoffensive: in short, nothing to write home about.

Although "Z Zegna" is descended from the same trio, it manages to avoid falling into the "fresh-clean-decent" trap, thanks to a meticulously calculated rigour that allows it to reach unrivalled heights of clarity, as well as formal composure and elegance.

The top and middle notes of "Z Zegna" unfold around citrus, rosemary and spices (nutmeg and white pepper), forming an accord that creates the effect of a perfectly ironed, crisp linen shirt, with a fruity zing that makes for an exciting opening. Iris, Cashmeran (a musky molecule with a green, foresty scent), a dry, crisp fraction of patchouli and vegetable musk form a wood-tinged accord taking "Z Zegna" into a solid, reserved, compact dimension.

The musky and ozonic notes are not overpowering, serving to bring a broad, open breath of invigorating fresh air reminiscent of snow-capped mountains glistening in the sun.

"Z Zegna" is one of the finest men's fragrances in its category: an oasis of calm, composure, style and distinction in a desert of excess and banality.

The aura "Z Zegna" projects around the wearer is perceptible at a distance of up to a metre; its clean, linear essence helps make it suitable even for the office, provided that just the right amount is applied. The persistence is excellent, indeed insuperable.

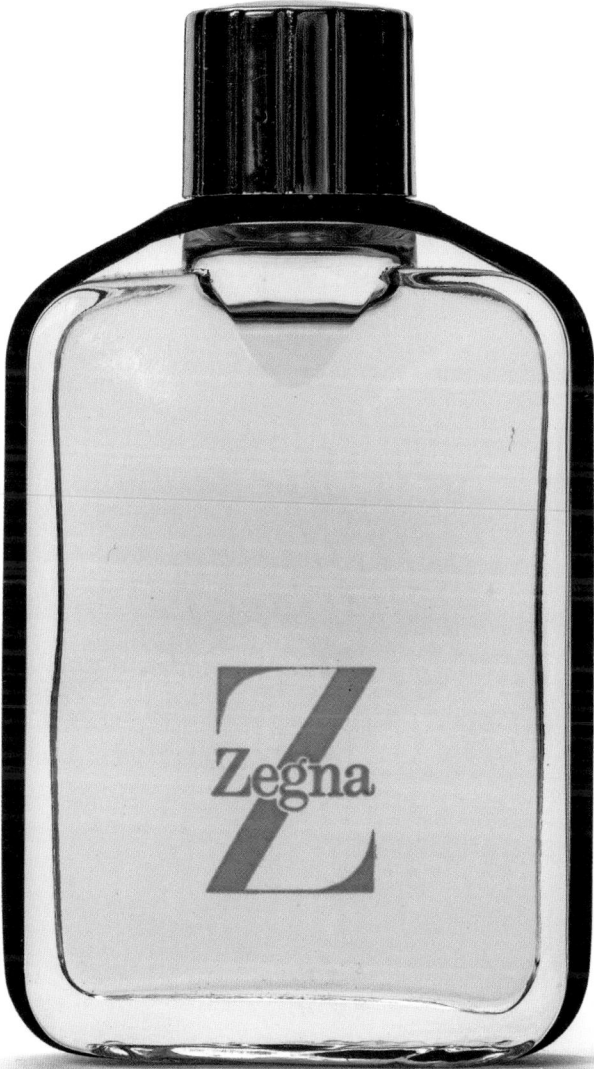

Bergamotto Marino

Brand: Gianfranco Ferré
Gender: unisex
Year of launch: 2006
Status: in production
Analyzed version: original edc
Author: Pierre Bourdon
Classification: ozonic citrus
Bottle design: Serge Mansau

At the beginning of the 2000s, the success obtained by alternative perfumery opened new opportunities in terms of both artistic expression and business. "Bergamotto Marino" is a testament to Ferré's interest in moving in a new, more engaging direction. Unfortunately, the market was not quite ready for a crossover of this kind, and may not have fully grasped the message: many perceived "Bergamotto Marino" as a step back into the past – while it was in fact an almost prophetic vision of the future of perfumery.

The name "Bergamotto Marino", together with the simple bottle, infact, evoke those of a number of independent brands for which the substance is more important than the form, and the vintage-tinged packaging is typical of a retro-style Cologne.

The formula revolves around three precious natural essential oils used in almost all traditional citrus colognes: neroli, jasmine and 25% marvellous bergamot from Calabria. Although these three main elements remain present throughout, the notes accompanying them take it into a bright, frothy, ethereal, contemporary dimension. The green nuances of the jasmine are bolstered by the lily of the valley, creating a floral accord that makes a gorgeous partner also for men's skin, while the ozonic notes, which remain delicate, add a sweet/sharp touch of melon. Towards the end, an ambergris/vegetable musk accord contributes texture and specific weight to the whole fragrance.

This creates the vigorous, extrovert and exhilarating effect of a classic Cologne, yet it's also subtle, sophisticated and contemporary; the quality of the composition and the materials is much closer to artistic perfumery than to an industrial fragrance, and this sensation is clearly perceptible.

"Bergamotto Marino" creates an aura of calm elegance around the wearer, without making its presence too keenly felt. It lasts for up to four hours on the skin, and this respectable duration places it mid-way between an Eau de Toilette and an Eau de Parfum, despite being a Cologne.

The composer, Pierre Bourdon (creator of many outstanding successes, such as "Kouros" by Yves Saint Laurent, "Dolce Vita" by Christian Dior, "Cool Water" by Davidoff, "Iris Poudre" for Frédéric Malle) has an exceptional talent for citrus fragrances; "Bergamotto Marino" by Ferré is a testament to both his respect for traditional scents and his desire to promote their beauty by bringing a skilfully innovative edge to them.

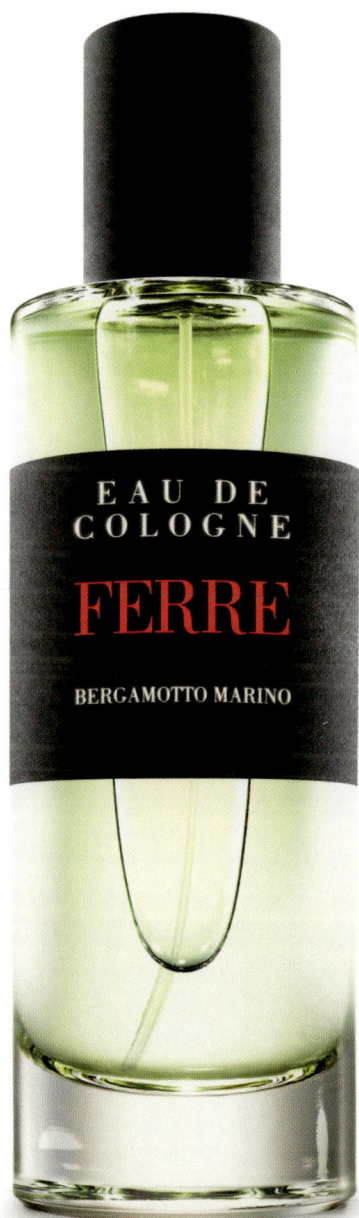

Paestum Rose

Brand: Eau d'Italie
Gender: unisex
Year of launch: 2006
Status: in production
Analyzed version: original Eau de Toilette
Author: Bertrand Duchaufour
Classification: woody floral

In 2006, the family that owned one of the most beautiful hotels in Positano, Le Sirenuse, decided to offer its guests a line of toiletries created specifically for the hotel. The composition of the fragrance was entrusted to a talented perfumer with a cutting-edge creative approach, Bertrand Duchaufour, who were to attract the attention of the international perfumery world just thanks to the perfumes created for Eau d'Italie. With "Paestum Rose", Duchaufour took an unusual approach to exploring the rose, giving it a uniquely original interpretation.

"Paestum Rose" opens with a fiery burst of spices, with black pepper, pink pepper, coriander, cinnamon and cumin forming a dry, pungent base, under which a floral sensation comes through gradually until it captures the attention. And when it does, the rose emerges in all its splendour! Lush and velvety-smooth, with an undertone of apricot (osmanthus), this three-dimensional rose is full and mature, tantalised and amused by the spices that revolve around it, paying tribute to its most vegetable aspect. As the base accord gradually rises up into the heart of the fragrance, the rose turns its attention to the woods (vetiver, cedar and patchouli) offering warmth and an extra fullness, while myrrh and incense make for a more "melting" whole. Towards the end, the rose fades to a sensual, floral shadow the wood notes continue to sigh after for a few hours. "Paestum Rose" is impressively intense, with very good projection and a duration of several hours.

It was a while since such a singular, interesting rose had been seen, and when it first appeared, the success of this perfume was such that it encouraged the owners of the hotel to continue their adventure in the world of perfumery.

The collaboration between the hotel and Duchaufour continued for several years, giving rise to such thrilling gems as "Baume du Doge", a spicy oriental featuring spices, resins and all sorts of heavenly elements, and "Jardin du Poète", which offers a whole new take on the aromatic facet, bringing a humid, sparkling, intensely Mediterranean touch to it.

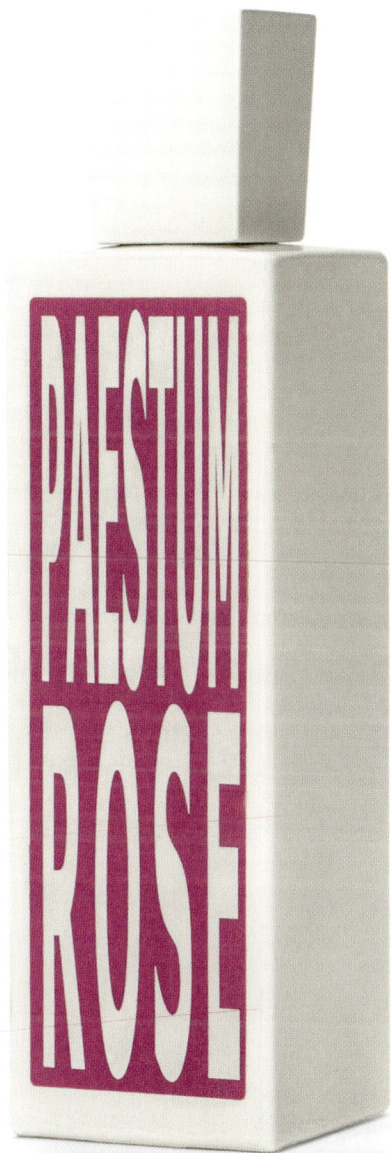

Light Blue pour homme

Brand: Dolce & Gabbana
Gender: masculine
Year of launch: 2007
Status: in production
Analyzed version: original Eau de Toilette
Author: Alberto Morillas
Classification: aquatic citrus
Bottle design: Alberto Gabba

Dolce & Gabbana entrusted the creation of "Light Blue" to one of the most prolific master perfumers, who with "Cologne" by Mugler (2001) had upgraded cologne to the 2.0 version, cleansing it of almost all its natural notes and plunging it into a rich bouquet of frothy white musks. Many fragrances by Morillas are possessed of a subtle, radiant light reminiscent of a steam bath, and a radiance able to fill an entire room, moving forth gracefully and gently, without making a song and dance about it. "Light Blue" is founded on a mix of this nature (white musk/dihydromyrcenol/calone), a cool, sharply clear, detergent accord that forms the base for half of the contemporary men's fragrances. In "Light Blue", the accord is introduced and accompanied at length by fresh, bitter citrus notes, an aromatic facet of juniper and rosemary, a hint of black pepper, and a musky base with incense. The resounding success obtained by "Light Blue" worldwide is due to the sensation of cleanliness and simplicity that runs right through it, which clearly tunes into the deepest yearnings of our chaotic, polluted Western society. The advertising images, featuring Bianca Balti and David Gandy half-naked amid the sea stacks, undoubtedly contributed to the success of "Light Blue": many consumers from abroad identified "Light Blue" as a "typically Italian" product precisely because of the commercial, although what the advertising transmits is not so much the true essence of Italy, but rather the stereotyped image of the *Bel Paese* abroad: beautiful women, citrus fruit, the sea and a traditional Italian melody. In any case, the advertising was consistent with the message transmitted by the name and the fragrance, which is something to be recognised and admired.

"Light Blue" is a simple, linear fragrance that does not develop to a great extent: its delicate projection does not invade the space around it, making it suitable for any occasion on which the wearer needs to feel clean and smart, without too much fuss.

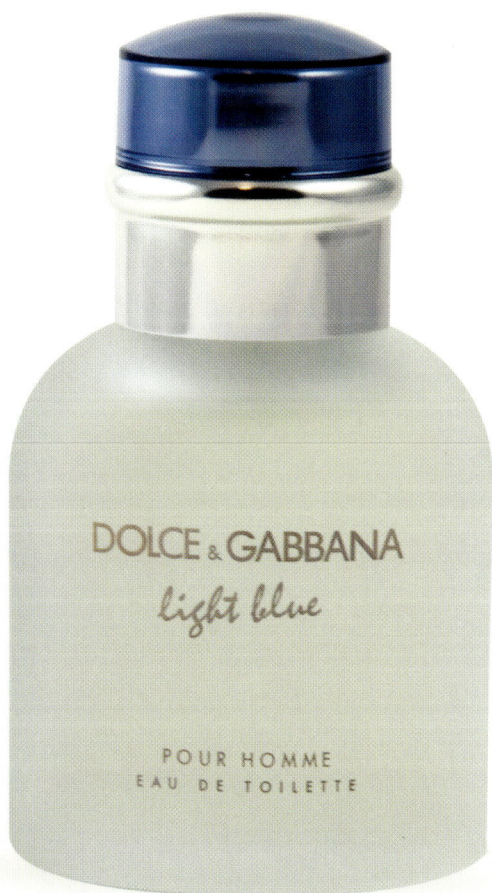

DOLCE & GABBANA

light blue

POUR HOMME
EAU DE TOILETTE

Infusion d'Iris

Brand: Prada
Gender: feminine
Year of launch: 2007
Status: in production
Analyzed version: original Eau de Toilette
Author: Daniela Andrier
Classification: powdery citrus

"Infusion d'Iris", one of the most successful fragrances launched so far by Prada, is the first example of a completely new category: powdery citrus. The molecular elements give "Infusion d'Iris" an unrivalled modern, radiant glow, while the natural elements enhance the whole and add character, just as a couple of carefully chosen accessories (sunglasses, a belt or a bag) can liven up a look you've worn countless times before.

An accord composed of vetiver, cedarwood, musks and an iris note spread a green, dry base, soft and powdery as a cotton wool cloud on which the fragrance can comfortably stretch right out. A green note of galbanum blows through the heart of the perfume, gathering up the woods from the base, together with a feather-light, perfectly pure neroli note. The top is a simple, timidly appealing mandarin, which brings a quiet, reserved gentleness right from the opening. The green undertone that runs right through "Infusion d'Iris" (formed by galbanum, cedar and vetiver), and the soft, powdery accord of musks and iris, are accents that add interest to a sophisticated, reassuring bouquet, with those clean, light qualities that are so popular with consumers all over the world and which have brought the perfume such extraordinary success. "Infusion d'Iris" has a duration of more than five hours, and a perfect radiance, enveloping the wearer in a delicate glow.

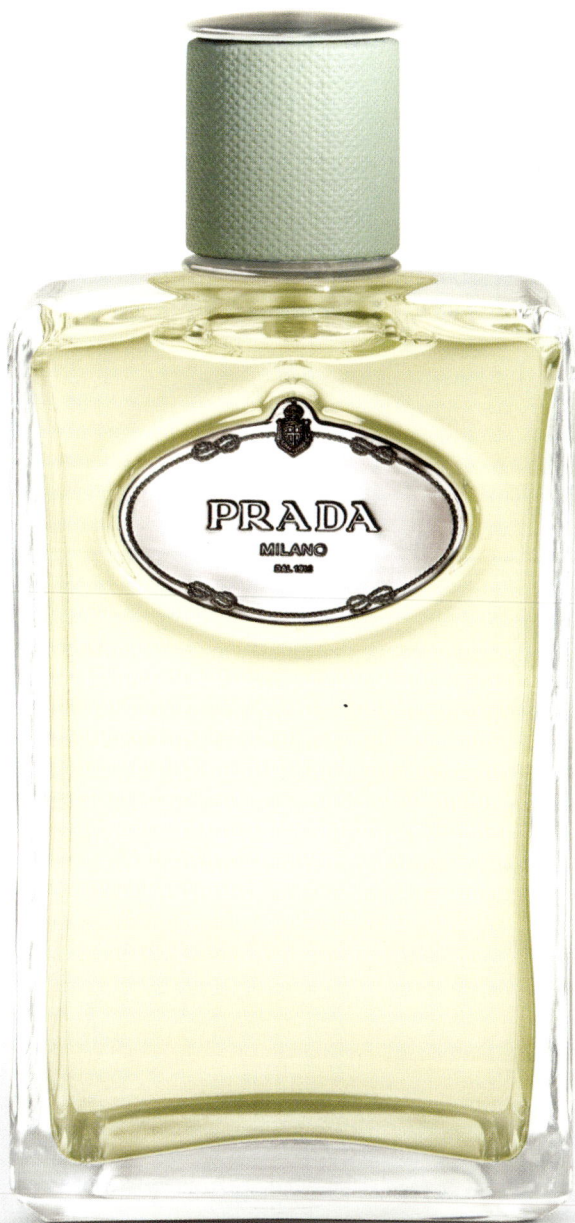

N°8 Opoponax

Brand: Prada
Gender: unisex
Year of launch: 2007
Status: discontinued
Analyzed version: original parfum
Author: Daniela Andrier
Classification: amber
Bottle design: Lalique

Long before artistic perfumery became a growing trend, Prada had launched an exclusive line of fragrances available only in the brand's own boutiques. The ten fragrances, which appeared between 2003 and 2009, were composed by Daniela Andrier of Givaudan, using the richest, most enchanting notes in perfumery, including orange blossom, violet, narcissus, leather and amber, benzoin, carnation, jasmine and opoponax, forming an encyclopaedic collection of scents of a rare, vibrant beauty. All the fragrances were composed of superb-quality materials, and the formulas were kept deliberately minimal, by subtracting element after element to free the starring notes from any embellishments or decorations traditionally associated with them in all their splendid, naked glory. This sort of approach naturally required not only natural materials of outstanding quality, but also a perfect command of the notes and an uncommon aesthetic sensitivity: Daniela Andrier has proved more than up to the task during her magnificent thirty-year career.

"N°8 Opoponax" obviously places the accent on the note of opoponax, a type of myrrh from Somalia, whose various facets are enhanced by the other elements in the formula – the bitter facet by the bergamot, the liqueur-like, sugary facet by the labdanum, the salty, shady one by the ambergris and the dry, the powdery one by the sandalwood.

The end result is magnificently warm, dense and raw, of impressive depth and intensity, with the elements bound together so closely that the individual notes are difficult to identify.

"N°8 Opoponax" is more an olfactory experience than a perfume, and cannot be fully appreciated without an open mind and a minimal amount of olfactory culture necessary to recognise the exceptional quality of the notes used. Since it is composed for the most part of heavy raw materials, "N°8 Opoponax" is a rather linear fragrance; after the first 15 minutes it takes to settle, it comes up to temperature and begins to spread with growing confidence for the following three hours. Since it is a parfum, its drydown lasts virtually forever. For its exclusive collection, Prada had ensured there was no expense spared, creating a product that could not be equalled – both the fragrance itself and the simply beautiful, sophisticated bottle designed by Lalique.

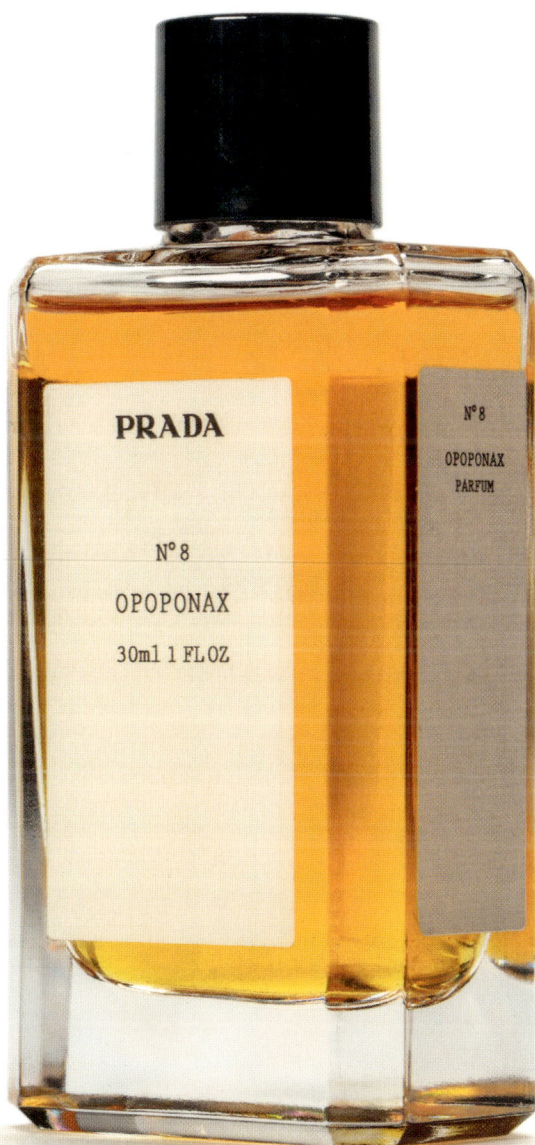

PRADA

N° 8

OPOPONAX

30ml 1 FL OZ

N° 8

OPOPONAX
PARFUM

Jasmin Noir

Brand: Bulgari
Gender: feminine
Year of launch: 2008
Status: in production
Analyzed version: original Eau de Parfum
Author: Carlos Benaim
Classification: floral oriental

From the name "Jasmin Noir", you might be expecting a fragrance dominated by the floral, green, creamy scent of jasmine, but "Jasmin Noir" is much more than a simple soliflore.

The formula revolves around an appealing musky/woody/gourmand base accord with a dry, sweet, exotic scent that is intriguing, although slightly flat and two-dimensional. The third dimension is brought in by the flowers, with gardenia and jasmine (the sambac variety, with a dense, indolic, animalic olfactory profile) literally "lighting up" the accord of almond, wood, tonka bean and vanilla with lush, green notes that shine brightly through, adding a feminine, dynamic sensation. The flowers in the heart accord bond in such a close embrace it is difficult to separate them, except for the key element of jasmine. Sambac jasmine – an absolute is used here, which is even more potent, narcotic and animalic than the essential oil – is a resounding note people either love or hate: for every individual who adores its decadent opulence, there are at least another two who detest it.

In "Jasmin Noir", Carlos Benaim manages to strike a perfect balance, adding just enough to give the fragrance a velvety, sensual, elegant allure, yet not enough to weigh it down and make it difficult to wear.

The moderate projection of "Jasmin Noir" makes it suitable for any occasion; despite the name, this is not a wild, nocturnal or dangerous fragrance – indeed it's a pleasant, extrovert perfume with an immediate appeal. Just as well, because there are plenty of disagreeably overpowering jasmines already, all of which could do with a touch of finesse. Moderation is a rare quality.

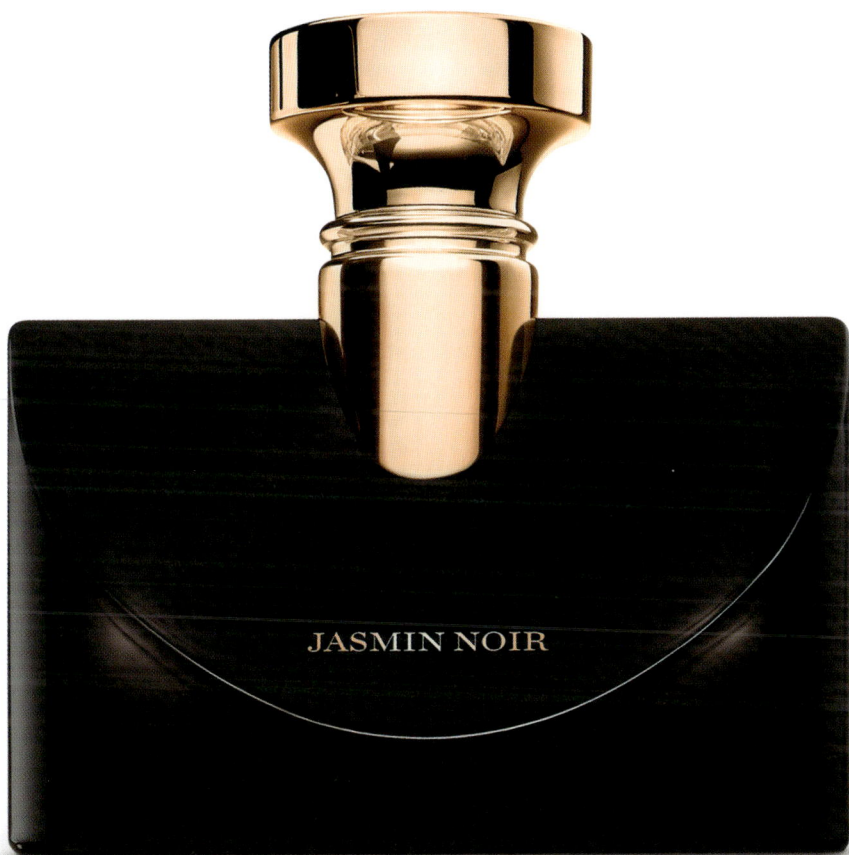

JASMIN NOIR

The One

Brand: Dolce & Gabbana
Gender: masculine
Year of launch: 2008
Status: in production
Analyzed version: original Eau de Toilette and Eau de Parfum
Author: Olivier Polge (IFF)
Classification: woody amber

At a time when most men's fragrances were experimenting with marine notes, musky-woody or clean-detergent notes (or a mix between two or more of these options), Domenico Dolce and Stefano Gabbana chose to venture in the opposite direction, launching a fragrance that marked a return to the rich olfactory structure of the classic ambers. The reason for this was simply that ambers are Stefano Gabbana's favourite. Generally speaking, when a project is aligned with a personal taste rather than budgetary expectations, the level of originality and distinction is more likely to be impressive; and that's just what happened here.

"The One" is an amber fragrance in grand style, enriched with a prominent tobacco component that brings a soft, material quality to the whole. The sweet, golden citrus opening has a subtle hint of orange blossom; basil and spiced notes of cardamom, ginger and coriander bring a touch of dynamism to the heart of the fragrance, binding with the cedar of the base with piquant, slightly powdery nuances. The ambergris brings a rounded touch to the composition, adding a dry, sweetly smoky note. "The One" seems lit up by the sun's rays and enveloped in a bronze-coloured silk cloak.

"The One" is a mature, self-aware man of sophisticated tastes, who appreciates full, rounded figures, preferably accompanied by a personality with rich nuances and interesting undertones. The projection and duration of the Eau de Toilette version of "The One" could have been wider and longer: it was a shame such a splendid fragrance could be enjoyed only by the wearer and the select few lucky enough to be allowed close! This is why it was joined in 2015 by the Eau de Parfum version, with a more marked projection and satisfying duration. Both versions were created by Olivier Polge, which at time "The One" was launched had numerous highly successful fragrances to his name.

A few years later, in 2015, Olivier Polge joined Chanel as the maison's new Maître Parfumeur: the fourth after Ernest Beaux (1921-1954), Guy Robert (1954-1974) and Olivier's illustrious father, Jacques Polge (1974-2016).

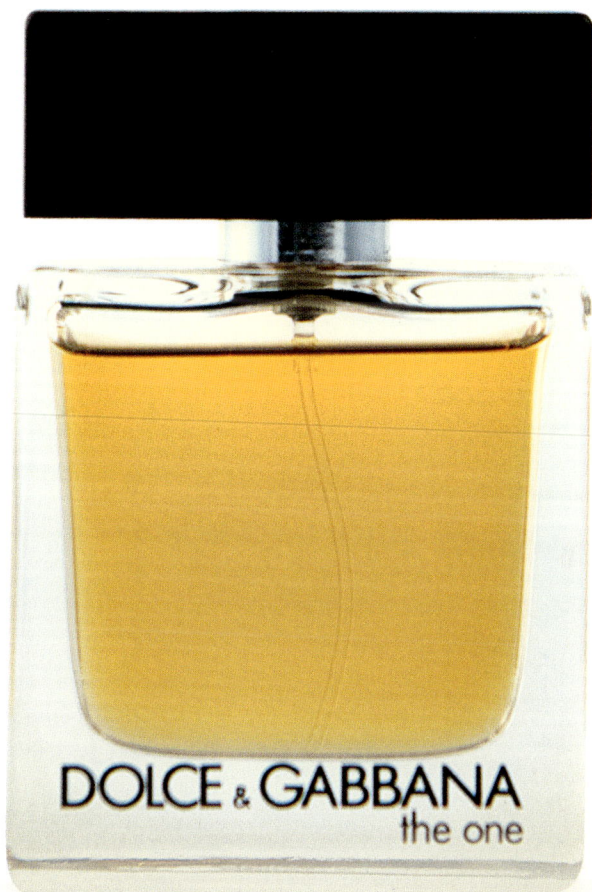

Bellissima

Brand: Blumarine
Gender: feminine
Year of launch: 2009
Status: in production
Analyzed version: original Eau de Parfum
Author: Sophie Labbé (IFF)
Classification: aquatic green floral

Within "Bellissima" by Blumarine beats a green, floral heart, with gentle, romantic tones that make it one of the most pleasant members of the aquatic floral family.

Orange, grapefruit and a touch of ginger open the floral accord, standing out against which is an appealing peony note, surrounded by crystal-clear aquatic notes. Cashmeran, vanilla and musks build a base for "Bellissima" to settle on after application, without adding an ounce of weight; the fragrance remains clear and focused all the time, with a surprisingly natural mood.

The composer, Sophie Labbé (winner of the prestigious Prix Coty in 2005) has a particular penchant for flowers, especially peony; her compositions are constructed with a light, exceptionally delicate touch, in which the material component has been removed in order to place the accent on their more ethereal, spiritual quality, giving the sensation of a floral whisper rather than actual flesh-and-petal flowers.

"Bellissima" has a moderate projection; it's a fragrance worn for the pleasure of the wearer rather than to impress the others. The lingering musky end note lasts for a few hours, creating a fresh, minimalist sensation.

Thanks to the square bottle crowned with a round top, together with the pinkish tinge of the liquid inside, the packaging of "Bellissima" is a textbook example of clean, simple lines and sophistication: a perfect reflection of the fragrance.

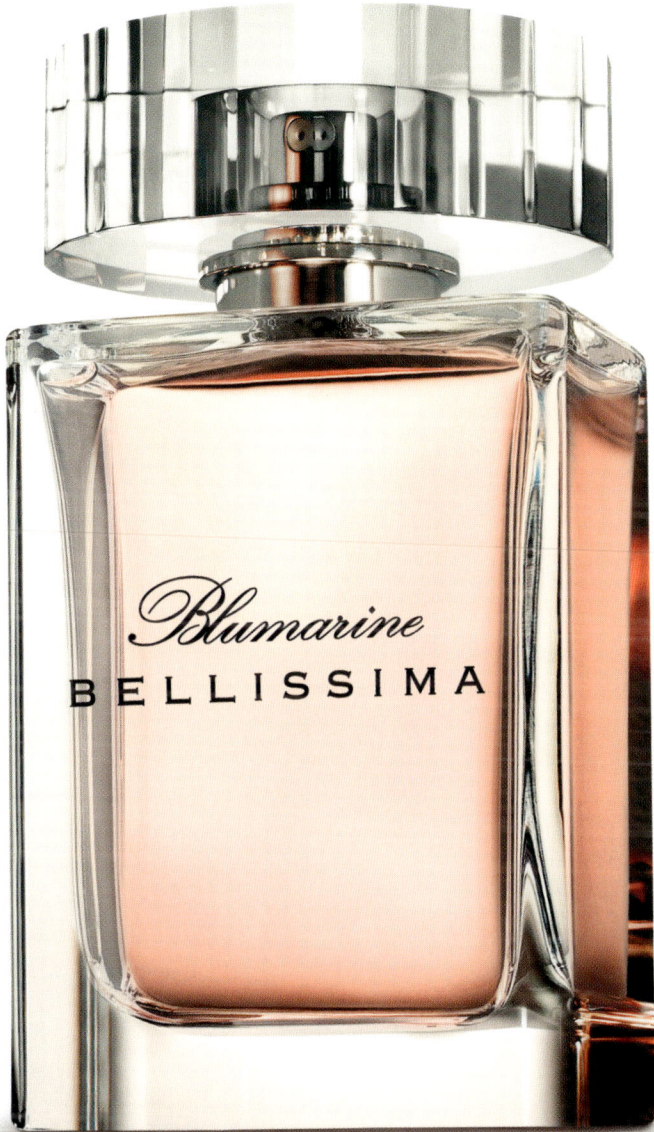

Black Afgano

Brand: Nasomatto
Gender: unisex
Year of launch: 2009
Status: in production
Analyzed version: original Extrait de parfum
Author: Alessandro Gualtieri
Classification: musky woody

In 2009, the world of artistic perfumery was shaken to its foundations by a raw, animalic perfume that smelled of dung, wood, spices, smoke and synthetic notes no-one had ever experienced before. "Black Afgano" was a major shock to the nose, and consumers were entranced by it. And it wasn't because of the name or the concept expressed by the brand (*"The perfumes I create are the story of my obsessions"*, said Alessandro Gualtieri about "Narcotic Venus", "Duro", "Nuda" and "China White"), but for the fragrance itself. "Black Afgano" leaps out of the bottle already complete, with the raw materials assembled in such a way that they create a linear, monolithic sensation. The fragrance does not develop significantly thereafter, although a few of its excesses soften a little around the edges after the first couple of hours.

The overall impression upon application is created by an astonishing amount of tobacco absolute, bonded to a woody bouquet of vetiver, patchouli, sandalwood and oud, a not-too-intense leathery accent, a few musks with woody facets, resins packed with character, such as incense and labdanum, and a subtle gourmand sensation afforded by a coffee note: A dry, thick, sticky *jus*, immersed in the darkest of shadows, brutal and vaguely disquieting.

Like the other fragrances in the Nasomatto line - all of them unusual, featuring splendid materials with a striking impact - "Black Afgano" is composed in accordance with the canons of the finest classic perfumery: so what is so original about this perfume is not the structure, but the notes used. The heart accord of "Black Afgano" had already appeared in "Duro" (launched a couple of years earlier); here, its roaring, irrepressible personality is taken to the extreme. Naturally, "Black Afgano" has been copied dozens of times - even by traditional perfumery - and our nose has become accustomed to such accords by now, so it is no longer the shock to the system it was in 2009. Nonetheless, it's worth getting to know one of the most courageous, innovative fragrances of our time, a stroke of creative genius that shaped a whole new taste. "Black Afgano" is an Extrait de Parfum, its extremely high concentration makes it assertive on the skin, almost to the point of arrogance, saturating the air around the wearer for a couple of metres; it should be dosed with intelligence, depending on the situation it is to express itself in. It lasts effortlessly for over 10 hours, a record that's hard to equal.

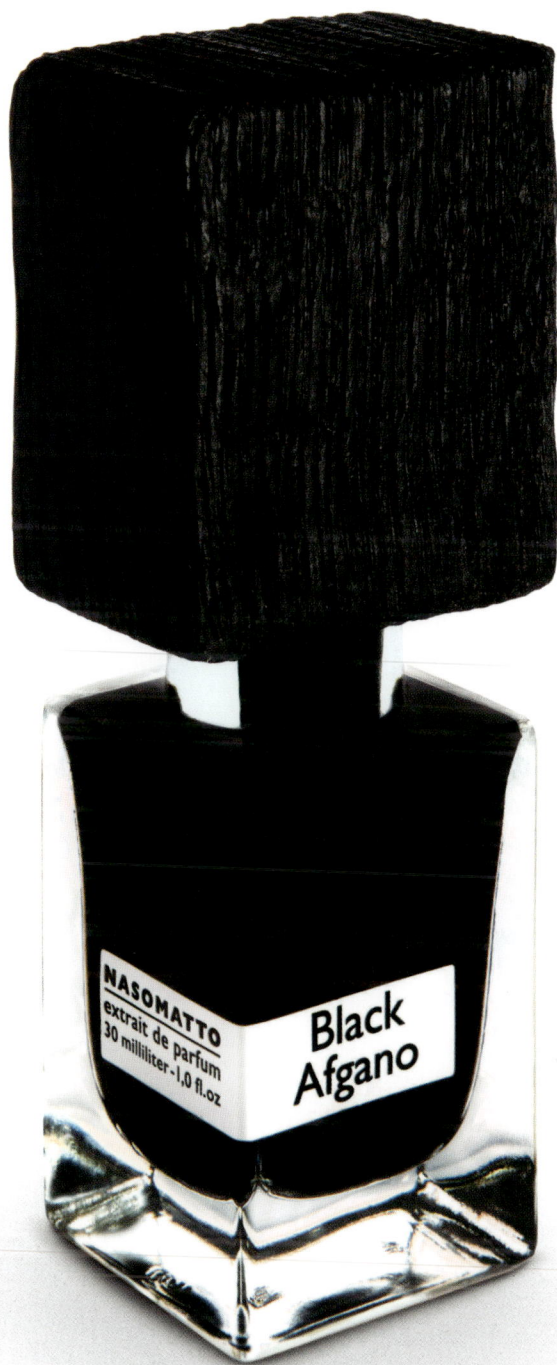

NASOMATTO
extrait de parfum
30 milliliter-1,0 fl.oz

Black
Afgano

Patchouli Nobile

Brand: Nobile 1942
Gender: unisex
Year of launch: 2009
Status: in production
Analyzed version: original Eau de Toilette
Author: Marie Duchène
Classification: woody
Bottle design: Nobile 1942

Italy's love story with patchouli continued in 2009 – exactly twenty years on from the launch of the legendary "Patchouly" by Etro – with another patchouli of outstanding quality: "Nobile's 1942". "Patchouli Nobile", by the young composer Marie Duchène, who made a name for herself with this fragrance, boasts an extraordinary balance, able to bring out the very best in the patchouli note, without ever being banal and predictable.

The dominant patchouli note maintains a gracious elegance, without ever betraying its true nature: warm, crisp and earthy, with a toasted/aromatic element added by the white pepper and guaiac wood. The patchouli unfolds in all its glory some ten minutes after application, when it is joined by the incense and an amber note enriched by sweet, very slightly powdery tonka bean. Towards the end, a surprising note resembling oak moss emerges, combining with the patchouli and creating a welcome, unexpected chypre effect, with an austere elegance closely reminiscent of the Grand Classics.

Dry and velvety, refined, perfectly modern yet classical at the same time, "Patchouli Nobile" received an enthusiastic welcome from aficionados of artistic perfumery from all over the world. "Patchouli Nobile" is not "hippy" enough to irk anyone, but it's still wise not to overdo it, because it creates an extremely lengthy, soft sillage. It has exceptional duration, lasting over eight hours.

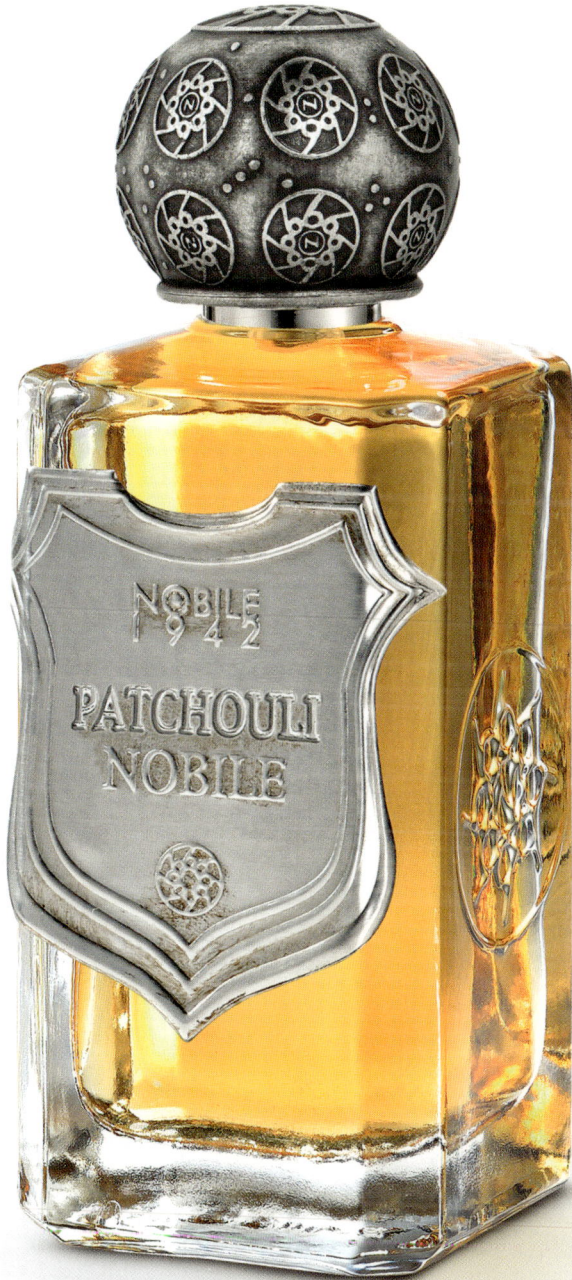

Versense

Brand: Versace
Gender: feminine
Year of launch: 2009
Status: in production
Analyzed version: original Eau de Toilette
Author: Alberto Morillas
Classification: musky citrus
Bottle design: Donatella Versace

When "Versense" made its appearance, feminine citrus fragrances enriched with musky nuances were thin on the ground. The citrus/musky facet had appeared a few years earlier with "Eau Belle d'Azzaro" (1995) and "V/E" by Versace (1998), followed by "Aromatonic" by Lancôme (1999), "Eau Parfumée au Thé Blanc" by Bulgari (2003), and in the same year, "Cristalle Eau Verte" (Chanel).
"Versense" has neither rich, sumptuous flowers nor a particularly impressive structure. It's neither excessively loud or showy, nor should it be: its aim is to act as a tonic, bringing a vibrant burst of energy to everyday life and a subtle, sophisticated, carefree glow to the wearer. Versense makes an excellent job of all this, thanks to its subtly refined bouquet of white musks, the style hallmark of Alberto Morillas for the last 15 years. In this fragrance, the musks have been applied with a light, airy touch, and the result is appealingly natural, less dense and "molecular" than other fragrances by the same composer.
"Versense" opens with a handful of green, vibrant citrus fruits that brings out the best in a splendid bergamot. The spicy facet of the bergamot is taken up by the cardamom, a cool, green, fairly pungent spice, which carries it into the heart of the fragrance, where it encounters jasmine, lily of the valley and fig, carrying forth the fresh, green sensation conjuring up a vision of wide open spaces and spring days.
The musky, woody trail of the end accord envelops the whole fragrance in a bright, sophisticated, slightly powdery sensation offering its joyful spirit a further boost. "Versense" is a sunny, sincere, bubbly fragrance, one of the finest in its category.
It offers the wearer a soft, discreet projection, with a versatility that makes it suitable for any occasion, and a duration of over four hours.

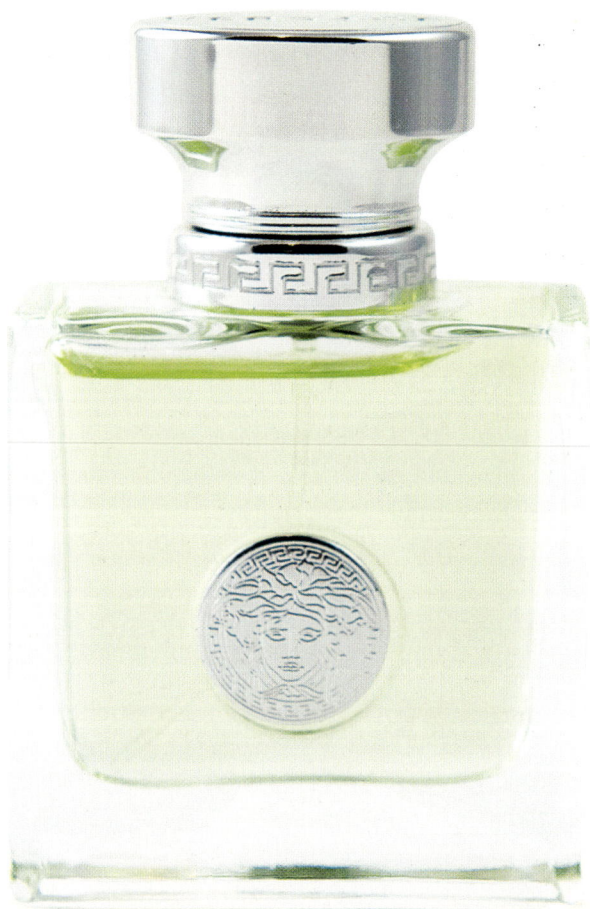

20
10

The Great Italian Perfumes of the 2010s

The decade in question was characterised by an underlying social unease that, at times, escalated into anxiety. Not only was it flagellated by natural disasters of huge proportions such as earthquakes, tsunamis and volcanic eruptions, but also by a series of bloody terrorist attacks perpetrated mainly in Europe, in which hundreds of people lost their lives.

No longer feeling safe, people began to change their habits, particularly with regard to consumption. The great e-commerce portals, like Amazon and Alì Baba, were set up, allowing consumers to shop 24/7 and have their purchases delivered – from anywhere in the world – directly to their homes.

Music and cinema also became available on demand, with Netflix and Streaming TV providing all kinds of entertainment at any time of the day or night. Even food became technological, with a wide range of apps enabling you to order any nationality of cuisine and have it delivered to your door in a matter of minutes. So consumers no longer needed to leave their homes, not even to go to the cinema or to a restaurant.

This was all facilitated by the spread of smartphones, devices with the power to provide a wide range of functions in a single tool: telephone, clock, internet, email, messaging services and, thanks to the apps that were continuously being developed to offer new functions, it is no exaggeration to say that we literally had the world in our pocket.

Social networks became notoriously popular; Facebook, LinkedIn and Instagram created personal and professional networks through which the user could connect with the entire world.

Also thanks to the development of these social networks, people started to feel increasingly less like "citizens of a country" and increasingly more like "citizens of the world"; reflections on the link between the environment and human activity prompted by World Forums on Climate Change started to increase ecological awareness, leading to more eco-friendly lifestyles (separate waste collection, choices of food and transport).

The urge to escape from an increasingly more complex and bewildering reality was most evident in the field of entertainment, with fantasy films such as *Avatar* and the saga of *Harry Potter* drawing massive crowds and making more money than any other film in the history of the cinema.

The trends of the decade

Having to contend with the new environmental awareness of many consumers, essence companies started to focus on workers employed in plant cultivation and essential oil processing plants, often located in Africa, India or other disadvantaged countries. Many, therefore, became involved in social policies designed to support the producers, protect their territories and promote their cultures and their local *savoir faire*.

Streams of new perfumes were launched, topping six hundred a year. Many of these were flankers, i.e. perfumes bearing the same name as fragrances already released, with a change in some notes or in the concentration. e.g. "Light", "Summer", "Black", "Eau", "Légère" versions.

Marketing was, to all intents and purposes, the predominant element in the launching of each new fragrance: from market segmentation to panel tests with consumers, every aspect was defined and planned to enable an exact estimate of the revenues obtainable in the different markets and hence determine the necessary investments.

Social networks enabled the fans of celebrities to come into contact with their idols, making the latter more influential than ever; capitalising on this phenomenon, many stars of the cinema, sport and music launched fragrances bearing their names (from Lady Gaga to Nicky Minaj, from Beyoncé to David Beckham, Justin Bieber and all the rest) targeting the new wave of consumers: the Millennials.

More demanding consumers, on the other hand, were intrigued by the possibility of wearing unique and exclusive fragrances: companies cottoned onto this trend, offering perfumes in limited editions (specifying the year the raw materials were collected), customisable (in terms of *jus* or packaging), vintage (re-editions of historic fragrances) and even tailor-made creations.

As regards composition, perfume houses discovered that consumers would decide whether or not to try a perfume on the basis of the *effluve* (i.e. by removing the cap and sniffing the spray nozzle). If they liked the smell, they would spray and try the perfume. Otherwise they would walk on. So the focus of the fragrances shifted from the heart of the perfume to the top note: the perfumes of this period had effervescent and explosive top accords – at the expense of base notes, which lost specific weight –, or displayed a linearity never experienced before, with top/heart accords dominated by the new musky molecules with their woody, floral, amber nuances, that remained unchanged for hours, on the skin as well as on the dispenser and the cap.

New extraction methods were developed (e.g. based on compressed carbon dioxide), which treated raw materials more delicately and respectfully, so that it became possible to obtain from the flowers – even the least cooperative ones – an essence that was purer and closer to the real scent of the living flower, while fractioning (i.e. the elimination, during distillation, of part of the essence collected) produced raw materials free of allergens and with more characteristic and distinctive nuances. As a whole, the olfactory notes lost specific weight and became more ethereal, purified, recreating the life breath of the plant, without its more carnal, rounded notes.

These developments led to a definitive division of the perfume market into two segments: that of traditional perfumery and that of artistic perfumery, which began such a strong trend that it led to the creation of hundreds of new "niche brands" throughout the world. In some cases, companies were genuinely interested in perfume as a means of expression, most often these were attempts to ride the crest of a strong, well-established, steadily growing trend.

Due to the differentiation of styles and interpretations proposed by independent perfumers all over the world, it is difficult to identify dominant trends in this period. Each and everyone could find a fragrance to reflect different aspects of their personality and lifestyle.

Against this backdrop, a trend that had originally made its appearance in the previous decade, made a comeback: unisex perfumes, suitable for both men and women. This trend evolved in the later years of the decade into *gender fluidity*, i.e. fragrances conceived for those who did not fall into the category of a single gender, but who could alternate between one or more of the coded ones (on the registration form for UCLA, the University of Los Angeles, there were as many as 19 quite distinct genders).

With regard to the fragrances created for a female target, the success of the gourmand formulas continued to grow: in fact, there were practically no perfumes "for her" that did not contain sweet, sugary or creamy notes of some kind.

Perfume for men definitely burst the boundaries of the traditional fougère, aquatic and woody fragrances, and was enriched with exquisite flowers and mouthwatering notes.

Italian perfumery

Italian fragrances continued to enjoy a wide appeal, spreading the reputation of *Made in Italy* products all over the world. The perfumes launched by Italian fashion designers were objects of desire that could generate extremely high profits, and stay steadily in the top ten on every international market, even though – or perhaps because – they were bearers of an international taste which the average consumer related to, irrespective of whether they lived in New York, Moscow, Dubai or New Delhi.

Bulgari, Prada, Versace, Trussardi, Marni and Bottega Veneta were among the brands that succeeded convincingly in combining the Italian touch with a contemporary feel, enjoying one success after another with innovative fragrances, satisfying in texture and with interesting details.

Following the successful example of Prada and Armani, who had already launched exclusive lines with limited circulation in the previous decade, since the 2010s most of the prestigious brands (such as Bulgari, Ferragamo, Versace, Gucci, Bottega Veneta) have been investing in new olfactory collections with "private", "exclusive", "atelier" or "couture" designations, available only in carefully selected stores, especially designed to transcend the greyness of the globalised average taste through more expensive and intriguing fragrances, contained in bottles with sophisticated designs, engaging names and *jus* which appear, on the whole, to be more closely aligned with the cultural heritage of the brands for which they are released. With their exclusive lines, the top brands still know how to surprise and dazzle the public.

Towards the end of the decade the defining line between artistic perfumery and traditional perfumery started to blur. A brand can, in fact, simultaneously enter the niche market with one line and the mainstream market with another; moreover, the panorama of the "niche" market is enriched every year by dozens of new brands, with such a speed and such an incredible number of new products that the public is beginning to lose enthusiasm and reflect increasingly more often on the real value of many fragrances. The public is beginning to feel nostalgic again for the beauty of certain fragrances of the past, "artistic" and "traditional" alike. The fans of vintage perfumery are rapidly gaining ground.

The year 2015 saw the launching of Miu Miu, the first perfume of this brand and the first formula to contain akigalawood, a new raw material obtained from the enzymatic digestion of patchouli, while Bulgari, the same year, continued its exploration of the nuances of tea with an equally innovative note of oolong in "Eau Parfumée au Thé Bleu".

New independent perfumers, often trained at Mouillettes & Co. in Italy and Cinquième Sens in Paris, started opening business alongside veterans who had already been in business for decades, getting themselves noticed through striking, original creations: Casamorati, Meo Fusciuni, Antonio Alessandria, Michele Marin, Masque Milano, Francesca dell'Oro, Nu_Be, Blood Concept, Uermì, Bogue, Francesca Bianchi, Profumum Roma, Homoelegans, Simone Andreoli, Filippo Sorcinelli, to name just a few.

Each of these Italian brands, whether in the artistic or traditional sector, demonstrated in its own way just how full of ideas and Beauty the Italian perfume sector still was, how much it still had to express through fine raw materials, olfactory richness, satisfying textures, strong concepts and, above all, a creativity that was not afraid to dare. And given the fact that Italian taste was so popular, why indeed should they not?

Candy

Brand: Prada
Gender: feminine
Year of launch: 2011
Status: in production
Analyzed version: original Eau de Parfum
Author: Daniela Andrier
Classification: gourmand amber

"Candy" is a surprising fragrance that can be interpreted on various levels, like one of those educational books which, read at the age of ten recounts an exciting adventure, read at thirty recounts the genesis of destiny, read at sixty offers a convincing explanation "... *on life, the Universe and everything*".

On a surface level, "Prada Candy" is a slightly burnt *crème caramel*, mouth-watering and tempting, not too sweet, ideal for current and former teenage girls who expect just that bit more from a *gourmand* fragrance.

On a slightly deeper level, "Prada Candy" is a splendid achievement that revolves around a note of benzoin, a mild and manageable raw material if used in small doses, with a tendency to run wild when overdosed. To my knowledge there is no other fragrance in contemporary traditional perfumery that contains so much natural benzoin, nor one giving it such a predominant role.

On an even deeper level, those who have been lucky enough to try the fragrances of Prada's exclusive line, offered until 2015 in the brand's boutiques, (all composed by Daniela Andrier), will recognise in "Candy" the "N°8 Benjoin" fragrance, which paid homage to raw, natural benzoin. A fierce and tender perfume, smoky, dry, bitter and as dense as chestnut honey, immersed in mellow yet dangerous shadow. In "N°8 Benjoin" there was no trace of caramel or musk to take the edge off the fragrance and make it "edible", because it targeted a different market segment from that of "Candy". "Prada Candy" is the sensible, well-mannered daughter of "N°8 Benjoin", and is, in any case, less frivolous and cloying than the name would suggest. The formula, in a nutshell, is only built on musk, benzoin and caramel. All heavy, dense and cloudy base notes that need a few minutes to heat up before manifesting themselves. The sweet/salty component of the benzoin is enhanced by the caramel note, the shady and subtly animalic component is reinforced by the musky note, while the smoky, evocative burnt leather part is one of the most captivating nuances of this resin. With "Candy", Prada has succeeded in giving a sophisticated, interesting edge to the ubiquitous modern gourmand trend. The lack of top and heart notes makes "Candy" a linear fragrance. When it reaches its optimal temperature it settles stably on the skin and for the following five hours its projection will be urbane but remarkably determined.

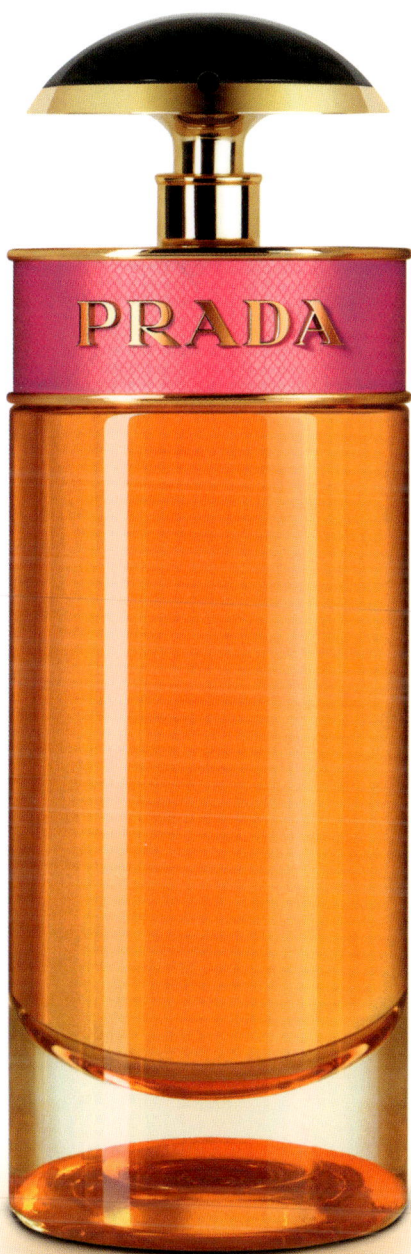

Bottega Veneta

Brand: Bottega Veneta
Gender: feminine
Year of launch: 2011
Status: in production
Analyzed version: original Eau de Parfum
Author: Michel Almairac
Classification: floral leather chypre
Bottle design: Thomas Maier

"Bottega Veneta" is one of those rare modern chypres that really deserve to be included in this legendary category. Although the vegetable musk it contains does not have the same dry, leathery, salty, haughty scent as the oak moss available until a couple of decades ago, the chypre accord is nonetheless convincing, forming the backbone of the whole perfume, giving it an understated finesse that whispers: *"Come closer!"*
The opening of "Bottega Veneta" is very short and graceful, with pink pepper and bergamot already well-blended with a green lily of the valley/jasmine accord, exuding discreet elegance. A few minutes from application, the chypre accord proceeds with patchouli, vegetable musk and a leathery note that adds three-dimensionality and bite to the whole. The overall effect is fairly linear and softly suffused with sweetness, bringing to mind the slightly powdery leather of Daim Blond by Serge Lutens, developed in an ultra-feminine key. "Bottega Veneta" is an extremely well-balanced perfume, enveloped in a sensuality with peaceful confidential aspects. It evokes serenity, solidity, sophistication, values totally in line with the brand that released it.
It lasts on the skin for over four hours, and has an extremely moderate projection, making it suitable for any occasion. Absolutely worth a try.

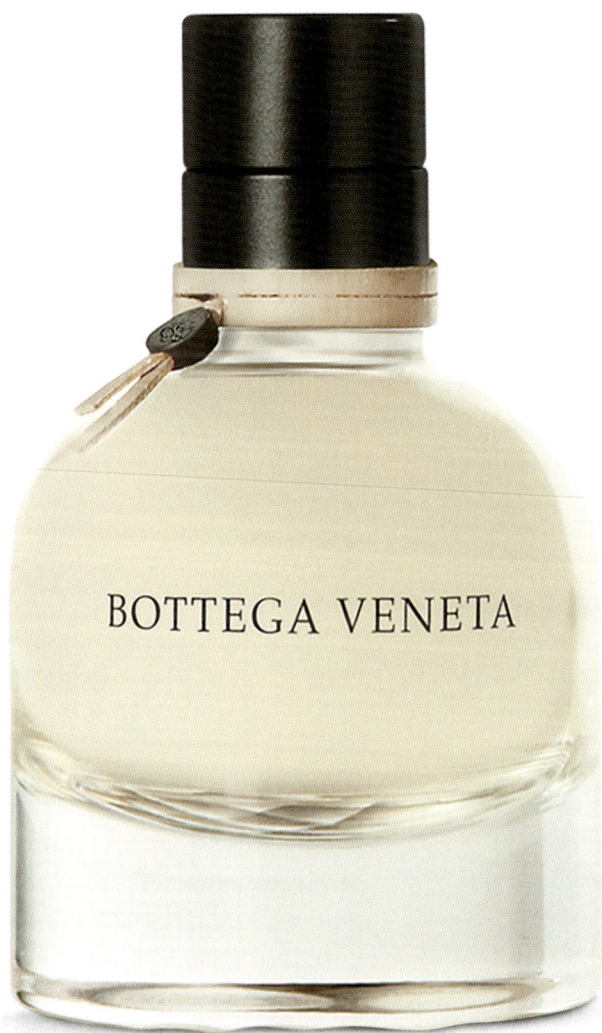

Potion

Brand: DSquared2
Gender: masculine
Year of launch: 2011
Status: discontinued
Analyzed version: original eau de parfum
Author: Annick Ménardo
Classification: aromatic woody

The founders of the brand Dsquared2, the twins Dean and Dan Caten, have strong Italian roots (their unabbreviated surname is Catenacci). And their brand was also developed in Italy. And although not all of their perfumes can claim to have an Italian soul, "Potion" can. Immediate, communicative, with a confidential and seductive tone, "Potion" projects outward in a compact, composed and instantly appealing way. The soft amber and woody base supporting the formula (cashmeran, patchouli, amber notes) adds body to a top/heart accord developed around rustic herbs (mint, angelica, thyme, gentian) evoking an aromatic green liquorice bonbon. A bouquet of spices (pepper and cinnamon) runs through "Potion" connecting top and base, warming the aromatic notes, giving them an interesting pungent counterpoint, and energizing the amber/woody base accord. Over it all hovers a hint of dry, subtly smoked incense, strongly reminiscent of the late lamented "Gucci pour Homme" of 2003. Potion, however, lacks the sculptural presence of "Gucci pour Homme"; its voice is more cordial, softened by an almost honeyed note that could attract a female target as well. It was composed by the great Annick Ménardo: the subtly ambiguous gourmand nuance and the dense velvety duskiness that characterise "Potion" are her most striking stylistic hallmark, making all her perfumes interesting, contemporary and vibrant. "Potion" does not contain marine notes, or aquatic notes in general, nor is it centred around a concept of cleanness and freshness, a choice that places it in sharp contrast with the vast majority of male fragrances on the market today. In contrast, its heart is alive with the best Italian perfumery of the 1990s: from "Moschino pour homme" (1990) to "Gucci Black" (1998) following on the heels of "By" (Dolce & Gabbana, 1997): splendid gems that have, unfortunately, long since disappeared, and which "Potion" – taken off the market a few years after its launch – is destined to follow to the Olympus of the "I'd like to but I can't any more" fragrances. In other words, the concept of "impermanence" explained to a perfume enthusiast: *"If you like it, buy it now, because tomorrow when you wake up it might be gone..."*.

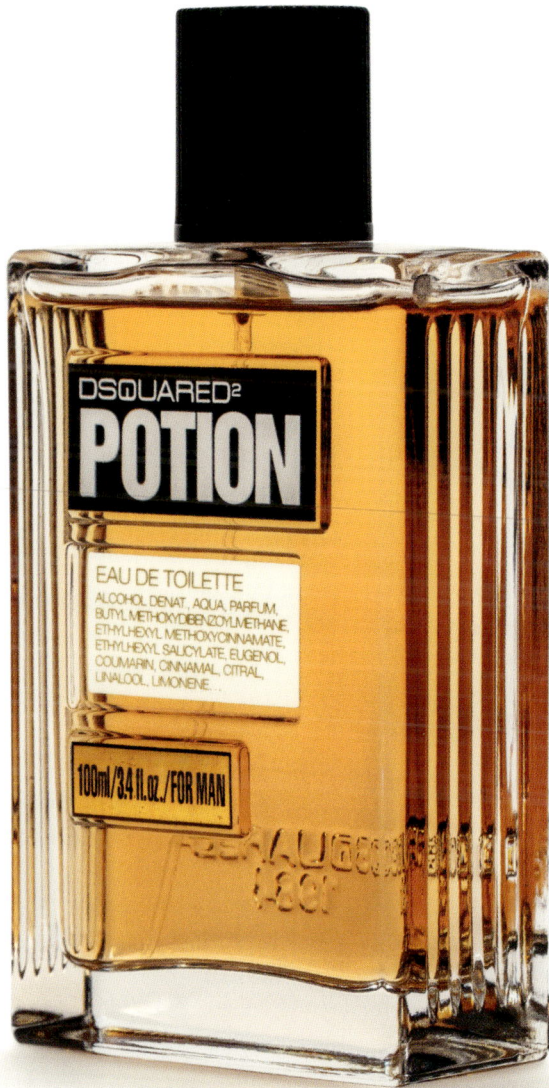

DSQUARED²

POTION

EAU DE TOILETTE

ALCOHOL DENAT., AQUA, PARFUM,
BUTYL METHOXYDIBENZOYLMETHANE,
ETHYLHEXYL METHOXYCINNAMATE,
ETHYLHEXYL SALICYLATE, EUGENOL,
COUMARIN, CINNAMAL, CITRAL,
LINALOOL, LIMONENE...

100ml/3.4 fl.oz./FOR MAN

Luberon

Brand: Maria Candida Gentile Maître Parfumeur
Gender: unisex
Year of launch: 2012
Status: in production
Analyzed version: original eau de parfum
Author: Maria Candida Gentile
Classification: aromatic floral

Until the arrival of "Kiki" (Vero.Profumo, 2009) and "Luberon", lavender was considered a traditional raw material, clean and inoffensive; it was contained in almost all Colognes and in many male fragrances, particularly in accords with other materials in the fougère family. Lavender was only allowed into women's perfumes in the smallest of doses, so as not to convey a dated feel or give too rustic an impression.

But "Kiki" and "Luberon" had the courage to dare and, playing with lavender in a new way, they have finally succeeded in giving it the leading role that it deserves. In order to give this raw material a longer life than that possible with a simple essential oil – a top note evaporating in less than an hour –, Maria Candida Gentile used, alongside the essential oil (green, aromatic, pungent), a very expensive absolute, with a three-dimensional effect thanks to which it finally reveals its more floral and vibrant, elegant and honeyed nuances, against an exquisitely comfortable undertone of warm hay. A dry, green, slightly smoky note of mate reinforces the green nuances of the essential oil, harmonising it with the oak moss base note, maintaining the structure upon which "Luberon" rests on green, dry, almost leathery tones. The result is a magnificent and absolutely natural fragrance, light-years away from the green angularity of English lavender fragrances; it conveys a velvety opulence exuding Italian-ness from every nuance.

"Luberon" is neither the best nor the most successful of the Maria Candida Gentile line: "Cinabre", "Hanbury" or "Barry Lyndon" (an opulent rose/incense, a baroque floral and an aromatic of rare richness) better convey the style and unparalleled talent of this Lady Perfumer who has not yet received the international acclaim that her talent deserves. I have included "Luberon" in this book because of its uniqueness, in its role as an otherworldly messenger, come to inform us that Queen Lavender cannot wait to show us what else she is still capable of. A must-have fragrance for those who are already inclined to love this note, and even more so for those who think they already know it, and perhaps hate it.

Despite having the intensity of a parfum, "Luberon" has a discreet projection that easily tops four hours which, for lavender, is like running the New York marathon.

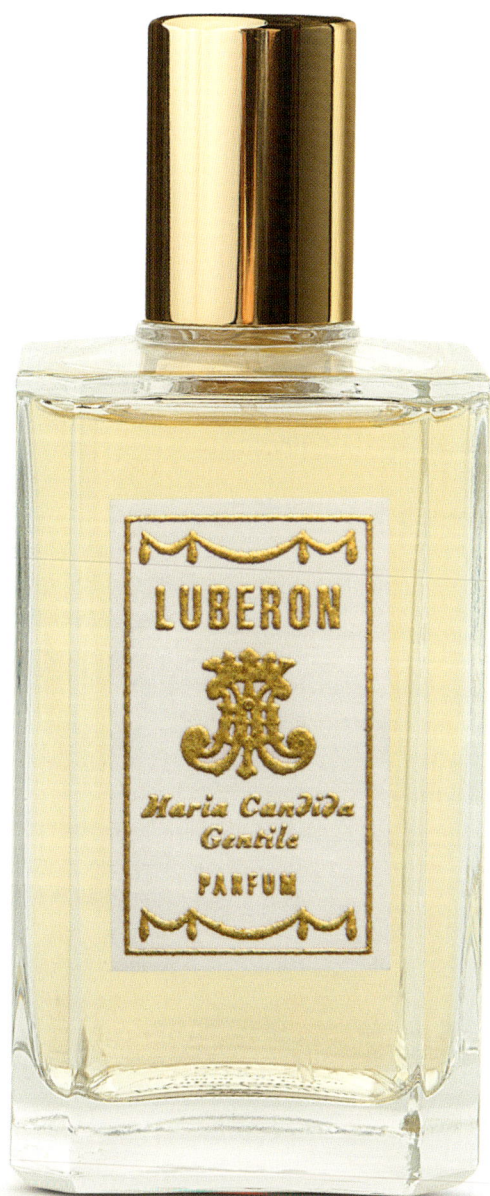

Oxygen

Brand: Nu_Be - renamed Oneofthose
Gender: unisex
Year of launch: 2012
Status: in production
Analyzed version: original Eau de Parfum
Author: Antoine Lie
Classification: musky woody
Bottle design: Francesca Gotti

The first five fragrances of the Nu_Be brand ("Oxygen", "Helium", "Carbon", "Hydrogen" "Lythium") drew their inspiration from the origins of the Universe, the primordial, formless gases from which all Life as we know it, and of which we are part, began.

"Oxygen" gives an extraordinary olfactory concreteness to an elusive sensation such as oxygen. Touches of saffron, frankincense and pepper, vetiver, white musk and an overdose of aldehydes suggest the clean, damp, fleeting smell of steam. A smell that is squeaky-clean, vivid, dazzling in its simplicity and yet cloudy, chalky, rough to the touch, with an artificial, plasticised component adding even more interest. "Oxygen" is built on contrasting sensations overlapping and dissolving one into the other in a continuous movement that never takes a precise shape, and results in a curious and interesting experience, unlike anything ever smelt before.

I have included "Oxygen" in this book as an example of extreme creativity, and research of new texture effects; although this research respects "wearability" criteria (in terms of the fragrance's overall pleasantness), "Oxygen" is nevertheless a challenging creature.

I'm sure that if I were asked to pilot a space shuttle around the Earth, there would be nothing I would rather wear. "Oxygen" was masterfully composed by one of the most renowned contemporary perfumers, Antoine Lie, the author of an endless string of astounding artworks (including "Secretions Magnifiques" composed for "Etat Libre d'Orange" and "XXLatex", created for the Italian brand Uermì [2014]). When Antoine Lie is given the opportunity to express himself freely, his subversive talent gives life to compositions out of any pre-established olfactory models and structures. In this case, Lie's genius is supported by the brand's desire to explore new paths, and the result is more refined and creative than almost all modern molecular perfumery. "Oxygen"'s etheric presence stays very close to the skin, lasting about three hours.

Its unusual packaging designed by Francesca Gotti -a pure, minimalist bottle emerging when you break the polystyrene box - is a splendid example of container-content coherence that evokes the concept of the brand to perfection.

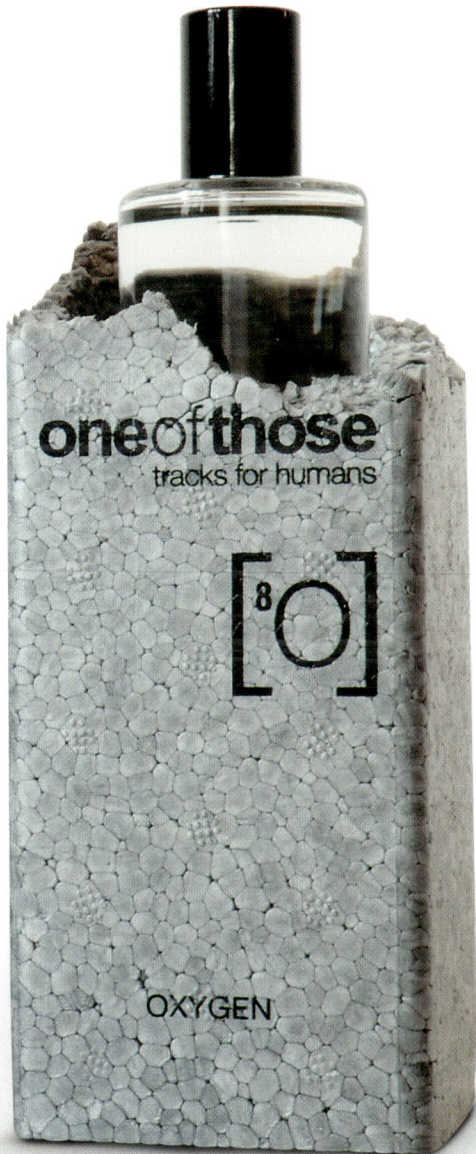

one of those
tracks for humans

[^{8}O]

OXYGEN

Eros

Brand: Versace
Gender: unisex
Year of launch: 2013
Status: in production
Analyzed version: original Eau de Toilette
Author: Aurélien Guichard
Classification: woody fougère
Bottle design: Donatella Versace

In the Pantheon of Ancient Greece, the God Eros symbolised lust rather than love. The kind of unbridled frenzy that led the gods and heroes in his thrall to chase madly after every maiden or wood nymph who happened to be in the vicinity (and who would gladly have done without such attention, considering how most of the stories turned out). Eros was often depicted as a beautiful, naked young man. So divinely and sublimely beautiful as to delight the gaze of both men and women.

The Versace fragrance bearing his name shares the same charming ambiguousness.

The opening of lemon, mint and green apple is lively, refreshing, tart and genderless. A few minutes later, the heart of the fragrance begins to unfold; a pink floral breeze with geranium and tonka bean brings "Eros" closer to a powdery-floral fragrance feminine. As soon as the vanilla of the base begins to emerge, binding with the mint of the top and the geranium of the heart, the fragrance turns into a fougère. Not a traditional fougère, but sufficiently fougère to suggest a male universe. After half an hour, the woody accord of the base (vetiver, cedarwood and vegetable musk) confirms this masculinity. The whole fragrance is enveloped in velvety Ambroxan, a relatively expensive synthetic molecule with the same salty, dry, musky, ambery scent as natural ambergris. Ambergris is a very hard to find raw material, possessing a different olfactory profile depending on how much time it spent floating in the ocean: Ambroxan is Ambergris' more accessible alter ego. In "Eros", Ambroxan wraps all the notes together and imprisons them on the skin indefinitely, with a projection powerful enough to fill a room.

Among all the fragrances that use Ambroxan brazenly and declare such use, "Eros" is one of the most interesting. More amusing than "Blue" (Chanel, 2010), more immediately appealing than "Sauvage" (Dior, 2015), "Eros" is nonetheless challenging to wear and not suitable for everyone. Joyful, carefree, extrovert, mischievous, a little vulgar, it is exactly the kind of fragrance that gets you noticed when you go clubbing: a sort of beam of a fluorescent spotlight. And believe me, this is not a flaw. Quite the contrary, it is one of its greatest qualities: in a market dominated by shoals of boring, totally uninspiring men's fragrances, totally uninspiring men's fragrances, "Eros" is like a diving holiday in the Maldives.

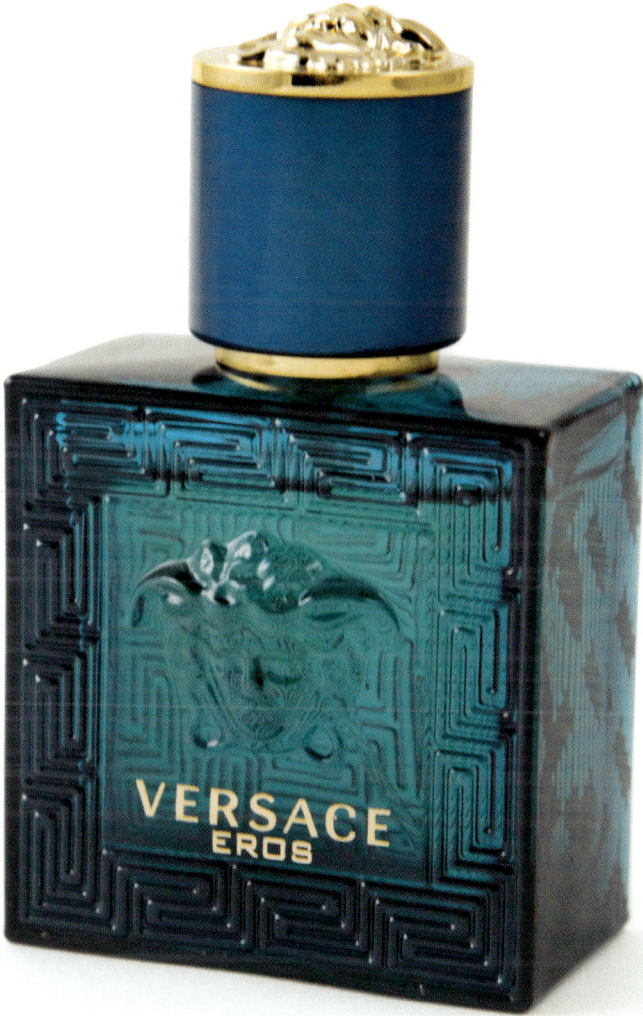

Marni

Brand: Marni
Gender: feminine
Year of launch: 2013
Status: in production
Analyzed version: original Eau de Toilette
Author: Daniela Andrier
Classification: woody floral

How it was possible to eliminate the specific weight from all the woods, flowers and spices in this fragrance is unknown to common mortals, with the exception of Daniela Andrier, its composer, who has created a small feminine jewel that is perfectly "focused", and yet painted with watercolour shades of rare delicacy and sophistication.

A vivacious bouquet with spicy nuances (black pepper, pink pepper, ginger, cardamom and cinnamon) accompanies the citrus top notes in a colourful and tantalizing sparkle.

Quarter of an hour after application, the spicy sensation gives way to a floral note resembling a rose, only perceptible on a transparent level, like one of the flowers floating on the water - along with Ophelia - in the famous painting by Millais. As the rose begins to fully express itself, it is joined by a note of incense contributing character and texture. This is the moment in which the *jus* acquires more specific weight and clearer contours, coming closer to other perfumes dominated by the rose/incense duo ("Trama", by Sonia Constant for Perle di Bianca and "Lyric" by Amouage). After half an hour, musk, vanilla and velvety woods bring Marni to a gentle whisper, reserved for those who have already been chosen and welcomed into its private sphere.

A self-assured, bright, serene, understated fragrance for a genuine, carefree wearer, ideal for all ages. Eloquently delicate, it spreads very little, but its presence can be perceived for at least three hours.

One of the most interesting Italian fragrances to have been released in recent years in traditional perfumery, don't miss the chance to try it, at least once.

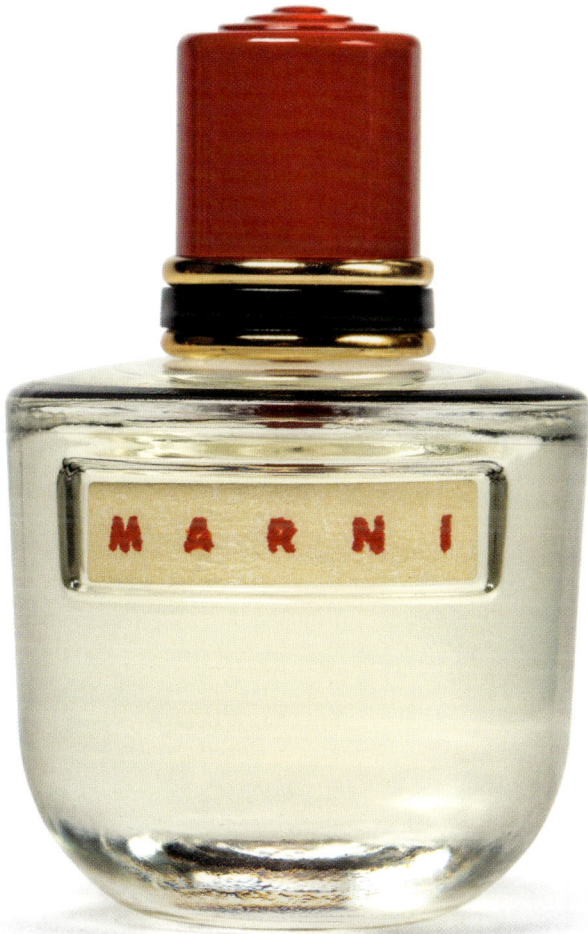

Eau Parfumée Au Thé Bleu

Brand: Bulgari
Gender: unisex
Year of launch: 2015
Status: in production
Analyzed version: Eau de Cologne
Author: Daniela Andrier
Classification: aromatic citrus
Bottle design: Thierry de Bachmakoff/Paolo Bulgari

Paradoxically, what makes "Eau Parfumée Au Thé Bleu" so particular and unusual is an accord that is a hundred years old. "Eau Parfumée Au Thé Bleu" opens with anise/lavender/violet/iris, a floral, green and sharp bouquet, endowed with a subtle and ethereal presence, like someone who is in the room, but not close by. You can see them in the corner of your eye, but they vanish under your direct gaze. This strange sensation, that makes you want to keep sniffing your wrists, creates a *trait d'union* between "Eau Parfumée Au Thé Bleu" and a legendary perfume: "Après L'Ondée" (Guerlain, 1906). It is probably difficult to bring the same notes together without evoking "Après l'Ondée" and, in fact, for fear of eliciting such a comparison, no-one does. With "Eau Parfumée Au Thé Bleu", Bulgari runs this risk, proving that paying homage to a Great Classic can indeed be done, if you know how to do it. What makes the difference – a huge difference – between "Après L'Ondée" and "Eau Parfumée Au Thé Bleu" is what stands between them – one hundred years of innovative raw materials. A dry, aromatic note of oolong tea and a bouquet of brilliant musks endow "Eau Parfumée Au Thé Bleu" with a dry, aromatic, invigorating, sharp personality, making it unquestionably contemporary – perhaps even a little ahead of its time. Behind "Eau Parfumée Au Thé Bleu" is Daniela Andrier, a master perfumer with incomparable sensitivity and sense of measure. A fragrance such as this, perfectly poised between hope and melancholy, smiles and tears, could not have been the work of anyone but her. "Eau Parfumée Au Thé Bleu" demonstrates that when there is vision, talent and desire for Beauty behind the creation of a fragrance, lessons from the past can be treasured and transformed into new creative lifeblood. When this happens, congratulations are in order. "Eau Parfumée Au Thé Bleu" spreads moderately but is clearly perceptible, particularly in the cooler months. The summer heat does not do it justice. Its four-hour longevity is a real record for a Cologne.

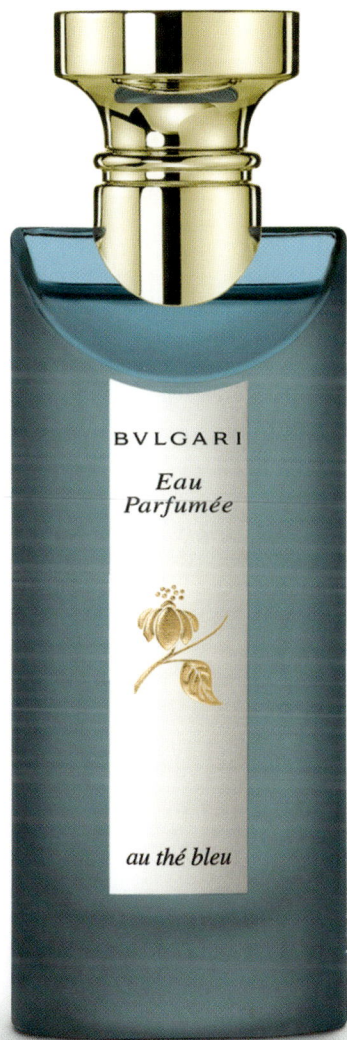

Miu Miu

Brand: Miu Miu
Gender: feminine
Year of launch: 2015
Status: in production
Analyzed version: original Eau de Toilette
Author: Daniela Andrier
Classification: floral

When Miu Miu was launched it did not resemble any other fragrance on the market. It had a vaguely retro vibration, yet resonated with a contemporary feel, bordering on the avant-garde.

Its composer, Daniela Andrier, who has been creating Miuccia Prada's perfumes for over fifteen years and who knows every aspect of her ironic and visionary aesthetic, has built it around a Givaudan raw material called Akigalawood, obtained from the enzymatic digestion of patchouli. A wood that is not whole, therefore, but carefully "fractionated" by a handful of enzymes that choose which part of the patchouli to digest and which part to leave behind. The substance is then washed in salt water et voilà, it no longer resembles patchouli, but has become a totally new material, dry, green, hazy, exotic, woody and very dense. Its unnaturalness is perceptible, yet it does not smell synthetic. Miu Miu opens with the most classic of classic accords: lily of the valley, rose and jasmine. This accord would take the fragrance thirty years back in time, were it not for its ever-so-light transparent aquatic note. The counterpart of the aquatic floral accord is the Akigalawood, which collects the green and dry aspects, adding its own sculptural component.

Although Miu Miu smells edgy, its floral heart beats in a demure, almost moving manner, like a quiet, still immature young girl. Adorable.

Miu Miu is also interesting for another reason: in general, perfumes have impact in the initial phases, toning down as the base notes emerge. Miu Miu works in reverse: its projection, delicate at the outset, increases progressively, and three hours after application, it can saturate the air around its wearer. Then it slowly tones down, for another five hours.

When a new material is patented, composers tend to overdose it, making it the main ingredient of the formula, so that the perfume will be original and recognisable. Following this phase, the note is added to the composers' standard palette and finds a good balance with the other notes in formulas created subsequently. From the launching of Miu Miu onwards, the fragrances built around Akigalawood have multiplied, but Miu Miu's bouquet remains nonetheless remarkable, balanced precariously between vintage and contemporary, glamour and understatement, personality and shyness, that is the many facets of a charmingly complex soul.

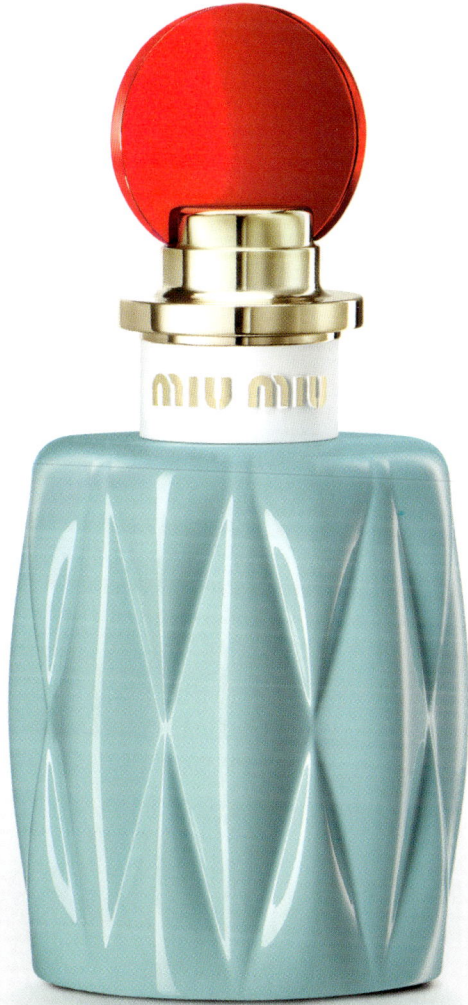

Tadzio

Brand: Homoelegans
Gender: masculine/unisex
Year of launch: 2016
Status: in production
Analyzed version: original Eau de Toilette
Author: Michele Marin
Classification: fruity ozonic

Sensuality is a frequent concept in perfumery. Sexuality, on the other hand, much less so. And Tadzio is an intensely sexual fragrance.

It tells of a boy of androgynous and callow beauty - delicate features and perfect skin. Creatures like Tadzio are destined to break more hearts before turning twenty one than we, mere mortals, could in an entire lifetime of revelling...

Tadzio pictures him as he emerges from the sea waters; the salt plays with his natural scent in a heady olfactory mix. He bites into a red fruit, juicy, forbidden, as he throws himself carelessly onto the sand, letting the sun kiss his white skin and tousled locks.

Tadzio - the reference is, of course to Thomas Mann's *Death in Venice* - is a strange fruity/ozonic hybrid, totally unclassifiable, which undoubtedly needed a good dose of courage in the making. It is insolent, scandalous, and yet intimate and innocent at the same time. This high-intensity polaroid is never confused or redundant, notwithstanding the quantity of notes and facets it contains. Quite the contrary, raw materials are well-disciplined, each serving its purpose perfectly in the creation of the story. Applauses go to Michele Marin, a young Italian author endowed with a touch both gentle and wild, who began his career creating a magnificent line of perfumed candles for the brand "Castello di Ama". "Tadzio"'s opening with bitter/green citrus notes (lime, orange, ivy), immersed in seawater (musk, note of cucumber) is followed by a tart, juicy sensation (blueberries and orange blossom); the dry base of patchouli, helichrysum and sweet myrrh adding texture and depth. "Tadzio" could never have been launched by a traditional brand, it is too disconcerting. Fortunately, artistic perfumery serves precisely this purpose: to entertain us with exciting perfumes that can tell us convincing stories.

And the Homoelegans brand is telling quite a few. To get into this book Tadzio had to compete with "Paloma y Raices", the love story between Frida Kahlo (Paloma) and Diego Rivera (Raices), and its poignantly beautiful dominant note of tuberose, and with "Quality of Flesh", a portrait of Francis Bacon, painted in the darkest and most brutal colours imaginable. "Tadzio" has excellent projection, and a duration of over six hours. Some find it fresh and breezy, while others find it is too thrilling to wear in public. In any case, it's a thrill that is well worth trying.

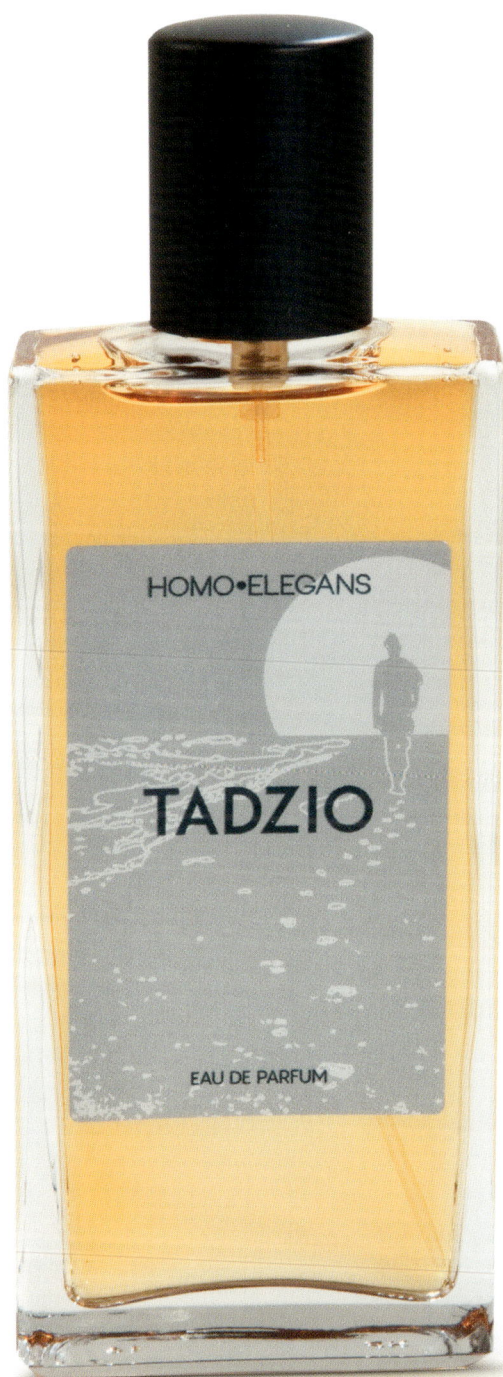

HOMO•ELEGANS

TADZIO

EAU DE PARFUM

Fleurs et Flammes

Brand: Antonio Alessandria Parfums
Gender: unisex
Year of launch: 2016
Status: in production
Analyzed version: original Eau de Parfum
Author: Antonio Alessandria
Classification: floral chypre

"Fleurs et Flammes", as the name implies, calls to mind fireworks of exuberant, coloured flowers.

Its citrus opening welcomes a green, dry note of galbanum, while the floral heart, the real engine of the perfume, begins to roar immediately below. As the minutes go by, the galbanum loses the company of citrus fruits to be joined by a beautiful lily, resounding, indolic, three-dimensional, carried in triumph by a handful of other flowers (rose, carnation and white flowers), in a generous and sophisticated accord reminiscent of the best women's perfumes of the 1980s.

The flowers are then flanked by benzoin, a hint of almond milk softening the whole, musk and dry woods taking the mind back a few decades once again, but the sensation still evades definition. Then the epyphany. It's a chypre! It is, indeed, an extremely rare example of a contemporary chypre. Although many perfumes released in recent years have been defined as chypres, there is no trace in them of oak moss (replaced by algae, vegetable musk or, more often, Evernyl), or of whole patchouli (only fractionated), or of natural flowers. Deprived of the densest and moodiest notes, the "modern chypres" can no longer express the sombre and restrained, tremendously sexy magic of the chypres of the past, and are forced to shine in the light of day, without chiaroscuro or narrative suspense.

In "Fleurs et Flammes", on the other hand, the opposites can be perceived, in all their wild and dazzling beauty. Dry, striking, exciting, "Fleurs et Flamme" recounts the eternal duel between Eros and Thanatos, Matter and Spirit, celebration and tragedy. "... *This perfume is a tribute to the Women of my family...*" confesses its creator.

"Fleurs et Flammes" is one of the most beautiful fragrances in the line produced by Antonio Alessandria, one of the most renowned Italian perfumers, who has devoted his life to perfumery, both traditional and artistic. While being absolutely contemporary, his perfumes are enriched by an ancient voice that vibrates in their soul, endowing them with an unparalleled elegance. In 2015, Antonio Alessandria was awarded the prestigious FiFi Awards for *Rudis*, composed for the brand Nobile 1942.

"Fleurs et Flammes" is a fragrance with a strong projection, reaching its peak half an hour after application. Its overall duration is good, with a musky and woody trail that lasts a few hours.

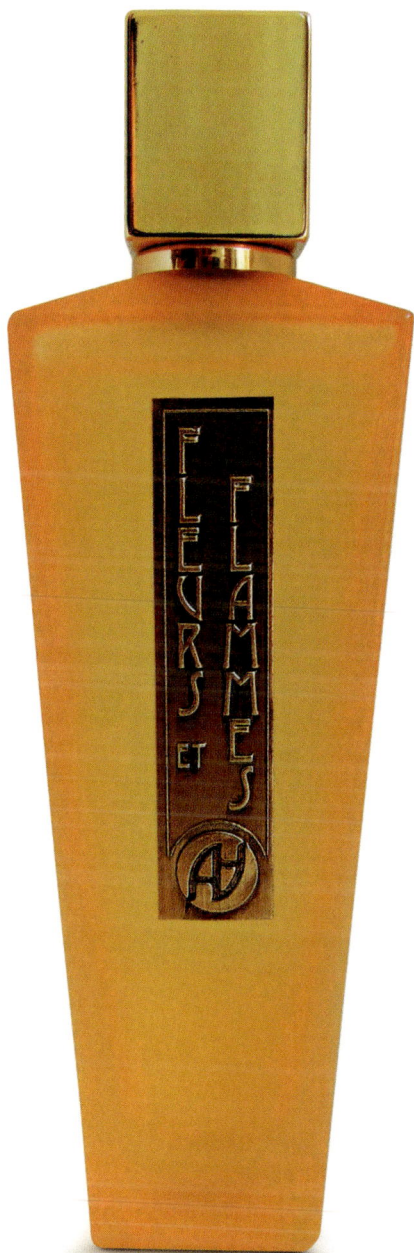

Bulgari Man Black Orient

Brand: Bulgari
Gender: masculine
Year of launch: 2016
Status: discontinued
Analyzed version: Eau de Toilette
Author: Alberto Morillas
Classification: floral oriental

The whole formula of "Gucci Man Black Orient" aims to achieve a satisfying olfactory fullness: the very word "Orient" evokes in its name Middle Eastern perfumery with its notes of spices, Tai'f rose and oud wood, to which the Arabs are very attached and which Europeans have learned to love as well.

"Bulgari Man Black Orient" slides on the skin with a sweet and spicy opening of cardamom and rum, combined with ripe fruit that leaves the scene as the heart notes emerge (tuberose and Tai'f rose, a very expensive variety of Damask rose with green and citrus nuances, grown exclusively on the Tai'f plateau near Mecca). Shortly after application, the wood, oud, leather and benzoin base notes open alongside the flowers in a warm, persuasive embrace, very deep and sensual, with the power to evoke sensations worthy of the best Arabian perfumery. Finally, a perfume with the right name!

The rose-tuberose accord, so rich and narcotic, may appear a gamble in a "masculine" perfume, and yet it is perfectly consistent with the "Oriental" concept, as well as providing the ideal counterpart to the oud/wood/leather base notes. Everything is very tightly knit with the notes working together superbly, and the result is a sensation of pure, concentrated luxury.

Dry, soft, warm, "Bulgari Man Black Orient" is that high-necked cashmere sweater reserved for evenings with friends, for cuddling on the sofa, for those moments when you simply want to feel good about yourself.

"Bulgari Man Black Orient" has a limited projection, and in this case the choice to keep it close to the skin is absolutely deliberate: if "Black Orient" raised its voice too much it would lose much of its class.

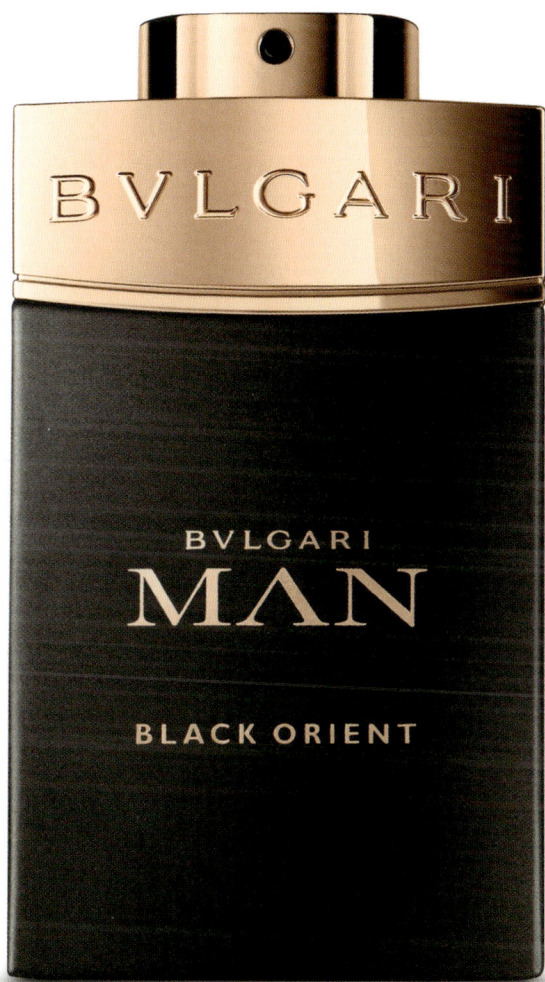

Trussardi Riflesso

Brand: Trussardi
Gender: masculine
Year of launch: 2017
Status: in production
Analyzed version: original Eau de Toilette
Author: Veronique Nyberg
Classification: woody oriental

Many men's fragrances by Trussardi are uncommonly consistent: they share complex structures supported by dense base accords, saturated with "masculine" nuances such as tobacco, wood, leather, smoky notes. Trussardi's ideal man is nonchalant, naturally elegant and self-assured, showing decisive, mature masculinity distinguished by a mix of irresistible characteristics. It is successful both in Italy and abroad, where he is perceived as the quintessence of "Italian-style" virility.

"Riflesso" is no exception to this rule: it is a woody oriental opening with a fruity-tart note of bergamot, apple and pink grapefruit, followed by a floral-green heart of geranium and violet leaves. Its woody (cedarwood), powdery (tonka bean) base revolves around a soft leathery nuance. The whole bouquet is energised by a handful of musks and a note of lavender, which spreads through the pyramid, bringing sobriety and reassuring elegance.

"Riflesso" is a fragrance that does not go unnoticed but it is so immediately pleasant and tempting as to be appreciated in any situation.

The general sensation evoked by "Riflesso" recalls another very successful woody amber fragrance released ten years earlier: "Yves Saint Laurent L'Homme". "Riflesso" could well be a younger brother, more relaxed, more entertaining. Who, basically, doesn't take himself so seriously.

And, of course, attracts more women.

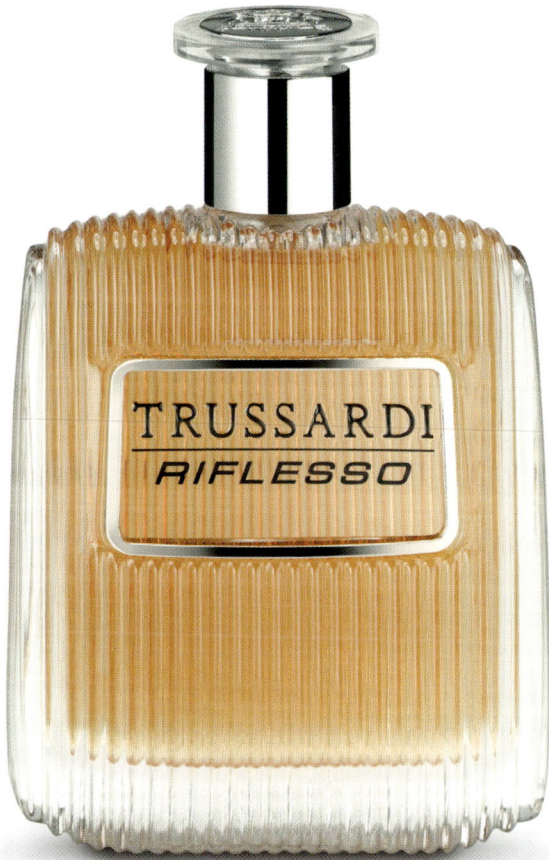

Cedro di Diamante

Brand: Perris Monte Carlo
Gender: unisex
Year of launch: 2018
Status: in production
Analyzed version: Eau de Parfum
Author: Luca Maffei
Classification: citrus

There is a lot more Italian-ness in this perfume - released for a brand that is officially based in Montecarlo - than in many other perfumes released for brands whose only Italian feature is their headquarter's address. First and foremost because Gian Luca Perris, founder and creative director, is Italian; so is the production and most of the raw materials. And the composer, Luca Maffei, is Italian too. In fact Maffei is currently the most sought-after Italian perfumer; his rich contemporary bouquets exude Italian-ness in every note: the 2.0 Italian-ness of the new generation, nourished by the lifeblood of the past, now ready to spread its wings to conquer the future.

But there's more! Capua, a long-established Calabrian company founded in 1880 and now a world leader in citrus essences, was also involved in the creation of this perfume: its innovative techniques of extraction, combined with a five-generations experience, make their citrus products the perfect benchmark for all other citrus essences.

At the heart of "Cedro di Diamante", a dazzling note of citron (used at 50%, that is half of the whole formula) is brightly resplendent. Its crystalline freshness is reflected and reinforced by a bouquet of lime, lemon and verbena extracted by compressed carbon dioxide (a process capturing the plant's most intimate and authentic essence) which highlight citron's greenest, freshest, most energizing aspect, a thirst-quenching sharpness joined by the slightest touch of innocent indulgence. A smack of cold, aromatic spices (pink pepper, cardamom ginger, Szechuan pepper) enlivens the citrus fruits, while the vegetable moss base supports the green feeling all the way through. Musks and iris add a powdery touch from the heart onwards, resulting in a longer duration of the citron than Nature would normally allow. "Cedro di Diamante" is an olfactory jewel as precious as it is rare: the presence of a large quantity of furocumarins inside the essential oil has pushed citron out of compliance with the safety standards imposed by European regulations. Eliminating the furocumarins, however, would mean depriving the essence of the three-dimensional complexity that makes it unique. We must thank Capua and its innovative molecular vacuum processing if we can enjoy citron again. "Cedro di Diamante" is perfect for all seasons, all occasions, and all ages; it spreads its brilliance with confidence for about an hour, then tones down into a spicy/dry/musky whisper lasting a good three hours.

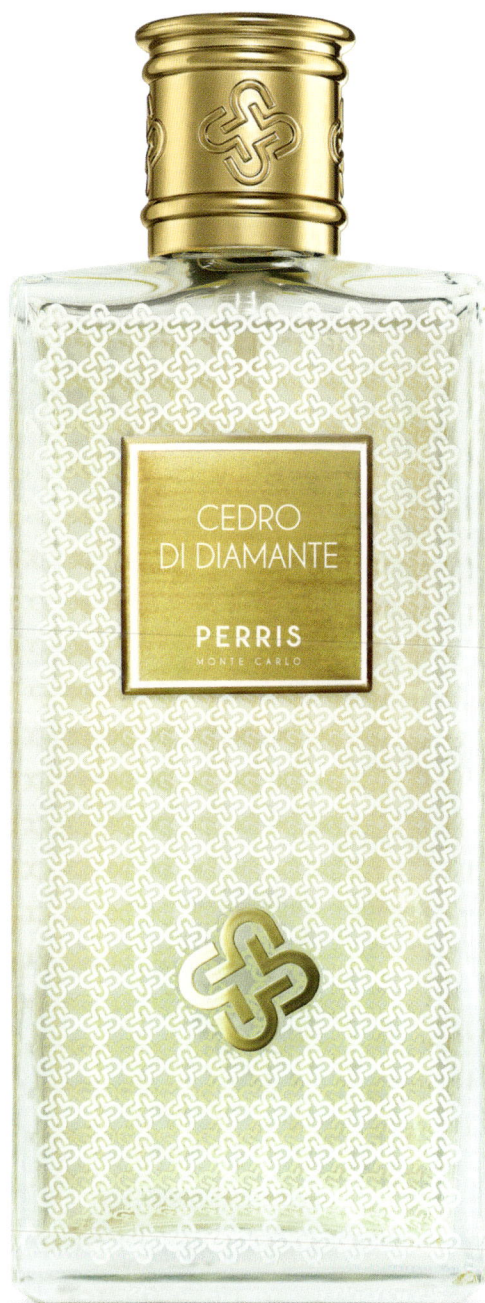

Memoire d'une Odeur

Brand: Gucci
Type: Unisex
First produced: 2019
Status: in production
Version analysed: Eau de Parfum
Author: Alberto Morillas
Classification: green floral

Green florals are like those precious emeralds inherited from a wealthy great-aunt, and immediately locked away in a safe. We never wear them because they are too precious and - alas! - passé... and yet they still mesmerise us, as memories of an opulent past. Suddenly, the brainwave: why not take them to the jeweller's, have them removed from their setting and transformed into something else? Set in a ring or pendant with a modern design, the emeralds could be enjoyed again! Gucci chose a little outdated green floral, and took it to one of the best jewellers in existence, Alberto Morillas, who transformed it into a refined minimalist, ultra-modern "signet ring" with a retro-vibe, that can be worn by anyone, of any age or gender, in any situation. The fragrance itself focuses on the clean, terse, frothy white musks typical of the Morillas's style joined by herbal notes of green meadow drying in the sun (freshly-cut grass, vetiver, mint). The opening lasts just a few minutes, then a warm, golden note of chamomile emerges, evoking natural landscapes immersed in the light of a summer sunset. A short-lived, dry accord reminiscent of a Pigato wine from the Ligurian Riviera adds a mineral, almost salty undertone.

The traditional top/heart/base evolution has been omitted in the interests of general linearity, which allows a longevity of six hours on fabrics and an intimate, rarefied voice, more suited to a family meeting than to a "fiesta loca".

The message conveyed by the name, bottle design, colour, fragrance and promotional images of "Memoire d'une Odeur" is extraordinarily consistent, helping to underline how Gucci has replaced the glamorous, eloquent fragrances of the past with a new, unusually understated direction which will puzzle the longest-standing fans of the brand. In fact "Memoire d'une Odeur" appeals a younger target, which feels uncomfortable with labels and stereotypes (even gender stereotypes); their desire for freedom is strong, as is the connection they feel with Nature. "Memoire d'une Odeur" is an homage to them.

Another round of applause for Gucci, for its ability to dare paths that others fail even to notice.

The beautiful green bottle is perfectly in keeping with its content, and is tribute to the iconic bottle of "Gucci Nobile".

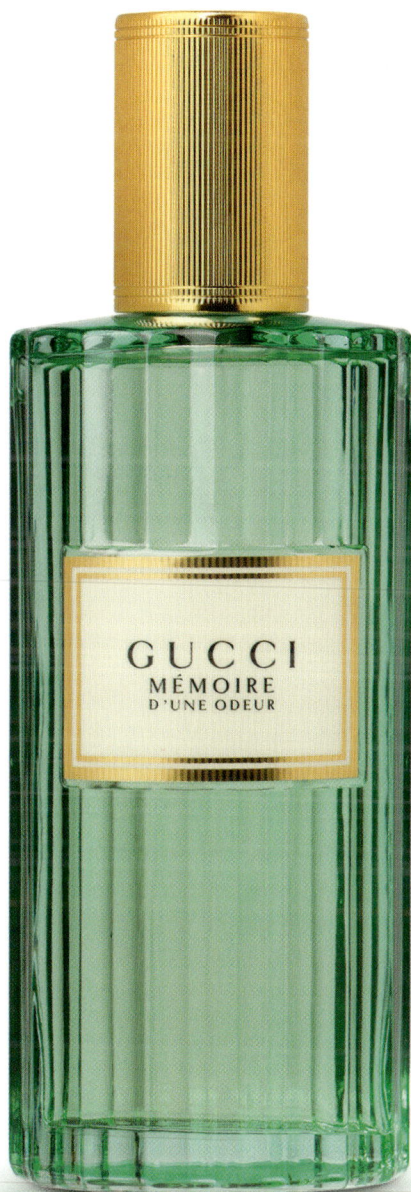

Interviews with the protagonists

When a consumer goes to a store and buys a perfume, he does so because something in that product has caught his imagination. Maybe the sophisticated bottle, maybe the marketing behind it, with all the trimmings of testimonials and TV commercials... Sometimes it is the fragrance itself that arouses interest. In any case, we rarely take the time to think about the whole process that transformed the "design of a new perfume" into a finished product, capable of getting noticed in the midst of many others shown on the shelves of shops. To get there, the whole product had to go through a series of long and rather complex production phases. Everything starts in the marketing office of the brand for which the fragrance will be released: every detail relating to the name, packaging, type of fragrance, market segment, etc. is evaluated and defined. The composition is then entrusted to a creation company. The creator, for his part, has undergone a professional training suitable for his task, and when he begins to create the fragrance he must be able to count on the most suitable raw materials. When the formula has been created, it must reach the consumer. In this case, a subcontractor is needed, i.e. a company that produces the necessary quantity, that bottles it and distributes it to stores. As for of bottling, there is the need of a glass company specialized in the creation of bespoke bottles, able to visually convey the values of the brand for which the fragrance is produced. Therefore, there are many workers involved and their synergy is of fundamental importance to grant the product the peculiarity and the pleasantness that will bring about its commercial success.

This chapter describes the perfume supply chain in Italy through the words of some excellent protagonists.

A chapter dedicated to the perfume supply chain in Italy described in the words of some of its uncontested leaders.

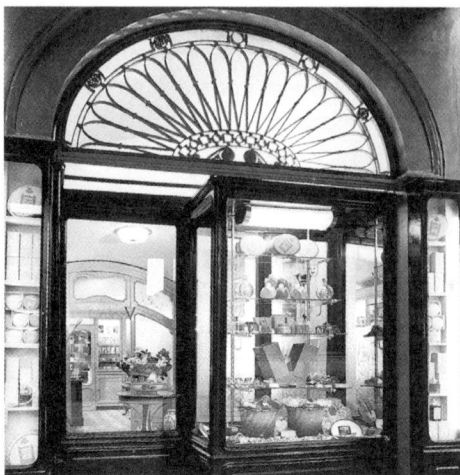

Tradition

Conversation with Carlo Pioli,
heir of the Borsari family

Can you tell us how the Violet came to be closely connected with the city of Parma?

The main reason behind the traditional association between Parma and the Violet was botanical.

This little flower, native to the Middle East, arrived in Parma in the mid-18th century thanks to the Bourbon family. In the renovated Botanical Gardens, the Bourbon family planted a number of of double-flowered violets belonging to a species with a particularly powerful scent, the *Viola odorata pallida plena* thereafter simply known as the Parma Violet: "Violetta di Parma".

When Marie Louise, the wife of Napoleon, arrived in Parma in 1815, she continued to cultivate this type of Violet, which she referred to, in the letters that have survived until today, as *"jolie petite fleur"* (pretty little flower) and was instrumental in the first research conducted to extract its essence. Throughout the 19th century, the Parma Violet was considered a symbol of beauty and seduction, enchanting poets and artists who celebrated it in their works. The name Violetta, given by Giuseppe Verdi to the heroine in "La Traviata", for example, became famous all over the world.

And the connection between the violet and Borsari?

Lodovico Borsari started his professional career as a shop boy in a barber's shop in Parma which, as tradition dictated, also produced cosmetics and perfumes. In 1870, wishing to create a fragrance that could symbolically represent the city and the flower, he started working on the creation of the perfume named "Violetta di Parma".

Many craft activities had existed in Parma, ever since the 1700s, originally connected with life at court, and they had gradually adapted to the requirements and circumstances of a city that had always been keen to project the best possible image of itself. So when Borsari set up his business, he found highly-qualified craft workshops already at his disposal for the production of elegant boxes and containers, printed using chromolithography, and of course, first and foremost, he found Vetrerie Bormioli, the glassworks that distinguished Borsari's production for over a century.

Borsari cooperated with the most important graphic artists and illustrators of his time, including Carboni, Boccasile, Volino and Nanni, with whom he worked continuously, coordinating the image of the various lines, designing posters, playbills and scented almanacs.

Through meticulous laboratory research (as proven by the various formulas that have survived unscathed) the perfume was then developed and refined: the composition interpreted the note of violet typical of the period, which was promptly adopted also by foreign perfume houses of the time (e.g. "Vera Violetta" by Roger et Gallet, 1892). The characteristic bright green hue of the jus is the natural consequence of the use of extract from *Viola odorata* leaves. In fact, the raw material suppliers still used the "enfleurage" extraction method.

The fragrance was then poured into glass and crystal bottles with exclusive lines and shapes, interpreting the evolution of style from Art Nouveau to Art Déco. The glass was finely cut with frosted bands, rendering the body of the bottle dynamic and enhancing the colour of the perfume. The caps were made of ground glass, as a natural complement to the whole. The packaging was impeccable, with a protective film around the neck of the bottle, sealed with a gold thread; the label, which generally depicted flowers or essential lines, was exquisite, with embossed print; the boxes had a complex design which highlighted the angles and the shape of the bottle, embellished with paper made with the most sophisticated techniques and printed in various colours.

Right from the outset, no expense was spared in terms of quality, research and marketing, in order to guarantee the success of the fragrance and enable it to compete with the products of the great Maisons.

In 1920, the exclusive store "Aurea Parma"

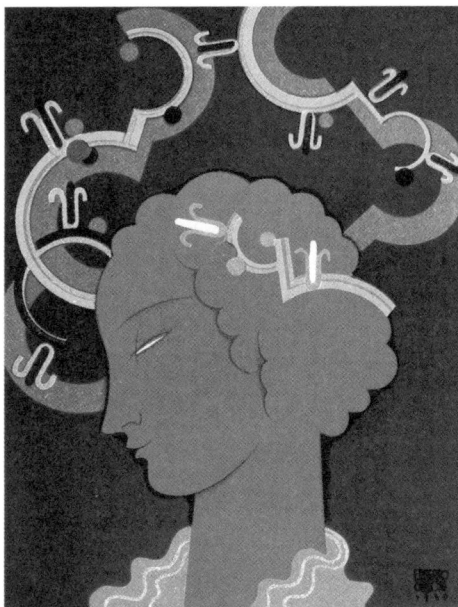

CAV•L•BORSARI&FIGLI
VIOLETTA DI PARMA

was opened and the tagline of "Violetta di Parma" became "*Il profumo distinto*" (the distinguished fragrance).

At the "Exposition Internationale des Arts Décoratifs et Industriels Modernes" held in Paris in 1925, Borsari, the only Italian company taking part, gained international recognition.

How is this historical heritage interpreted, and what is in store for it in the future?

Today the institution named Parma Color Viola is responsible for the promotion of this tradition, describing the theme of the violet in all of its expressions: botanical, olfactory, cultural and traditional.

The long-established shop "Color Viola", with its original decor in the Art Nouveau style of the 1930s, still sells bottles of vintage "Violetta di Parma", in addition to a large range of violet-based products such as sweets and home fragrances.

In the Giardino Ducale of Parma, with the project "Il posto delle Viole" (the place of the violets) we are cultivating double-flowered Parma violets in age-old greenhouses, the same plants that were grown in the Botanical Gardens in the mid-1700s.

In Spring, when the violets are in bloom and in September, when they go back into their greenhouses, we organise theme-based exhibitions, olfactory research and botanical drawing activities.

Also as part of the events for "Parma Italian Capital of Culture 2020", we will be in the forefront with an exhibition dedicated to the first 150 years of "Borsari 1870".

Training
The licensee company

Conversation with Emanuela Rupi, President of Mouillettes & Co.

You have worked in Florbath, Firmenich, Creations Aromatiques and Morris, covering all the most fascinating roles in the sector, both on the customer and the supplier side: Fragrance Development Manager, Marketing Evaluator, Brand Manager. And now you have become a trainer for Mouillettes & Co.

How did your career begin?
My career began when I joined Florbath in 1982. This was a really special moment for the Italian perfume sector: we take the fashion-perfume combination for granted now, but it actually took off in this period.

Florbath was enjoying a resounding success with a very sophisticated line of bath foam: glass bottles with cork stoppers, containing coloured, perfumed bath foam

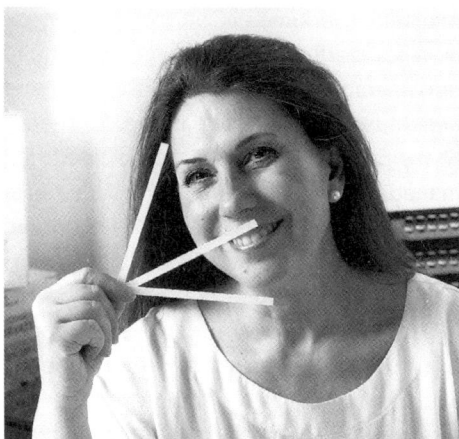

with essences based on a single theme: vanilla, rose, tuberose, orange blossom...

My first job was in the Production Department where I learned the more technical jobs such as filtering, packaging and labelling, under the direction of Giulio Alberto Sanguinetti, an intelligent, good-natured, extremely scrupulous man, who was also in charge of selecting the new fragrances to be launched on the market, and was considered by the entire perfume sector as one of the best Italian professionals of the time.

From Production I was then moved to Quality Control and eventually to the Laboratory itself.

Another important figure in Florbath was Riccardo Sanguinetti: it was thanks to him that the company signed the first licensing contracts to produce the first perfume by Krizia (the famous "K", composed by Maurice Roucel), Fendi and, later, Fiorucci.

In the meantime, thanks to Roure, I had started studying raw materials, which enabled me to acquire technical skills essential for my work but, even more important, it gratified me at a personal level, because I had had a passion for perfume ever since I was a child and was the proud owner of a collection of several hundred miniature perfumes! Cultivating my passion for perfume had led me to acquire considerable knowledge of the perfume market, without even realising it. Thanks to my curiosity and my little bottles I had managed to memorise an incredible number of perfumes, knowledge that proved to be extremely useful when Giulio Alberto Sanguinetti agreed to let me work with him in Product Development. When a proposal came in from an essence company, it was easy for me to determine whether the fragrance could be considered original or whether I had "already smelt" it elsewhere. Additionally, from the moment I joined the company we would have a blind test each morning on commercially available perfumes. I would have to analyse and memorise them, and learn to recognise them. I have kept up this habit, which began in Florbath, for over thirty years now (when I arrived in the office this morning the test strip was already on my desk as usual!) and it has enabled me to analyse every nuance in this sector.

Would you tell us about the Italian adventure in the perfume sector?

While Florbath was acquiring the licences that enabled it to become an international company, my evaluation responsibilities allowed me to work with all the essence companies, during which I learned a great deal. And of course, I made myself known. Soon, job offers started to arrive, but for quite some time, I didn't take them into consideration.

But when Florbath was taken over by Sanofi, I decided to consider an offer from Firmenich. I was asked to come to Milan by Roger Schmidt, who was the manager of the subsidiary at the time. He suggested that I spend a few days in the company before making a decision,

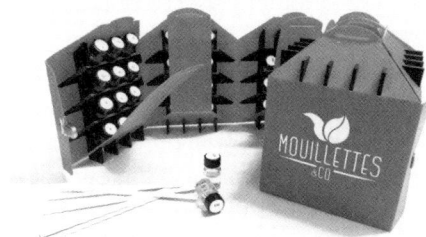

in order to fully understand the role that I had been offered. It was such an exciting experience that I decided to leave Florbath.

I joined Firmenich in 1988 in my new role as Marketing Evaluator and my job was to back up the sales staff in the development of projects received from Italian customers, while working in close contact with colleagues in the creative department (Alberto Morillas, Jacques Cavallier, Annick Ménardo...). A major figure for me in the company was Angela Lui. She covered the role of sales manager for alcohol-based perfume, but she also had incredible technical and olfactory knowledge. Firmenich was a multinational with numerous subsidiaries all over the world, which succeeded in working synergetically on projects notwithstanding the distance, thanks to the possibility to carry out its role in these production sites in the various countries. This made it possible not only to get to know the colleagues, but first and foremost, the different markets, so that colleagues – in my particular case the *evaluatrices* – could be interchangeable when the need arose. So I spent long periods at the headquarters in Geneva, and in the production sites in Paris, New York and Barcelona. It was an amazing period and, from a personal standpoint, it was extremely challenging. I consider Firmenich as a sort of University course. The experience I acquired in those seven

INTERVIEWS WITH THE PROTAGONISTS Training

years allowed me to gain a more complete vision of the sector.

In 1994, I decided to accept the job offer I received from Marco Maffei, Manager of the Italian subsidiary of Creations Aromatiques, in a sales role, following alcohol-based perfume customers. Having worked for so many years in Florbath, I had a very good understanding of customers' needs and timescales, so I felt ready to accept the challenge of such a new role. Together with the creative team of Creations Aromatiques (Christine Nagel, Michel Almairac...) we produced some important Italian fragrances for Fendi, Mila Schön, Versace, Krizia, Biagiotti and many others.

Four years later, Riccardo Sanguinetti of Florbath told me that Giulio Alberto was about to retire, and he needed someone with in-depth knowledge of the fragrances. So he asked me to come back.

After so many years of globetrotting, the idea of being able to return to Parma pleased me immensely, not to mention the unexpected opportunity of taking on the role that had been my mentor's: perfume development. I still remember the first project I worked on: it was the first Fiorucci perfume, composed by Christine Nagel.

Looking back a few decades later, I can say that the Italian perfume experience was an exceptional and exciting adventure, and I feel happy and lucky to have been part of it. I had exceptional teachers, to whom I owe a great deal.

Back then it was possible to do things that seem impossible today.

When I was developing the perfume for Fiorucci or Krizia, I met Elio Fiorucci and Krizia personally... There was an exchange of creativity, of Italian genius, that is much more difficult to find nowadays.

On the basis of your experience, what was the key factor that enabled the Italian perfume sector to become a world leader in the industry?

Creativity was the quality most appreciated in our sector. When an Italian Brand would summon the essence companies for the launching of one of its perfumes, everyone would flock, and composers were delighted to work on Italian perfumes because they could give free rein to their creativity. This guaranteed high-quality, innovative but, above all, original perfume because designers would license their brand to companies specialising in the development and marketing of perfumes. While reserving the right to the "last word", they would entrust the work to entrepreneurs and professionals with notable experience in the field. This meant that the perfumes really did reflect the style, values and aesthetic vision of the designer, becoming ambassadors of the brand worldwide.

The quality of the Italian perfumes of the 1980s and 1990s were totally on the same level as internationally-renowned brands such as Dior, Chanel and Yves Saint Laurent. A typically Italian aesthetic imprint is perceivable in the perfumes of Armani, Versace, Coveri, Krizia, La Perla and Fendi, and this made them attractive to the Italian public, who identified with them, but also to an international public, who were enamoured of Italian-made products.

How did you come into contact with artistic perfumery?

In the year 2000 Gucci took over Sanofi Beauté, of which Florbath was a part. Gucci moved everything to Florence, but it was not interested in keeping the licences for the Krizia and Fiorucci perfumes, so another of Parma's long-established companies stepped in: Morris. "Florbath Profumi di Parma" shut up shop in 2000. Yet again, I received job offers from essence companies in Paris.

Working abroad for so many years had given me a privileged vantage point and a personal maturity that I might not have acquired otherwise. However, in the end I decided to choose Parma, my hometown: concrete, down to earth, with a deep appreciation of common sense and quality of life. Characteristics that make it unique. Okay, so it's also a little provincial, but where's the harm in that? Particularly if we look at its business acumen, which is in no way inferior to that of the great metropolises.

I carefully assessed the offer from Morris, which already had the perfume licences of brands such as La Perla, Sergio Tacchini, Genny and Ferrari and with the addition of the Krizia and Fiorucci licences, it needed to consolidate its staff. I joined the company in a dual role, that of Fragrance Development Manager for corporate brands – I was extremely proficient in this area – and that of Brand Manager for certain brands, and this was something totally new for me. Once more, I had met another star in the firmament of Italian perfumery, Giovanni Borri. Once more, an entrepreneur was willing to invest in me, giving me the opportunity to learn a new role in which I would be able to broaden my knowledge.

In the last four years, I was given the marketing responsibility for the development of a sector whose growth appeared promising: niche perfume products.

Florbath had sold us the Italian distributorship of the brands Penhaligon's and Piguet, and my job would be to help expand the brand portfolio. Morris signed distribution contracts with Laura Tonatto, BOIS 1920, Ineke and Etat Libre d'Orange. I worked at Morris for ten years. Another great school, full of professionals from whom I learned a lot.

So now we've reached the present...how did your collaboration with Maria Grazia Fornasier and Mouillettes & Co. begin?

Maria Grazia Fornasier was the first woman in Italy to manage a subsidiary of an essence company. She was the one who opened the subsidiary of Mane – a prestigious, long-established French company producing essences and fragrances – in Milan. In a world with only men at the top, this lone woman attracted attention. And I was watching her from a distance. Then Maria Grazia was CEO of Takasago Italia for 10 years, and the time finally came for us to really meet each other. At the end of the '90s, she was a fragrance supplier and I was the customer. Over the course of time, mutual admiration and respect drew us closer together. Then, once again, Maria Grazia decided to take on a difficult challenge by opening the first Italian company of olfactory training and consulting: she founded Mouillettes & Co. in 2004.

When she asked me if I wanted to work with her I thought about it often but I didn't feel ready until 2012, when I started to work for Mouillettes & Co. as an external consultant.

After a while, Maria Grazia asked me to join the company in a more active role and I liked the idea. I brought my product development experience to Mouillettes & Co. thanks to which it could further broaden its range of services. But what I received in return enriched me beyond belief. Training is a very specialised area which I had never dealt with before, and I had no idea that I would have liked it so much. I discovered that being given the chance to transmit to others the wealth of experience that I had gained over all those years was hugely gratifying to me on a deep personal level, and this was something that greatly surprised me.

Training is generosity. Giving today's professionals, but even more important, the new generations, the opportunity to acquire knowledge to elevate their professional status is essential.

Today Mouillettes & co is an SRL (Limited Liability Company). In addition to Maria Grazia and myself, there are two other major figures, Sara Ravo who, after having acquired great expertise in retail, joined us in 2014, and Elena Scotti, who has been at Maria Grazia's side since 2004. Every day you learn something new from someone. In my case, I can say that Maria Grazia has been my latest great school!

As a professional who knows this field inside out, what, in your opinion, is in store for the Italian perfume sector?

Italian brands are strong all over the world, the "Made in Italy" concept is still an extraordinary driver for development, but globalisation has unified average taste on an international level and nowadays the big multinationals expect an immediate and surefire profit from perfumes. It is my sincere hope that the future will bring back the courage to launch fragrances that represent the Italian spirit, that mix of sensuality, elegance, luxury and creativity that has always distinguished us.

For this to happen, companies will have to start investing in training, they will have to remember the true value of those skilled and proficient professionals who would be happy to teach the trade to young people, helping them grow and develop their talents.

Creativity

Conversation with Maurizio Cerizza, Perfume Composer

Maurizio Cerizza is the first great Italian perfume composer of the modern era, and his exceptionally long career began when appreciation for Italian-made products was at its height. He has composed dozens of successful perfumes for Roccobarocco, Sorelle Fontana, Mavive, and Atkinson's, as well as for various brands of artistic perfumery (Boellis, Pineider, Calé, Onyrico).

You have over four decades of experience as a composer. That's a very long career! How have you nurtured the joy of composing all these years?

By doing things that make sense to me. If a project doesn't make sense to me, if it doesn't bring me anything new, if it doesn't challenge me or fascinate me, I leave it to others. I don't do anything mechanically, just for the sake of doing it. This is part of my idea of freedom! And for composing, freedom is important.

Where do you draw inspiration for your compositions?

Nature is always a great inspiration: I still remember a long walk in Favignana I took twenty years ago. I was alone by the sea, and I was surrounded by fig trees that were emanating a fabulous fragrance. When I went back to the laboratory at the end of my holidays, I composed a perfume for men with scents of the sea and figs, one of the first, in actual fact, to contain that note. Nautilus by Mavive.

Observing the world and immersing yourself in Culture are also highly inspiring experiences, which can give rise to new associations of ideas and stimuli. But to

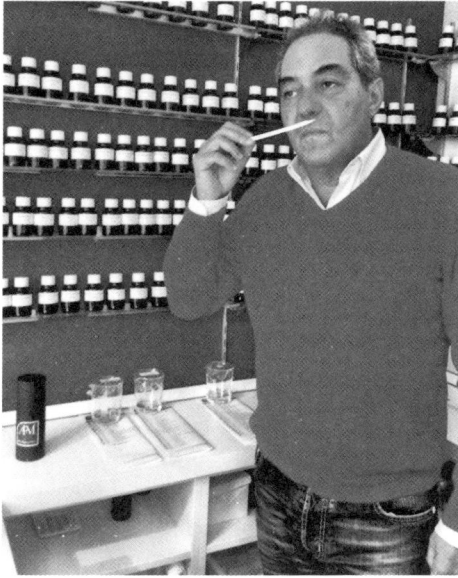

overdose certain notes in order to obtain special effects to surprise the public. Unfortunately, placing the emphasis on a single note risks upsetting the balance of a composition. It's important to "listen" to the formula, understand if it can take the overdosed note, and if so, what is the absolute limit that can be reached without upsetting the balance. And take a step back.

How can sensitivity be developed to such a degree?

With age! When I was young, I had to run masses of tests to reach a satisfying result. Now I don't need nearly so many. To learn to make the raw materials communicate with each other, you have to study them in depth, in thousands of different formulas. Today, thanks to the experience I have gained over the years, I know how they will behave before I use them. But I still haven't stopped learning: to grow in this profession, you should never stop applying yourself and studying seriously. It's fundamental. Twenty years is the absolute minimum, but it's only when you get to thirty that you start to realise that all your efforts have allowed you to develop independent thought and something close to freedom of expression.

"*I have good technical knowledge, but when I paint I forget it*" said Kandinsky. Surely that is what experience is for, is it not?

be able to recognise and grasp the inspiration, you have to cultivate your soul, be open, learn new things. It's the work of a lifetime.

How do you express your Italian-ness in the perfumes you compose?

Wearing scent is an intimate act, prompted by the way you feel. So is composing. The fragrances I create are Italian because I am Italian, and Italian culture permeates everything I do. We have the largest cultural heritage in the world, with tens of thousands of artistic masterpieces of inestimable value. And they are not hidden. They are available to anyone wishing to discover them, in every corner of Italy. And it's clear that having been born here and having always breathed this air, this is perceptible in what I create. My fragrances are powerful and communicative, but always balanced; they express an idea of elegance and harmony that derives from my being Italian. Even when I seek originality, I never lose sight of proportion.

For example, today there is a trend to

You experienced the *Made in Italy* explosion of the 1980s and 1990s first-hand. What was it like working in the Italian perfume sector at that time?

Marvellous, creative, a real adventure. We all felt that we were taking part in something big. In the 1980s and 1990s, I was a novice and I was eager to share in that

INTERVIEWS WITH THE PROTAGONISTS Creativity

atmosphere. There was excitement, ideas, courage, in a much freer, more relaxed dimension. As colleagues, we shared everything: not only at work, but also socially. I am a very sociable person and I cultivated friendships with colleagues at that time that are still strong today.

How has the perfume sector changed over the last twenty years?
The whole world is racing ahead at breakneck speed! So the contemporary perfume sector is a system that moves at a frenetic pace, and demands are pressing. Before a project arrives on a perfumer's desk, all aspects have already been taken care of: IFRA recommendations, Regulatory aspects (i.e. *fragrance policies adopted by different countries*), availability of raw materials, Marketing. In other words, all the accompanying issues. The perfume only enters the scene at the end. Although it's a very different environment from the one I grew up in, it wouldn't make any sense to try to slow down this crazy rat race. Instead, you just have to internalise it, while striving to be true to yourself.

Is it possible to maintain your creative freedom intact in an environment like today's?
Of course! When a composer sits down to work, his/her idea is not to give the customer the fragrance requested, but to make the fragrance requested a small masterpiece. This is achieved through technique and sensitivity, but above all with the freedom to say no, the freedom to carefully choose projects that you believe in, and in which you can express something truly authentic.

Production chain
The producer of natural raw materials

A conversation with Gianfranco Capua

Capua 1880 is a leading company in the production and working of citrus essential oils (bergamot, tangerine, lemon and sweet orange). Now at its fifth generation, Capua 1880 exports its products to 54 countries; over eighty people work in its two seats located in Campo Calabro and San Gregorio.

Can you tell us the history of your company?
Ours is a wholly familiar history. We began in 1880, five generations ago, with the technique of absorption "through sponge down" to collect bergamot essential oil, a procedure evolving over three generations, turning the manual technique of the beginnings into an industrial procedure. The passage of the company from my father Domenico to me, in the 1980s, brought about a substantial change: I immediately perceived the opportunities we would have by leaving the commodities-standard market, which made quality too univocal, to focus on research. I started by introducing new qualities, then I dedicated myself to the innovation of extraction and process methods, which allowed me to create completely new products. Bergamot, for example, changes colour and smell every week of ripening, so I started to implement a qualitative differentiation of the extraction. Later, as the rules governing the use of citrus essential oils became progressively more restrictive, I tried to transform the challenges they posed to me into product peculiarities. I have included some technologies for the separation of natural contaminants, for example by subjecting bergamot to

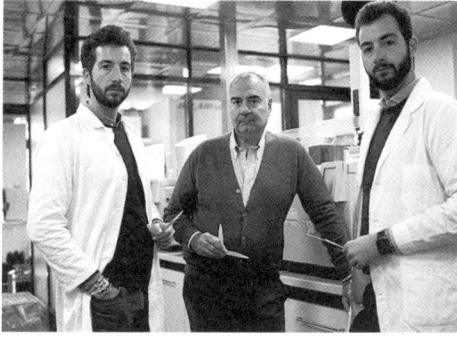

molecular treatments capable of eliminating furocoumarins (which have phototoxic elements being potentially harmful to health) and make it perfectly compliant with regulations, as well as unique.

Who is Capua today?

Today Capua 1880 is the main collector of interest as for citrus notes. The Maitre Parfumeurs from all over the world visit us regularly, proposing interesting challenges both in terms of cultivation and of production processes which should grant essential oils that meet their needs for novelty, distinction, uniqueness. They ask us for increasingly diversified technical procedures specifically tailored to their needs, and in this way they push us to constant research and innovation.

We collaborate with the Agriculture Faculty of the Mediterranean University in Reggio Calabria, and the Pharmacy Faculty of the University of Messina, with which we have launched research doctorates, as well as systems and analytical methods.

In the last three years we have implemented a new technique that allows us to extract odorous substances even from the aqueous phases of the fruit, that is, from its juices. This new product, called NatProFile, is enjoying enormous success, because it is stable, performing and extremely powerful (it contains a one hundred- and-fifty-times

higher concentration of aromatic elements than that of fresh juices), characteristics that are in great demand both in the food industry and in perfumery. The olfactory profile of the NatProFile product is different, and it is a diversity that perfumers appreciate so much.

We also bought thirty-two hectares of land on the Ionian Coast, and created a "Citrus Farm" where we planted several botanical varieties. We enjoy doing grafts and hybrids to see if we can come up with something interesting. Meanwhile, it is an educational place, where we show how to plant, prune and harvest. Our guests are delighted to walk through our gardens, because they can touch the whole process from sowing to harvesting fruits, and understand the extraordinary value that the natural product brings with it.

From your privileged observatory, how did the natural raw materials market change in recent decades?

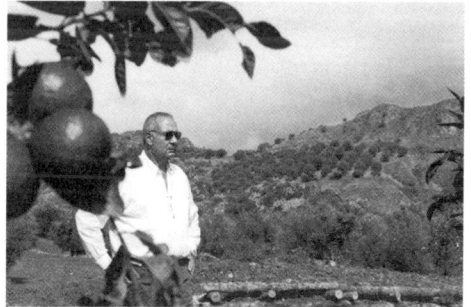

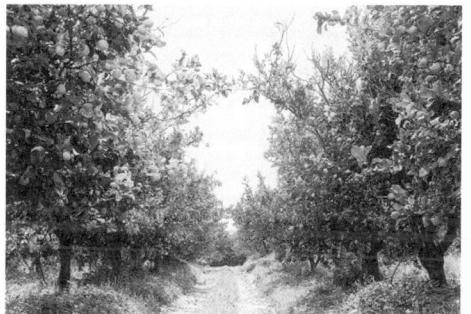

INTERVIEWS WITH THE PROTAGONISTS Production chain

From the 1980s onwards – when we supplied customers such as Morris, Adam, Paglieri, Vidal – the market has undergone great changes. The most important concerns the acquisition of Italian brands by large multinational groups: today, a percentage close to 80% of Italian perfumery brands are licensed by foreign companies.

Today's consumers seem oriented towards natural products; how do the "green" trend affect the raw material market?

The interest shown by consumers in the natural raw material has urged the multinationals accordingly; many have understood that Nature represents a trump card in today's market, and now use it in greater quantities – obviously choosing the most appropriate features for the final product in which it will be inserted. They come to discover first-hand how the essences they insert in perfumes of their brands are processed, and then offer consumers information in this regard, enhancing the work of those who produce the natural material.

The demand has therefore got back to a strong growth, and I have the feeling that it will continue to grow further.

How do you see the evolution of contemporary perfumery?

The trend that I seem to notice most is the return to a less abstract, more "figurative" perfumery, focused on the main ingredient. What differentiates the perfumes launched by the different brands is the way in which this protagonist is used, that is the style, that strong component linked to the corporate identity.

In reality, what is missing is the desire to dare, to take risks; Italian perfumers often prefer to follow trends rather than create them. For example, the olfactory profile of a bergamot or a tangerine undergoes important variations according to the different stages of ripening on the plant and the extraction techniques. The Maitre Parfumeurs are very interested in all these variations, they come to study them directly on the field to understand the added value they can give to their compositions. For example, when Ferré decided to launch his Bergamotto Marino in 2006, Pierre Bourdon came to visit the bergamot fields. For this perfume he selected an area near the sea, to get an olfactory profile in which the ozonic component was perceptible from the start. We welcome creators from all over the world every day... only Italians are missing!

Italian perfumers seem no longer interested in talking to producers of raw materials, and they let their competitors obtain all those wonderful aspects of natural variability that create new fashions and make creations unforgettable.

There are few brands with a strong Italian identity that constantly ask for raw materials from our land, and are fully supported in this choice, also due to the excellent feedback that the market recognizes them worldwide.

So what should Italian perfumers do to regain their identity?

Italian perfumery has a great history behind it. Although they have sold their licenses, brands could use their discretion to obtain more consistent raw materials to strengthen an identity that, in fact, belongs to them.

One day I dream of seeing Armani, Trussardi, Dolce & Gabbana (Stefano and Domenico), and Versace strolling through our gardens to discover the origins and varieties of raw materials, and to choose the ones they wish to use for their fragrances. It would be an event bringing further prestige to Italian visibility and to the corresponding natural territory that we represent in the world.

Italy is a country with a great tradition in the production of raw materials for perfumery. How do you see the future of the business area in which Capua is operating?

The productive vocation in this field is still growing. Above all since the sector is no longer relegated to the supply of essences-commodities but, thanks to the push given by multinationals with their big brands on the one hand, and by the Maitre Parfumeurs on the other, it is now able to produce botanical specialties, with precise features of extraction and territory. The interchange between the world of creation and the production capability has promoted an innovation that continues to create new opportunities. Potentially, it could go on expanding for a long time to come. To give an example, until a few decades ago bergamot mainly entered men's perfumery or colognes, but today it is an important ingredient in all fine perfumery, even for women.

Which are the most requested products on the market today?

The most requested type of product is the one with the highest technical content: if bergamot is the flagship of our production, it is true that we obtain extraordinary results also with tangerine in its many varieties (green, yellow, red), blood oranges, lemons... In the end, it is not a question of the most popular kind of citrus fruit, but of a technology capable of making the most of the wonderful gifts of nature.

Which product are you most proud of?

The one that I still have to create!

Which is your company's trump card?

The complete mastery of the sector in which we operate: when we are contacted by perfumers and research centres, they are struck by our ability to understand their language and their exigencies, and to respond in line with their expectations. Especially with regard to rules, which become more stringent every day. We have technical skills able to comply with regulations and at the same time produce exactly what the customer requires.

Do you think there is an Italian Style in perfumery?

More than a real Italian style, I would speak of Italian characterizing notes. That is to say those raw materials that – grown here by us – have always been used and are ever more characterizing the world of perfumery. Citrus fruits, of course, are the first that come to mind as they are typical of the Italian identity.

How do you see Capua 1880 in the future?

At present the company is in the hands of my sons Rocco and Giandomenico, who have been working with me for eight years now. The legacy that I leave in their hands is the passion for this profession and all my expertise, gained over a lifetime.

In October 2019 I became Cavaliere del Lavoro; during the awarding I could speak with President Mattarella, and I remember I told him that one of the most difficult tasks of us entrepreneurs is to instil in the new generation passion and pride for the peculiarities of our territory.

Production chain
The glassware company

Conversation with Federico Montali, Marketing and Business Development Manager of Bormioli Luigi.

Bormioli Luigi represents Italian excellence in the glassware sector: over a thousand people work in its twenty moulding lines with five furnaces, located in two plants (Parma and Abbiategrasso). The company produces a total of 250 million pieces per year, which are exported all over the world.

Can you tell us how the company "Bormioli Luigi" was founded?

The Bormioli family has been handing down the secrets of the art of glass-making from generation to generation since the 17th century. The business was undoubtedly founded even earlier, but the first reliable information we have dates back to the 1600s. Originally located in France, the Bormioli family moved to Italy, constructing glass-making furnaces at every stage of its journey: in Altare (province of Savona), Fidenza (province of Parma) and in Parma, where it settled permanently in the 1800s. So it was in the city of Parma that the company consolidated its business and took on the definitive identity with which we are all familiar today.

In 1946, Mr. Luigi Bormioli, an engineer to trade, decided to break away from the main branch of the company to found a production plant in his own name, i.e. "Bormioli Luigi SpA". Luigi's aim was to establish himself as a specialised glassware manufacturer, making objects that, at that time, were the most technically challenging, advanced and difficult to produce, in order to enter a niche market that was of no interest to the other members of the Bormioli family.

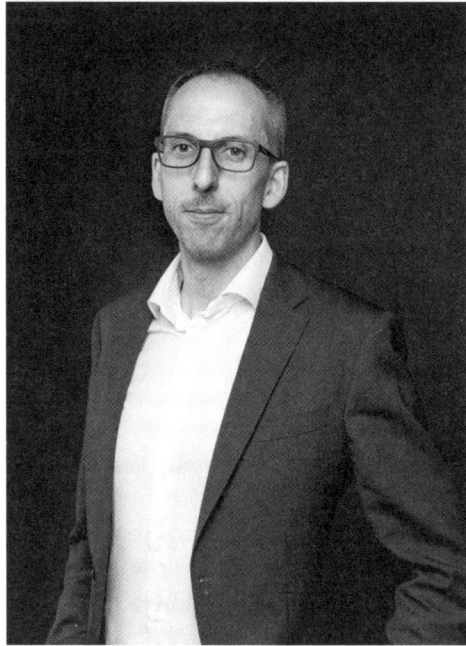

Today, the company is still firmly in the hands of the Bormioli family. Can you tell us how things have developed over the past decades?

Right from the outset, the company started specialising in bottles of different types. In the 1960s, it diversified into tableware for the home and the "horeca" (hotel, restaurant, catering, etc.) sector, while in the 1980s it launched a business branch dedicated to luxury perfumes. This began with the production of bottles for some French brands, followed by Italian brands (Euroitalia, Ferragamo, Angelini, ICR, etc.), and today it has achieved international fame, manufacturing products that are sent to every corner of the world.

The current CEO is Mr. Alberto Bormioli, son of the founder and an engineer like his father Luigi, born in the year that the company was founded. Alberto Bormioli followed in the footsteps of his father with the same aim: to provide the most innovative, excellent glassware that technology could produce.

The fact that the company is still the property of the family today, is a unique and invaluable advantage, guaranteeing continuity and constant product innovation. In fact, the glassware industry requires heavy investment and long-term programming, because the glass melting furnace is extremely expensive, its construction is long and complex and once it has been put into operation, it cannot be switched off. This characteristic differentiates the glass sector from all other industries, the machinery of which can be started and stopped according to production requirements. But when the furnace has been put into operation and starts to produce the glass, this process must continue non-stop: the load can be varied, but the process generates such high costs that these have to be covered by production.

In order to feed the furnace with a regular and constant production load, the business must be managed on the basis of medium-to long-term objectives. The fact that Bormioli Luigi is a family business and is not an investment fund (which usually compels Managers to attain short-term objectives on a three- or four-monthly basis) is an important advantage because it guarantees that the activity will be supported by a forward-looking management, to the benefit of production continuity and programming.

Can you give us an idea in figures of the value of Bormioli in the perfume sector?
Over the last twenty years, the turnover of Bormioli Luigi has more than tripled: from a figure of approx. fifty million euro in 1999, we rose to one hundred and eighty million in 2018, a figure that ranks us as leader on the Italian market and a top player on the global market, in which we have a twenty to twenty-five percent share. The glassware market for the luxury perfume sector is worth approx. two billion euro on a global level. It includes very few companies, all of which are European. In fact, the concentration of the perfume market (with dozens of brands owned by just a few multinationals, such as Coty, LVMH, L'Oréal, Estée Lauder) has led to a similar concentration in the glassware market as well.

What are the key factors of Bormioli's success?
To achieve results of this level, it is vital to have a forward-looking mentality and the capacity to accept any kind of technical challenge customers may bring, and then turn it into a standard process, to which competitors have to adapt if they want to stay in the market. But it is also necessary to keep investing in state-of-the-art technology, both in terms of glass and in finishing processes, without forgetting that it is the skill of the technicians that makes it possible to achieve excellence in our products. For us, it is of paramount importance to invest a lot also on human resources: first and foremost on training to enable our staff to grow and specialise; but that's not all, we are doing all we can to keep them in the company, and not lose them after we have trained them.

Where does the creativity for a bottle of perfume come from?
The design of the product is dictated by the customer. The company presents us with the design of the bottle that it wants to make and we perfect it, transforming the drawing into a finished container, ready to hold the perfume. For us, technical challenges give us the chance to grow; a segment of the market expects us to create things that are difficult to make,

which require complex processing and custom-tailored processes. We have the capacity to respond to their needs because we are flexible, strongly oriented towards innovation and hence able to adapt our production to the customer's needs, while others struggle to do so. Without our know-how, for example, a bottle like that of "Idôle" by Lancôme would never have been made, because we are practically the only ones able to produce such thin glass.

What could Italian companies do to promote our excellences more effectively on foreign markets?

In non-European countries such as China, for example, Italian and French products are considered equally luxurious. So it is not a question of the product. Also because often the quality of the Italian product is actually higher. But the French are much better than we are at teaming up to promote French-made products as the very height of luxury and exclusivity. We are not as good as they are at working together to promote our products with the same energy!

What challenges will the future bring? How will you face them?

In the future we shall continue to focus on innovation, flexibility and agility.
As far as innovation is concerned, we shall continue to offer our customers the technologies and products of tomorrow, because those made today are already six months old: in fact, when we develop a new bottle, it takes about six months of study and implementation to go from the design to the finished product.
In order to be able to design and create products that will make a difference in the future, a "Research & Development" Department able to devise new solutions

is of paramount importance. Like Inside Coating, for example: an internal lacquering of the glass, for decorative purposes, able to withstand contact with the perfume. The black, red and pink versions of "Armani Sì" apply this very technique, as do "Narciso Rodriguez" and "Dange-Rose" by Blumarine. When we proposed it to customers a few years ago, it was a completely new feature, with the power to make the difference in terms of the perceived luxury of the product. Now it has become a standard that all our customers can request. Nevertheless, a great deal of research had to be done, followed by medium- to long-term development work, in order to be able to provide it with all the necessary safety and quality requirements.
Another innovative technique that we have just developed is called *Prisma* and it consists of the application, under vacuum, of very thin layers of metallic salts that create iridescent reflections on the bottle depending on the angle of observation. This effect has been used for the "Flowerful" version of "Amo Ferragamo".

As for agility, being agile means being able to respond quickly to the demands of a market which, with the success of social media and the advent of influencers, has become unpredictable. A photo posted on Instagram by a successful influencer may result in the public shifting demand from one product to another. And in some cases, this can produce a peak of a hundred thousand requests for a given product, to be fulfilled instantly. Adapting to such an unpredictable market can be complicated, but it is also an interesting challenge. A challenge that forces you to rethink the way you produce and prioritise flexibility: in production, in decoration and in the management of human resources. Flexibility means being able to produce large quantities of bottles - even small ones - at the drop of a hat. If, for example, an order arrives for a few tens of thousands of bottles, but it is not yet clear whether they are to hold an eau de parfum or an eau de toilette, you need to have the flexibility to prepare everything else and then decorate the bottles at the last moment. And not everyone is equipped to do this.

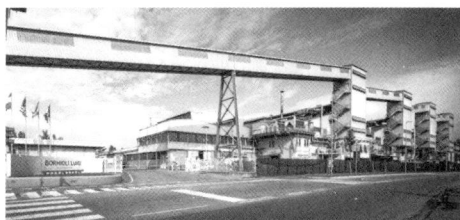

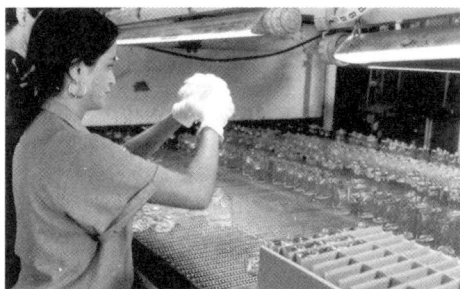

Can you already glimpse future trends in the packaging of products?
One of the most visible is the average weight of the bottles, which has been growing steadily in recent years. The thicker the glass in a bottle, the greater the perceived luxury; this perception is correct because the thicker the glass, the more it costs. But it is also true that some particularly expensive and artistic bottles are made of very thin glass, whose processing is technically more challenging and difficult, involving higher costs. "Idôle" by Lancôme, for example, is packaged in a bottle so thin and light that the thickness of the glass is almost imperceptible, so that the packaging practically disappears, displaying only the essence it contains. This signals a new direction, expensive, heralding an essential type of luxury, less ostentatious and more in line with the concepts of eco-sustainability gaining ground in our sector. From an ecological perspective, glass has a huge advantage over other materials, especially plastic, due to its chemical inertia. Glass is inherently chemically stable and this makes it the best material for the food and perfumery sectors. Moreover, it is infinitely recyclable: unlike plastic whose polymer chains deteriorate when continuously recycled, glass does not deteriorate when it is recast, even a thousand times over. The trend of eco-sustainability, within

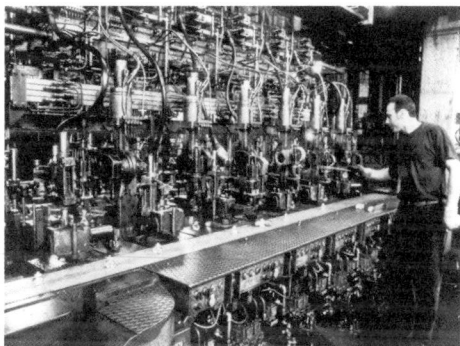

our specific market, has not yet been regulated by a specific framework; for the time being, the demand for particularly thin glass is still dictated by a precise aesthetic choice, rather than the desire to reduce packaging materials.

What characteristics do the bottles commissioned by Italian brands have?
The demands of the European market, particularly those of the Italian and French markets, are pretty much aligned, both aesthetically and in terms of quality, and there are no significant differences in the packaging of the perfumes. American customers, on the other hand, prefer slightly

more eye-catching bottles, while the Arab world, a great consumer and producer of perfumes, is very fond of gold and precious details, which make their bottles richer and more extravagant, while still maintaining a certain elegance.

Production chain
The subcontractor

*Conversation with Ambra Martone,
ICR Board Member and President
of the Accademia del Profumo.*

In its production facility of over fifty thousand square metres, ICR produces eighty-five million perfumes for thousands of brands around the world. These figures are growing steadily, which places the ICR among the top players in the luxury perfume sector in Europe. What are the origins of this success?

ICR was an offshoot of Marvin, the pharmaceutical company founded by my grandfather, Vincenzo Martone, in the 1940s. Marvin was specialised in the manufacturing of antibiotics and over-the-counter pharmaceuticals. However, the development of the company convinced my grandfather to use his technical know-how as a pharmacist also to promote the beauty sector, by opening other business branches related to cosmetics. He developed a make-up line, a perfume line and a skincare line. My grandfather was the first in Italy to understand the importance of providing anti-allergenic skincare products.
It was my father Roberto who had the insight, in the 1970s, to specialise in luxury perfumes.
Italy at that time still had a sort of "inferiority complex" compared to France: although there were skilled workers qualified to carry out the various production phases of a quality product, the perfumes were still commissioned and produced in France... and even their names were usually French! My father founded ICR (Industrie Cosmetiche Riunite S.p.a.) with the express intention of concentrating in a single company all the services related to the launching of a perfume: from creation to packaging, bottling, logistics and distribution.
It was the right idea at the right time, because at the end of the 1970s some emerging fashion designers promoting the *Made in Italy* drive, were considering branching into perfume and needed a reliable partner to produce their fragrances. ICR's first cooperation projects in this sector were with Romeo Gigli, Renato Balestra, Nazareno Gabrielli, Nicola Trussardi and Gianni Versace and very soon ICR had become the benchmark for all Italian brands which wanted to launch their own perfume: Bulgari, Salvatore Ferragamo, Emanuel Ungaro, Roberto Cavalli, Blumarine, DSquared2, Pomellato, Gai Mattiolo...
Since then, ICR has authored countless successes, thanks to which it has grown and developed to become a reference at a European level. But that's not all: the acquisition of Chinese, Arab and Russian customers has given us the opportunity to come into contact with other realities beyond Europe, further expanding our reference market.
And for the future we are also focusing on developing our own artistic perfume brand dedicated to the Marvin family, with fragrance lines for the home and for body care, LabSolue and Acqua Adornationis.

How is such incredible success maintained?
By having the insight to predict and set market trends, and by not skimping on

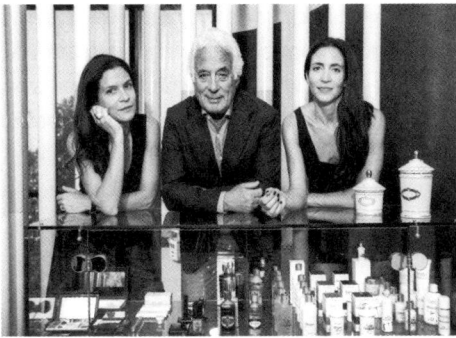

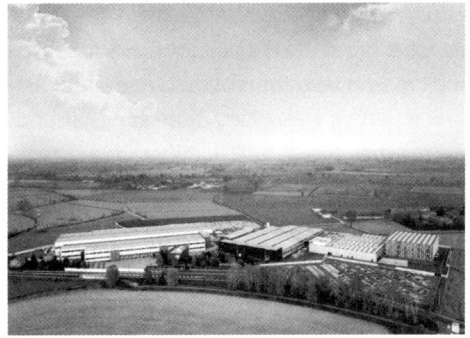

investment: you need to be prepared at all times, otherwise you find yourself already out of the market.

For example, at the end of the 1980s, my father had already figured out how our company would be likely to develop in the 1990s, so he began expanding all of the facilities: the headquarters, production plant and warehouses were all moved into larger buildings, in Lodi. In 2017, a new production unit was set up alongside the already existing one.

Thanks to these investments, we are now able to manage, in their entirety, all the various phases in the development of a project, whether it be for perfumes, perfumed bath lines or amenities for hotels and airlines, conducting the complete process of creation, production and logistics in-house, from the development of the formulas and the packaging, to shipping all over the world. We produce eighty-five million bottles a year, for Altaia, Angelini Beauty, Blumarine, Bulgari, Collistar, Eau d'Italie, Emanuel Ungaro, Gai Mattiolo, Gianfranco Ferré, Intimissimi, Laura Biagiotti, Lord, OVS, Salvatore Ferragamo, Shaka, Tezenis, Trussardi... their success is also ours.

But calling them customers doesn't render the idea. We have been working alongside some of them for thirty, forty years... Over time synergies and strategies have been developed and shared, creating bonds that transcend the customer-supplier relationship.

ICR is still a family business. How do you all manage this complexity?

Upline of any other consideration, there is a unifying long-term vision shared by the whole family. In any case, the corporate roles are clear and quite distinct, so as to avoid overlapping and confusion for those with whom we work. My father is the President, and my sister Giorgia and I are on the Board of Directors. She takes care of Marketing and IT, and I deal with production and logistics. Additionally, our various departments (logistics, quality, planning, etc.) are run by highly-qualified managers. We believe that skill and experience are fundamental for the growth of the company, and spending time and money in the recruitment of the best professionals and in the development of our human resources is a priority for us.

How do you view the future of ICR?

The perfume sector is running in two directions: on the one hand, we see growth in the best seller lines, which are characterised by high production volumes and speedy service; on the other, we are witnessing the development of a more artistic demand, characterised by craftsmanship and custom-tailored products. ICR has invested in both trends: on the one hand, with the expansion of the production plant and the purchasing of increasingly more technological and automatic machines, including collaborative robots; on the other, with the creation of the Atelier, a production space that offers an alternative way of working, from the composition of the fragrances to the possibility to produce very small batches, and to customise them down to the tiniest detail. In addition, in 2014, we opened the first Hotel à Parfums, which is housed in the old Milanese headquarters of our perfume factory, a structure which we had already converted into the Magna Pars Event Space (a charming space for some of the most prestigious events in Milan). The Hotel has forty suites that offer guests an unforgettable experience, starting from the olfactory check-in, during which the guest is invited to our perfume laboratory to choose a suite, on the basis of its fragrance. From that moment on, guests can feast their sense of smell during our olfactory aperitifs and dinners "à Parfums" and at the spa, with a series of treatments to choose from, all accompanied by different fragrances. We have noticed that the Hotel à Parfums is very popular with the world of fashion and design... but also with families, who appreciate the unusual spaciousness of our suites. Most of our guests are Italian, but a fair percentage also comes from France, the United States, Russia and China. But we're not stopping here: in November we'll be opening another 20 new suites and we've got 20 more planned for the year after that.

You have been President of the Accademia del Profumo since July 2019. Can you tell us something about this new assignment?
It was a great honour for me to accept the Presidency of the Accademia. Besides being a prestigious institution, the Accademia

has a deep emotional significance for me: many beautiful memories of my childhood are linked to the Accademia del Profumo Award, such as the big boxes of perfumes belonging to the finalists, which my father would bring home to explore. The chance I have been given today to direct the development and promotion of the Award is a real pleasure and a great challenge for me, and I am committed to continuing in line with what has been done so far, with the aim of raising its level and its prestige even more.

How do you view the future of the Accademia del Profumo?
My relationship with the Accademia del Profumo began five years ago, when I joined the steering committee to work on projects aimed at developing the culture of perfume in Italy. We organised local and national events in order to arouse public interest and promote the value of Italian perfume, involving the whole supply chain. In the future, I would like to bring even more glamour and energy into the Accademia's initiatives. I am particularly interested in cultural projects with the power to generate interest in the public both virtually and on social networks, and through events and fairs that already exist around the country and which could become yet another channel through which to promote Italian perfume and its supply chain.

How would a person who has Perfume in her name, in her heart and in her family DNA define the essence of Italian-ness in perfume?
Perfume is an expression of the same aesthetic sensitivity that pervades most of our everyday lives: from the beauty of our cities, to our food and clothing choices, to the design that distinguishes products *Made*

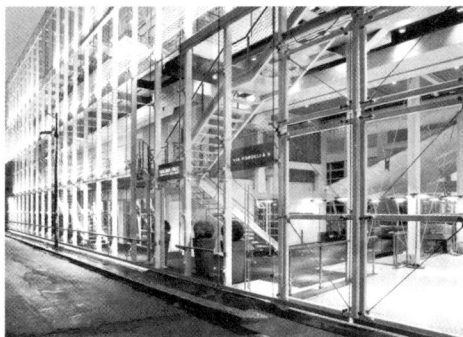

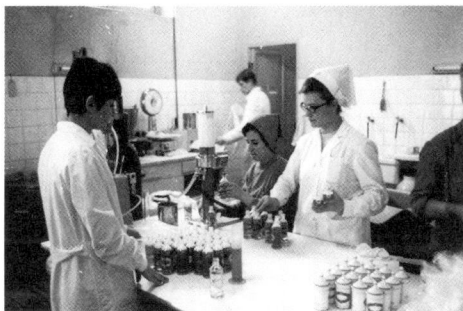

in Italy. Being surrounded by a culture of Beauty from our earliest years, it is second nature to us to express it in the perfumes that we create and to seek it in the clothes that we wear. Italian perfumery is also an embrace between Know-How, i.e. the excellence and genius of our craftsmanship, and Sentiment. We are a passionate people: we thrive on emotion and we love real fragrances with strong personalities, that make us stand out from the rest.

Production chain
From raw materials to creative fragrance compounds

Interview with Anthony Moellhausen, Chairman of Moellhausen S.p.A.

Moellhausen is a leading company in the creation of fragrances. Founded over fifty years ago, it is a historic reference for raw materials of the perfume sector at worldwide level. Can you tell us how Moellhausen was born?

Although the surname Moellhausen comes from Germany, my family is a melting pot of different nationalities and cultures: German, French, Italian and Turkish. In fact, at the beginning of the 1900s, my family lived in Izmir, Turkey, and this is where my father Eithel was born. He was of German nationality, but his mother was French. My mother, on the other hand, was born in Rome, to an Italian father and a Greek mother.

In 1910, when Ataturk seized power, foreign residents were stripped of their wealth and property, and obliged to leave the country. At the age of twenty-seven, my father was entrusted a diplomatic assignment in Rome, where he remained till after the end of the Second World War.

At the beginning of the 1950s, his meeting with Giovanni Mastracchi – engineer and successful Italian manufacturer of cosmetic products and toothpastes – was a turning point. Mastracchi gave my father the opportunity to join E.M.A. (Essenze e Materie Aromatiche) – a company with seat in Imperia which imported raw materials and essential oils for the perfume and cosmetics sectors from France – as foreign business contact-person, also in consideration of his uncommon mastery of five languages. In view of this new job, the whole family moved to Imperia and, in the 1960s, the growth of Mastracchi's enterprise aroused the interest of the first multinational cosmetics companies, so much so that Unilever even offered to purchase it.

In the meantime, my father has established close ties with Aurelio Cerizza. They both took over E.M.A. in 1964.

Entering the new company as a partner, my father was responsible for raw material trading, while Cerizza dealt with the

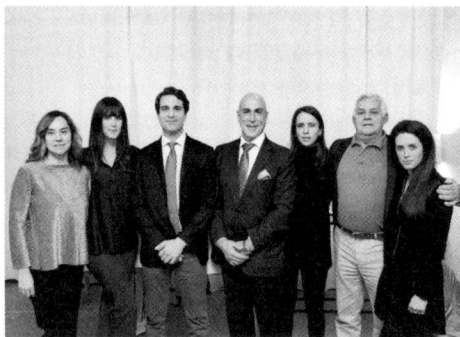

composition of formulas for perfumery and cosmetics. After a few years they parted ways and, while Cerizza founded his own business focusing on composition, my father began to specialize more and more in international trading, also getting distribution rights of products by Haarmann & Reimer and Dragoco, two of the most prestigious companies expanding in those years. In the mid 1960s, Italy appeared on the international market for the first time, thanks to a number of renowned brands that were requiring refined fragrances for their products. This opportunity was seized by companies such as the ones of my father and Cerizza, which could therefore develop further.

In 1967, my father decided to close E.M.A. and to open another company under his own name. So he founded Moellhausen which, with my daughters, my niece and my nephew, is now in its third generation.

Today, Moellhausen is headquartered in Milan, with industrial facilities and offices around the world, and is considered a world reference in the fragrance sector. Acknowledged as one of the most highly qualified industrial partners, Moellhausen works alongside the most selective brands in the perfume and beauty sectors, participating with its know-how and the most diversified raw materials in the creation of products with a high olfactory impact.

A great result! But let's go back to the second generation. Tell us something about yourself and your brother, Luca.

My brother Luca and I joined the company when we were around twenty years old, and Moellhausen was still small, with about half a dozen employees. We both started "from scratch," initially providing unskilled labor: my father made us unload trucks filled with raw materials or used us to filter essential oils (once I managed to flood a whole warehouse!).

Gradually, we were given positions of responsibility in different areas, but smoothly complementary: Luca focused more on chemistry, aroma chemicals and industrial dynamics, whereas I was more interested in natural derivatives. I found the complexity of their supply chain particularly challenging, and I developed the citrus products branch – derivatives of orange, bitter orange, bergamot, lemon, etc.

In the meantime, the world was undergoing landmark changes that were to revolutionize our way of doing business: the advancement of technology, with the advent of personal computers and the Internet, made it possible to develop better, more precise methods for dealing with flavor and fragrance materials. At the same time, markets were becoming increasingly accessible, utterly expanding business opportunities.

During the Formula 1 races, I happened to notice that the dirty but romantic mechanics of the 1960s had been replaced by professionals with steadily more sophisticated technology, whose millimetric adjustments could determine the outcome of a race. Suddenly I realized that Moellhausen could strive to get the same level of technology and efficiency.

So we decided to invest in hydroalcoholic perfumery of the highest quality. The

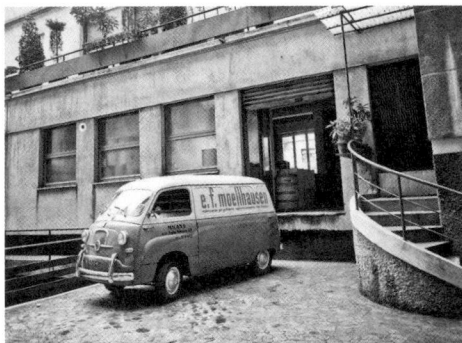

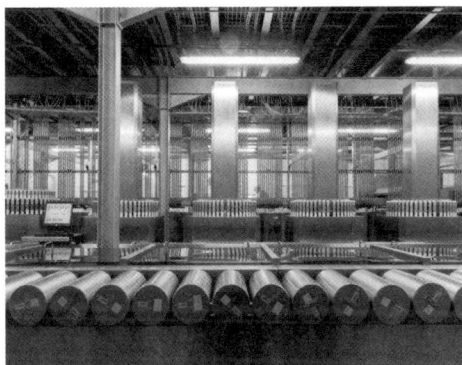

How has the perfume sector changed over the last twenty years?

Technological innovation has led to changes in many of the processes, making them faster and more efficient. Thanks to the modern GCMS systems, for example, we can run spot checks and routine controls which would once have been unthinkable, such as a systematic examination of genuineness and absence of undesirable substances – allergens or otherwise.

Legal provisions have also changed. If, from one side, the work of perfume manufacturers has become rather complicated, it is anyway true that end-consumers must be able to rely on products which do not put their health at risk. After all, even in the past, the imposed limitations have certainly never prevented great perfumers from creating legendary perfumes...

As for legendary perfumes and changes in taste, once upon a time there were the so-called "evergreen scents", timeless fragrances whose identifiability was some sort of signature scent of the person wearing them. But today it is the public that makes the difference, and it no longer seems to be interested in this kind of perfumes.

Consumers have discovered their sense of smell as a way to convey emotions, so instead of investing in a single perfume "forever," they prefer to create a collection of different fragrances that will satisfy their need for originality and exclusivity.

functional perfume industry already had at its disposal a large number of companies specialized in formulations for soaps and detergents, products containing fairly common raw materials. But with our background so centered on the finest raw materials, we had the potential to focus on a much more specific sector, to which we were sure to be able to offer a product of flawless quality.

Over the last twenty years, the speed with which technology and ICT have developed has transformed Moellhausen into a highly automated company: the raw materials are classified, selected and mixed using amazingly autonomous tools and robots.

It is, of course, a much less romantic environment than it used to be, when the perfumer would sit in a laboratory at an organ, surrounded by vials and scales, and everything was made by hand!

On the basis of your experience, what make Italian perfumes different from those produced in other countries?

I am sure that the perfume culture of a nation is rooted in its food culture. Those lacking in gastronomic culture – who eat carelessly, without attention, without creativity – do not usually have a great understanding of perfume. For instance, spices make Middle Eastern cuisine rich and exciting, and this richness is also reflected in the Middle Eastern idea of perfume. In Italy, as in France, the variety of gastronomic delights, the creativity of certain dishes or wines form the basis for understanding and appreciating the perfumes we create in our country.

For us, as Italians, this is even easier because our territory is full of plants with extraordinary fragrances such as laurel, myrtle, bergamot and sweet orange, broom, mint, helichrysum and Roman chamomile. Even Centifolia rose! Creativity in perfumes is not the only pride in Italy. Our land is ideal for growing the plants from which the most sought-after raw materials in the world are extracted.

What is the key to the success of Italian perfumery?

Italian perfumery, whose popularity exploded from the 1970s through the 1990s, gained international attention thanks to a mix of culture and creativity that companies already very experienced in the sector knew how to capitalize on and guide towards success.

Nowadays it seems that history is repeating itself: the mainstream luxury perfume sector appears to be almost totally monopolized by the French and the only way to overturn this situation seems to lie in generating an extreme luxury, imbued with a culture, an individuality and a creativity that only artistic perfumery can express. The small Italian brands and independent perfume composers are demonstrating their ability to put Italy right back on the international marketing map. And as was the case forty years ago, their ideas are welcomed by those with a strong background in this field who have the experience to make them successful.

The technology that Moellhausen presently holds, for example, means that small companies can be provided with the same excellent service as larger companies, enabling them to compete on an absolutely identical quality level.

So what are Italians lacking in order to obtain the visibility and allure of companies in other countries?

Italy is naturally drawn to luxury. Not only in the fashion sector, but just look at the world of design, motors, the excellence of our food and wine... Our drive to create originality and exclusivity is the same force that propels us towards individualism, and this is a characteristic that the whole world envies us. This, however, is also our greatest limitation, because it prevents us from taking joint action. This individualism prevents us from working as a team, from having a general vision that would enable us to promote our products more efficiently through a shared effort.

Can you describe us Moellhausen today?

Fifty years from its foundation, Moellhausen represents the Italian challenge to an international market dominated by French and Swiss giants, a sort of state-of-the-art "boutique factory" that customers can come to either for a single raw material or for the creation of an entire line of fragrances, complete with marketing strategy for its market launch.

Our quality system complies with ISO 9001:2015 standard; our warehouses stow over 2700 raw materials, all immediately available and stored under nitrogen blanketing. This avoids oxidation while preserving the olfactory characteristics of the ingredients.

We currently import from 75 countries and export to 72 and, although this international approach places us side by side with the multinationals, we are keen on remaining a small company. This is a carefully considered choice, consistent with our pursuit of excellence: above and beyond our actual financial gain, for us it is a question of pride to be able to offer our customers products with cutting edge quality.

How do you intend to face future challenges?

As I mentioned earlier, the third generation of Moellhausen – represented by my niece, my nephew and my daughters Michelle and Dominique, both perfumers – has already joined the company, igniting it with an enthusiasm and creativity that are helping us enter more and more international markets. Our family history is based on the mixing of different cultures. We are curious by nature and travel a lot. This rich and varied cultural background is our trump card, it is reflected in our work and allows us to be key players in countries whose consumers have a significantly different cultural background from the western one.

In addition to creativity, we shall also continue to focus on innovation and excellence. I am convinced that we can only compete with the overwhelming power of the French companies by offering a better quality product, controlled, certified and perfect in every respect. This is how we will grow as a global player in this market.

Brands
Artistic perfumery

Conversation with Massimo Nobile and Stefania Giannino, founders and creative directors of the artistic perfume brand Nobile 1942

The brand Nobile 1942 is now well-established worldwide. Your rich fragrances with their Italian soul have been enchanting not only the European public but also Russia, the Arab world and the USA for almost twenty years now. How did you start in the perfume sector?

Massimo: I grew up in the midst of the prestigious brands represented by my father and those sold by my mother in her perfume shop, an exquisite salon that attracted excellent customers from far and near. As I grew, my dream to become an engineer crumbled because I was so enthralled by this environment. So after finishing school, instead of going to university, I decided to start working right away as a representative of emerging brands. I grafted long and hard until I finally made it as a representative for Chanel. But the higher I rose, the more this exclusive environment into which I was born seemed to lack emotion. And when you work without emotion, in my opinion, it's better to have the courage to hand in your notice and start from scratch, even if you have a family and children – or indeed because of it. This was the real trigger for me: my responsibilities as a father and a husband. So I decided to create my own brand. The Niche perfume sector, with its elegant modes of expression and its cultural awareness, had a very high chance of success, and the example of Acqua di Parma was opening up new opportunities for those who did not want to work with the multinationals. Both Stefania and I were excited by this idea.

Stefania: When Massimo asked me to work with him on a project to create a brand of perfume, with the aim of increasing the appeal of Italian elegance and taste all over the world, I instantly accepted. I said yes instinctively. I felt that the time had come to demonstrate how Italy too had something to say in the field of artistic perfumery. Right from the outset, our goal was to create a project that would last over time, unrelated to trends and fashions, both from an olfactory and aesthetic perspective. And in actual fact, we have never chosen olfactory themes on the basis of the fashions of the moment! In our fragrances we express ourselves and the things we love: beauty, *joie de vivre* and the elegance typical of Italy.

Massimo: And so, at the beginning of the 2000s we founded Nobile 1942, a great challenge in an industry which, at that time, would cut you off short with no time to explain, if the perfume had little or nothing to say. Although it was really difficult at the start, I didn't lose hope: my family had taught me that all goals are attainable if you are determined enough.
And the results finally started to appear. Created in a small pioneering company, Nobile 1942 has now been growing for fifteen years in sales and in respect, both in Italy and abroad, conveying the glamour and elegance typical of Italian perfumery. This is a result that we are very proud of and which drives us to work even harder.

How has niche perfumery changed over the last twenty years?
Stefania: In 2004, when our project began, we were alongside long-established brands such as L'Artisan Parfumeur, Annick Goutal, Piguet and some Italian brands like Tonatto and Villoresi. There were only a few of us working to produce something creative and original, in a very small market segment.

Massimo: The artistic perfumery sector was like a club: its atmosphere was velvety, impalpable. There was the club of the noses, the club of the perfumers and that of the critics, and the shop owners were all cultured and had very clear ideas... It was a world teeming with creativity, and the desire to discover and invent new things for the sheer passion of doing so, without ever

looking at a clock. Year after year, interest began to grow around this niche thanks to the word-of-mouth of satisfied customers, and the numbers began to rise faster and faster. When we started out, the environment was pervaded by a strong ethos, but in recent years hundreds of new brands have emerged, driven only by business and numbers. Then the niche began to arouse the interest of the multinationals: L'Oréal was the first to acquire a niche brand, followed by LVMH, P&G, Estée Lauder and Puig...

What are the characteristics that distinguish Italian perfumery?
Stefania: The Italians are great users and connoisseurs of perfume. Italy has a large community of enthusiasts, and a distribution channel that is much more highly developed than elsewhere. But the factor that really makes our perfume stand out is what distinguishes Italian-made products in general: creativity. We are a nation of artisans, full of ideas and with a long history behind us. We are lucky enough to have great insight and interesting contents to develop. And we are also a nation of individualists, always in pursuit of elegance and exclusivity!

What factor should Italy focus on to promote "Made in Italy" perfume in the best possible way?
Stefania: The expressive opportunities of the niche have greatly stimulated the sector's industry, while innovations in mining techniques have broken new creative ground, causing enormous ferment. The perfume production chain has been growing further in recent years but there is still a lack of production plants for compounds, and essential oil production plants could also be increased. The problem is that there is a lack of expertise specific to the processing techniques. I think the time has

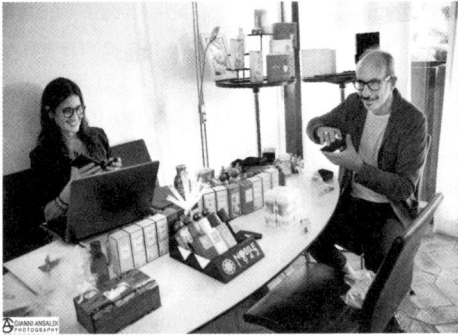
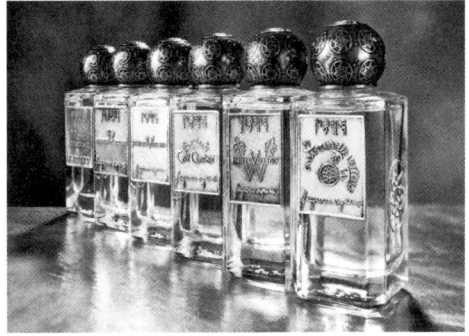

come to expand the perfume culture, which currently stops at empirical knowledge, because we don't have the tools here to take it further. To do so, we are forced to go to schools in other countries. If we want our perfume sector to be accorded its true value, we need to set up university training schools. This is the main difference that exists between Italy and France.

What in your opinion does the future of artistic perfumery hold?

Massimo: I think that in the future the niche perfume sector will run along two main lines: on the one hand, distribution will be expanded and become more "commercial": the brands will be displayed in splendid corners inside Department stores, Concept stores and well-stocked perfumery chains. On the other hand, there will be an even more "niche" perfume sector: small artisans and family brands with a production style built on research and personality and driven by a passion for artistic creation.

Stefania: I am also convinced that in the future there will be room for people like us, who believe in perfume as a form of art. It's going to be long, hard road for anyone starting today - as it is for those who have been on the market for years - with no possibility to take short-cuts. Risks have to be taken, different, innovative paths forged in

order to gain credibility. It will be arduous, but value will be rewarded, in time.

And with regard to Nobile 1942? What challenges will you have to face?

Stefania: Our choices have always been guided by consistency and authenticity and we intend to continue along these lines in the future. The challenge of Nobile 1942 is therefore to succeed - notwithstanding the growth of the sector - in keeping faithful to our dream of creativity and craftsmanship, while remaining a family-run business. We're counting on being joined by our daughters in the near future!
Massimo: I'm not afraid of the future. I have the sensation that the Italian perfume sector is gaining ground, also on an international level; the challenge is to stay on the right road, that of professionalism, ethics and culture. We want to keep providing solutions for those who have a passion for perfume and are constantly on the lookout for exciting fragrances. We appeal to a market segment that has studied over the past years, has become informed, attended courses and become master of its own choices. We cannot and we must not fail to live up to their expectations! We won't bother anyone, and we certainly won't tread on the toes of the multinationals: and if things go as we expect, they'll be the ones working hard to keep their business!

10, Corso Como > 1999 > 10, Corso Como > ♀
10, Corso Como > 2010 > 10, Corso Como Uomo > ♂
401 è Amatrice > 2018 > 401 è Amatrice > ⚥
V Canto > 2015 > Alibi > ⚥
V Canto > 2015 > Amans > ⚥
V Canto > 2015 > Cor Gentile > ⚥
V Canto > 2015 > Ensis > ⚥
V Canto > 2015 > Irae > ⚥
V Canto > 2015 > Kashmirie > ⚥
V Canto > 2015 > Magnificat > ⚥
V Canto > 2015 > Mastin > ⚥
V Canto > 2015 > Mea Culpa > ⚥
V Canto > 2015 > Mirabile > ⚥
V Canto > 2016 > Cicuta > ⚥
V Canto > 2016 > Lucrethia > ⚥
V Canto > 2016 > Mandragola > ⚥
V Canto > 2017 > Arsenico > ⚥
V Canto > 2017 > Stricnina > ⚥
V Canto > 2018 > Cianuro > ⚥
V Canto > 2018 > Curaro > ⚥
V Canto > 2018 > Ricina > ⚥
V Canto > 2018 > Stramonio > ⚥
V Canto > 2019 > Fili > ⚥
V Canto > 2019 > Posi > ⚥
Abaton Bros > 2004 > Blazer > ⚥
Abaton Bros > 2004 > Gessato > ♂
Abaton Bros > 2004 > Tailleur > ♀
Abaton Bros > 2004 > Tubino > ♀
Abaton Bros > 2008 > Fieno Donna > ♀
Abaton Bros > 2008 > Fieno Uomo > ♂
Abaton Bros > 2011 > Il Chinotto in Fiore > ⚥
Abaton Bros > 2017 > Chinotto Dark > ♂
Abaton Bros > 2017 > Chinotto Gourmand > ⚥
Abaton Bros > 2018 > Fior di Chinotto > ♀
Abdes Salaam Attars Perfumes > 1980 > Bazaar > ⚥
Abdes Salaam Attars Perfumes > 1989 > Acqua Santa (Holy Water) > ⚥
Abdes Salaam Attars Perfumes > 1989 > Notte African (African Night) > ⚥
Abdes Salaam Attars Perfumes > 1989 > Cuoio Tartaro (Tartar Leather) > ♂
Abdes Salaam Attars Perfumes > 1989 > Legno di Nave (Sea Wood) > ⚥
Abdes Salaam Attars Perfumes > 1989 > Muschio di Quercia
   (Oakmoss) > ⚥
Abdes Salaam Attars Perfumes > 1989 > Tasneem > ⚥
Abdes Salaam Attars Perfumes > 1989 > Tè delle Isole > ⚥
Abdes Salaam Attars Perfumes > 2008 > African Queen Black
   Panther > ♀
Abdes Salaam Attars Perfumes > 2008 > African Queen Pink Panther > ♀
Abdes Salaam Attars Perfumes > 2008 > Hindu Kush > ♀
Abdes Salaam Attars Perfumes > 2010 > Balsamo della Mecca
   (Mecca Balsam) > ⚥
Abdes Salaam Attars Perfumes > 2010 > Colonia dell'imperatore
   (Cologne de L'empereur) > ♂
Abdes Salaam Attars Perfumes > 2010 > Cuba Express > ⚥
Abdes Salaam Attars Perfumes > 2010 > Elle > ♀
Abdes Salaam Attars Perfumes > 2010 > Fiore della Notte
   (Night Blossom) > ⚥
Abdes Salaam Attars Perfumes > 2010 > Frutti Paradisi > ⚥
Abdes Salaam Attars Perfumes > 2010 > Green Tea > ⚥
Abdes Salaam Attars Perfumes > 2010 > Grezzo (D'Eleganza) > ⚥
Abdes Salaam Attars Perfumes > 2010 > Gringo > ♂
Abdes Salaam Attars Perfumes > 2010 > Mona Lisa > ♀
Abdes Salaam Attars Perfumes > 2010 > Morning Blossom > ⚥
Abdes Salaam Attars Perfumes > 2010 > Persona > ⚥
Abdes Salaam Attars Perfumes > 2010 > Rose des Bois > ⚥
Abdes Salaam Attars Perfumes > 2011 > Oud Caravan N. 1 > ⚥
Abdes Salaam Attars Perfumes > 2011 > Oud Caravan N. 2 > ⚥
Abdes Salaam Attars Perfumes > 2011 > Oud Caravan N. 3 > ⚥
Abdes Salaam Attars Perfumes > 2011 > Sharif > ⚥
Abdes Salaam Attars Perfumes > 2012 > Acqua di Angelica > ⚥
Abdes Salaam Attars Perfumes > 2012 > Flanel Rain Forest > ♂
Abdes Salaam Attars Perfumes > 2012 > Oasis > ♀
Abdes Salaam Attars Perfumes > 2012 > Palermo Don Corleone > ⚥
Abdes Salaam Attars Perfumes > 2012 > Tawaf > ⚥
Abdes Salaam Attars Perfumes > 2012 > Afghan Charas >
Abdes Salaam Attars Perfumes > 2012 > Arabia > ⚥

Abdes Salaam Attars Perfumes > 2012 > Attar Maulana > ♂
Abdes Salaam Attars Perfumes > 2102 > Bambini > ⚥
Abdes Salaam Attars Perfumes > 2012 > Casablanca > ⚥
Abdes Salaam Attars Perfumes > 2012 > Chillum > ⚥
Abdes Salaam Attars Perfumes > 2012 > Rose Heart > ♀
Abdes Salaam Attars Perfumes > 2012 > Tabac > ⚥
Abdes Salaam Attars Perfumes > 2012 > Tambour > ♂
Abdes Salaam Attars Perfumes > 2012 > Tartar Leather > ♂
Abdes Salaam Attars Perfumes > 2012 > Tcharas > ⚥
Abdes Salaam Attars Perfumes > 2013 > Lake Flower > ♀
Abdes Salaam Attars Perfumes > 2015 > Amber Chocolate > ⚥
Abdes Salaam Attars Perfumes > 2015 > Amber Jasmine > ⚥
Abdes Salaam Attars Perfumes > 2015 > Amber Oud > ⚥
Abdes Salaam Attars Perfumes > 2015 > Amber Rose > ⚥
Abdes Salaam Attars Perfumes > 2015 > Feromone (Pheromone)
   pour Femme > ♀
Abdes Salaam Attars Perfumes > 2015 > Feromone (Pheromone)
   pour Homme > ♂
Abdes Salaam Attars Perfumes > 2015 > Gipsy Queen > ♀
Abdes Salaam Attars Perfumes > 2015 > Milano Café > ⚥
Abdes Salaam Attars Perfumes > 2015 > Oud Laos > ⚥
Abdes Salaam Attars Perfumes > 2015 > Sensemilla > ⚥
Abdes Salaam Attars Perfumes > 2015 > Venezia Giardini Segreti > ⚥
Abdes Salaam Attars Perfumes > 2016 > Aalacho N. 1 > ⚥
Abdes Salaam Attars Perfumes > 2016 > Aalacho N. 2 > ⚥
Abdes Salaam Attars Perfumes > 2016 > Cuoio dei Dolci > ⚥
Abdes Salaam Attars Perfumes > 2016 > Ihram > ⚥
Abdes Salaam Attars Perfumes > 2016 > Il Giglio di Firenze > ⚥
Abdes Salaam Attars Perfumes > 2016 > Prima Rosa > ⚥
Abdes Salaam Attars Perfumes > 2018 > Chocolate Spicy (Maya) > ⚥
Acca Kappa > 1997 > Muschio Bianco > ⚥
Acca Kappa > 1998 > Glicine > ♀
Acca Kappa > 1999 > Cedro > ♂
Acca Kappa > 1999 > Libocedro > ♂
Acca Kappa > 2003 > Calycanthus > ♀
Acca Kappa > 2004 > Hibiscus > ♀
Acca Kappa > 2004 > Mimosa > ♀
Acca Kappa > 2004 > Wisteria > ♀
Acca Kappa > 2010 > Blue Lavender > ♀
Acca Kappa > 2012 > Giallo Elicriso > ♂
Acca Kappa > 2012 > Giardino Segreto > ♀
Acca Kappa > 2013 > Green Mandarin > ⚥
Acca Kappa > 2013 > Virginia Rose > ♀
Acca Kappa > 2014 > Black Pepper & Sandalwood > ⚥
Acca Kappa > 2014 > Tilia Cordata > ♀
Acca Kappa > 2014 > Vaniglia Fior di Mandorlo > ⚥
Acca Kappa > 2014 > White Moss > ⚥
Acca Kappa > 2016 > Idillio > ♀
Acca Kappa > 2016 > Ode > ⚥
Acca Kappa > 2017 > Fior d'acqua > ♂
Acca Kappa > 2019 > Mandarin & Green Tea > ⚥
Acca Kappa > 2019 > Myscent > ⚥
Acca Kappa > 2019 > Sakura Tokyo > ♀
Accendis > 2015 > Accendis 0.1 > ⚥
Accendis > 2015 > Accendis 0.2 > ⚥
Accendis > 2015 > Aclus > ⚥
Accendis > 2017 > Lucepura > ⚥
Accendis > 2017 > Lucevera > ⚥
Accendis > 2018 > Fiorialux > ⚥
Accendis > 2018 > Luna Dulcis > ⚥
Acqua del Garda > 2015 > Itinerary I > ♂
Acqua del Garda > 2015 > Itinerary II > ♀
Acqua del Garda > 2015 > Itinerary III > ♀
Acqua del Garda > 2015 > Itinerary IV > ♀
Acqua del Garda > 2017 > Gelsomino Assoluto > ♀
Acqua del Garda > 2017 > Intenso d'agrumi > ♂
Acqua dell'Elba > 1999 > Classica Men > ♂
Acqua dell'Elba > 1999 > Classica Women > ♀
Acqua dell'Elba > 2000 > Bimbi > ⚥
Acqua dell'Elba > 2002 > Blu Men > ♂
Acqua dell'Elba > 2002 > Blu Women > ♀
Acqua dell'Elba > 2005 > Sport > ♂
Acqua dell'Elba > 2010 > Arcipelago Men > ♂
Acqua dell'Elba > 2010 > Arcipelago Women > ♀

Acque di Italia > 2015 > Tabacco e Bergamotto di Taormina > ♂
Acque di Italia > 2017 > Legni Chiari di Lipari > ♀
Acque di Italia > 2017 > Legni Scuri di Vulcano > ♂
Acque di Italia > 2017 > Muschio del Trentino > ⚥
Acque di Italia > 2018 > Acqua di Venezia > ⚥
Adrienne Vittadini > 1994 > AV > ♀
Adrienne Vittadini > 1999 > Adrienne Vittadini > ♀
Adrienne Vittadini > 2002 > Venezia > ♀
Adrienne Vittadini > 2003 > Capri > ♀
Adrienne Vittadini > 2012 > Amore > ♀
Adrienne Vittadini > 2013 > AV Glamour > ♀
Aeon > 2016 > Aeon 001 > ⚥
Aequalis > 2015 > N. 1 > ♂
Aequalis > 2015 > N. 2 > ♀
Aequalis > 2015 > N. 3 > ♀
Aequalis > 2015 > N. 4 > ♀
Aequalis > 2015 > N. 5 > ♀
Aequalis > 2015 > N. 6 > ♂
Aequalis > 2015 > N. 7 > ♂
Aequalis > 2015 > N. 8 > ♀
Aequalis > 2015 > N. 9 > ♂
Aequalis > 2015 > N. 10 > ♂
Aequalis > 2015 > N. 11 > ♂
Aequalis > 2015 > N. 12 > ♂
Aequalis > 2015 > N. 13 > ♂
Aequalis > 2015 > N. 14 > ♀
Aequalis > 2015 > N. 15 > ♀
Aequalis > 2015 > N. 16 > ♀
Aequalis > 2015 > N. 17 > ♂
Aequalis > 2015 > N. 18 > ♀
Aequalis > 2015 > N. 19 > ♀
Aequalis > 2015 > N. 20 > ♀
Aequalis > 2015 > N. 21 > ♂
Aequalis > 2015 > N. 22 > ♂
Aequalis > 2015 > N. 23 > ♂
Aequalis > 2015 > N. 24 > ♂
Aequalis > 2015 > N. 25 > ♂
Aequalis > 2015 > N. 26 > ♀
Aequalis > 2015 > N. 27 > ♂
Aequalis > 2015 > N. 28 > ♂
Aequalis > 2015 > N. 29 > ♀
Aequalis > 2015 > N. 30 > ♀
Aequalis > 2015 > N. 31 > ♂
Aequalis > 2015 > N. 32 > ♀
Aequalis > 2015 > N. 33 > ♂
Aequalis > 2015 > N. 34 > ♀
Aequalis > 2015 > N. 35 > ♀
Aequalis > 2015 > N. 36 > ♀
Aequalis > 2015 > N. 37 > ♀
Aequalis > 2015 > N. 38 > ♀
Aequalis > 2015 > N. 39 > ♂
Aequalis > 2015 > N. 40 > ♀
Aequalis > 2015 > N. 41 > ♀
Aequalis > 2015 > N. 42 > ♀
Aequalis > 2015 > N. 43 > ♀
Aequalis > 2015 > N. 44 > ♀
Aequalis > 2015 > N. 45 > ♀
Aequalis > 2015 > N. 46 > ♀
Aequalis > 2015 > N. 47 > ♀
Aequalis > 2015 > N. 48 > ♀
Aequalis > 2015 > N. 49 > ♀
Aequalis > 2015 > N. 50 > ♀
Aequalis > 2015 > N. 51 > ♀
Aequalis > 2015 > N. 52 > ♀
Aequalis > 2015 > N. 53 > ♀
Aequalis > 2015 > N. 54 > ♀
Aequalis > 2015 > N. 55 > ♂
Aequalis > 2015 > N. 56 > ♂
Aequalis > 2015 > N. 57 > ♂
Aequalis > 2015 > N. 58 > ♂
Aequalis > 2015 > N. 59 > ♀
Aequalis > 2015 > N. 60 > ♂
Aequalis > 2015 > N. 61 > ♀
Aequalis > 2015 > N. 62 > ♂
Aequalis > 2015 > N. 63 > ♀
Agatho Parfum > 2019 > 195 A.C. > ⚥
Agatho Parfum > 2019 > Adone > ⚥
Agatho Parfum > 2019 > Castiamanti > ⚥
Agatho Parfum > 2019 > Fauno > ⚥
Agatho Parfum > 2019 > Giardinodiercole > ⚥
Agatho Parfum > 2019 > Rossopompeiano > ⚥
Alberta Ferretti > 1993 > Femina > ♀

Alberta Ferretti > 1995 > Parfum de Nuit > ♀
Alberta Ferretti > 2009 > Alberta Ferretti > ♀
Alchimista > 2015 > Enapay > ⚥
Alchimista > 2015 > Nefertiti > ♀
Alchimista > 2015 > Nefertum > ♀
Alchimista > 2015 > Quasar > ⚥
Alchimista > 2016 > Makalu > ⚥
Alchimista > 2019 > Cocos Island > ⚥
Alessandro Dell'Acqua > 2001 > Alessandro Dell'Acqua > ♀
Alessandro Dell'Acqua > 2003 > Alessandro Dell'Acqua Man > ♂
Alessandro Dell'Acqua > 2005 > Woman in Rose > ♀
Alessandro Della Torre > 2001 > Alessandro Della Torre > ♀
Alison Oldoini > 2013 > Black Violet > ♂
Alison Oldoini > 2013 > Cuir d'Encens > ♂
Alison Oldoini > 2013 > Marine Vodka > ♂
Alison Oldoini > 2013 > Oranger Moi > ♀
Alison Oldoini > 2013 > Rhum d'hiver > ♂
Alison Oldoini > 2013 > Rose Profond > ♀
Alison Oldoini > 2014 > Chocman Mint > ♂
Alison Oldoini > 2014 > Crystal Oud > ♂
Alison Oldoini > 2016 > Diafana Skin > ♀
Alison Oldoini > 2019 > Ambra Guaiac > ⚥
Alison Oldoini > 2019 > Bourbon Oud > ⚥
Allegri > 1991 > Allegri > ♀
Alta Manifattura Cosmetica > 2018 > Absolute Orchid > ⚥
Alta Manifattura Cosmetica > 2018 > Intensely > ⚥
Alta Manifattura Cosmetica > 2018 > Nude > ⚥
Alta Manifattura Cosmetica > 2018 > Pure Amber > ⚥
Altaia > 2015 > By Any Other Name > ♀
Altaia > 2015 > Don't Cry for Me > ⚥
Altaia > 2015 > Yu Son > ⚥
Altaia > 2016 > Ombù > ⚥
Altaia > 2017 > Tuberose in Blue > ♀
Altaia > 2018 > Purple Land > ⚥
Altaia > 2019 > Wonder of You > ⚥
ALV Passport – Alviero Martini > 2017 > Capri > ⚥
ALV Passport – Alviero Martini > 2017 > Firenze > ⚥
ALV Passport – Alviero Martini > 2017 > Roma > ⚥
ALV Passport– Alviero Martini > 2017 > Taormina > ⚥
ALV Passport– Alviero Martini > 2017 > Venezia > ⚥
Alviero Martini – 1ª Classe > 2004 > Geo Donna > ♀
Alviero Martini – 1ª Classe > 2004 > Geo Uomo > ♂
Alviero Martini – 1ª Classe > 2005 > Flags Donna > ♀
Alviero Martini – 1ª Classe > 2005 > Flags Uomo > ♂
Alviero Martini – 1ª Classe > 2007 > 1ª Classe Incenso from Asia > ♀
Alviero Martini – 1ª Classe > 2007 > 1ª Classe Man > ♂
Alviero Martini – 1ª Classe > 2007 > 1ª Classe Sandalo from Oceania > ♂
Alviero Martini – 1ª Classe > 2007 > 1ª Classe Woman > ♀
Alviero Martini – 1ª Classe > 2007 > Geoblack Man > ♂
Alviero Martini – 1ª Classe > 2007 > Geoblack Woman > ♀
Alviero Martini – 1ª Classe > 2010 > Urban Safari Man > ♂
Alviero Martini – 1ª Classe > 2010 > Urban Safari Woman > ♀
Alviero Martini – 1ª Classe > 2012 > Urban Safari a City Story > ♀
Alviero Martini – 1ª Classe > 2012 > Urban Safari a Jungle Story > ♂
Amaranthvs > 2017 > Terrae di Siena > ⚥
Angela Ciampagna > 2015 > Aer > ⚥
Angela Ciampagna > 2015 > Ducalis > ⚥
Angela Ciampagna > 2015 > Hatria > ⚥
Angela Ciampagna > 2015 > Kanat > ⚥
Angela Ciampagna > 2015 > Liquo > ⚥
Angela Ciampagna > 2015 > Nox > ⚥
Angela Ciampagna > 2015 > Rosarium > ⚥
Angela Ciampagna > 2016 > Faun > ⚥
Angela Ciampagna > 2016 > Ignes > ⚥
Angela Ciampagna > 2018 > Laetitia > ⚥
Angela Ciampagna > 2018 > Materia > ⚥
Angela Ciampagna > 2018 > Miracula > ⚥
Angelo Caroli > 2016 > Amore Nero > ⚥
Angelo Caroli > 2016 > Innamorata > ⚥
Angelo Caroli > 2016 > Liquirizia Nera > ⚥
Angelo Caroli > 2016 > Magnifico Patchouli > ⚥
Angelo Caroli > 2016 > Olio Emozionale > ⚥
Angelo Caroli > 2016 > Sette Agrumi > ⚥
Angelo Caroli > 2016 > Tuberosa Nera > ⚥
Angelo Caroli > 2016 > Viola > ⚥
Angelo Caroli > 2018 > Ambra Oud > ⚥
Angelo Caroli > 2018 > Incenso Indiano > ⚥
Angelo Caroli > 2018 > Orchidea Nera Oud > ⚥
Angelo Caroli > 2018 > Rosa Nera Oud > ⚥
Angelo Caroli > 2018 > Sandalo Imperiale > ⚥
Angelo Caroli > 2018 > Tabacco & Vanilla > ⚥
Anna Dello Russo > 2010 > The Scent of Anna Dello Russo > ♀

Anna Paghera > 2017 > Azzurro d'Ibla > ♀
Anna Paghera > 2017 > Bianco Ninive > ♀
Anna Paghera > 2017 > Blu d'Arabia > ♀
Anna Paghera > 2017 > Giallo di Tebe > ♀
Anna Paghera > 2018 > Arancio di Tangeri > ♀
Anna Paghera > 2018 > Turchese di Nila > ♀
Anna Paghera > 2019 > Rosso di Cipro > ♀
Anna Paghera > 2019 > Verde di Kent > ♀
Antica Barberia Colla > 2015 > Colonia N. 0 > ♂
Antica Barberia Colla > 2015 > Colonia N. 1 > ♂
Antica Barberia Colla > 2015 > Colonia N. 4 > ♂
Antica Barberia Colla > 2015 > Colonia N. 9 > ♂
Antica Erboristeria e Spezieria San Simone > 2017 > Via Maggio > ♀
Antica Erboristeria e Spezieria San Simone > 2017 > Via Pian dei Giullari > ♂
Antica Erboristeria e Spezieria San Simone > 2017 > Via Torta > ♀
Antica Erboristeria e Spezieria San Simone > 2018 > Via dei Bastioni > ♂
Antica Erboristeria e Spezieria San Simone > 2018 > Via dei Calzaiuoli > ⚥
Antica Erboristeria e Spezieria San Simone > 2018 > Via dei Tornabuoni > ♂
Antica Erboristeria e Spezieria San Simone > 2018 > Via della Vigna > ⚥
Antica Erboristeria e Spezieria San Simone > 2019 > Via della Ninna > ⚥
Antiqua Firenze > 2017 > Antiqua > ♀
Antiqua Firenze > 2017 > Dea Sutra > ♀
Antiqua Firenze > 2017 > Fico Fiorentino > ⚥
Antiqua Firenze > 2017 > Miss Tuberosa > ♀
Antiqua Firenze > 2017 > Notturno di Rosa > ♀
Antiqua Firenze > 2017 > Oasi di Agrumi > ⚥
Antiqua Firenze > 2017 > Presente & Futuro > ♀
Antiqua Firenze > 2017 > Sogno a Firenze > ⚥
Antiqua Firenze > 2017 > Stella di Mare > ♀
Antiqua Firenze > 2019 > Emozioni > ♀
Antonio Alessandria > 2014 > Nacre Blanche > ♀
Antonio Alessandria > 2014 > Noir Obscur > ⚥
Antonio Alessandria > 2014 > Nuit Rouge > ♀
Antonio Alessandria > 2015 > Fleurs et Flammes > ♀
Antonio Alessandria > 2016 > Eperdument > ♀
Antonio Alessandria > 2017 > Gattopardo > ♀
Antonio Alessandria > 2018 > Fara > ♀
Antonio Alessandria > 2019 > Dies Aurorae > ♀
Antonio Croce > 2017 > Ardente > ♀
Antonio Croce > 2017 > Incantevole > ♀
Antonio Croce > 2017 > Meraviglia > ♀
Antonio Croce > 2017 > Perfetta > ♀
Antonio Croce > 2017 > Sofisticata > ♀
Antonio Croce > 2017 > Straordinaria > ♀
Antonio Croce > 2017 > Unica > ♀
Antonio De Curtis > 2007 > Antonio De Curtis > ♂
Antonio De Curtis > 2009 > Malafemmena > ♀
Antonio De Curtis > 2015 > Principe > ♂
Antonio Fusco > 2005 > Antonio Fusco > ♀
Antonio Fusco > 2005 > Uomo > ♂
Antonio Visconti > 1975 > Coeur de Vanille > ♀
Antonio Visconti > 2005 > Akaba > ♀
Antonio Visconti > 2010 > Alhambra > ♀
Antonio Visconti > 2010 > Bal Masqué > ♀
Antonio Visconti > 2010 > Black Tear > ♀
Antonio Visconti > 2010 > Bois de Gayac > ♂
Antonio Visconti > 2010 > Clair de Lune > ♀
Antonio Visconti > 2010 > Esprit Libre > ♀
Antonio Visconti > 2010 > Extrait de Cedrat > ♀
Antonio Visconti > 2010 > Fleur de Lys > ♀
Antonio Visconti > 2010 > Fleur de Nuit > ♀
Antonio Visconti > 2010 > Fleur et Feuille de Jasmin > ♀
Antonio Visconti > 2010 > Glam Flower > ♀
Antonio Visconti > 2010 > Juicy Flower > ♀
Antonio Visconti > 2010 > La Divina Tubereuse > ♀
Antonio Visconti > 2010 > Le Sens du Plaisir > ♀
Antonio Visconti > 2010 > Musk de Roi > ♀
Antonio Visconti > 2010 > Rebel > ♀
Antonio Visconti > 2010 > Rose Sauvage > ♀
Antonio Visconti > 2010 > Rose Supreme > ♀
Antonio Visconti > 2010 > Sea Island > ♀
Antonio Visconti > 2010 > Silver Wood > ♀
Antonio Visconti > 2010 > Soir de Mer > ♀
Antonio Visconti > 2010 > Tabarom > ♂
Antonio Visconti > 2010 > Temps d'hiver > ♀
Antonio Visconti > 2010 > Terre de Feu > ♀
Antonio Visconti > 2015 > Foliage > ♀
Antonio Visconti > 2015 > Oud Maharaji > ♀
Antonio Visconti > 2015 > Oud Mohave > ♀
Antonio Visconti > 2015 > Oud Nomade > ♀
Anucci > 1989 > Anucci Men > ♂
Anucci > 1990 > Anucci Femme > ♀

Anucci > 1990 > Dalini > ♀
Aqua di Jesolo > 2014 > Lungomare > ♂
Aqua di Jesolo > 2014 > Rosso Veneziano > ♀
Aqua di Jesolo > 2014 > Voglio Vivere Così > ♀
Aqua di Ponza > 2009 > Aqua di Ponza > ♀
Aqua di Ponza > 2015 > Aqua di Ponza Profumo > ♀
Aqua Flor > 2016 > Meltemi > ♀
Aqua Flor > 2017 > Orphyca > ♀
Aqua Flor > 2017 > Aenigma > ♀
Aqua Flor > 2017 > Ambra > ♀
Aqua Flor > 2017 > Aoud > ♀
Aqua Flor > 2017 > Aphrodisya > ♀
Aqua Flor > 2017 > Azar > ♀
Aqua Flor > 2017 > Bakarika > ♀
Aqua Flor > 2017 > Bakhur > ♀
Aqua Flor > 2017 > Beirout > ♀
Aqua Flor > 2017 > Belladonna > ♀
Aqua Flor > 2017 > Berbere > ♀
Aqua Flor > 2017 > Bergamotto di Calabria > ♀
Aqua Flor > 2017 > Brisas > ♀
Aqua Flor > 2017 > CD > ♀
Aqua Flor > 2017 > Derwish > ♀
Aqua Flor > 2017 > Don > ♂
Aqua Flor > 2017 > Empereur > ♂
Aqua Flor > 2017 > Flamboyant > ♀
Aqua Flor > 2017 > Frenesia > ♀
Aqua Flor > 2017 > Hussar > ♀
Aqua Flor > 2017 > Jalousie > ♀
Aqua Flor > 2017 > Jasmin > ♀
Aqua Flor > 2017 > Kale > ♀
Aqua Flor > 2017 > Kodo > ♀
Aqua Flor > 2017 > La Habana > ♀
Aqua Flor > 2017 > Mediterranea > ♀
Aqua Flor > 2017 > Mistura > ♀
Aqua Flor > 2017 > Monna Lisa > ♀
Aqua Flor > 2017 > Myrrah > ♀
Aqua Flor > 2017 > Oltremare > ♀
Aqua Flor > 2017 > Rais > ♀
Aqua Flor > 2017 > Rosa Damascena > ♀
Aqua Flor > 2017 > Rosae > ♀
Aqua Flor > 2017 > Rugiada > ♀
Aqua Flor > 2017 > Spleen > ♀
Aqua Flor > 2017 > Sultan > ♀
Aqua Flor > 2017 > Tzigana > ♀
Aqua Flor > 2017 > Zagaria > ♀
Aqua Flor > 2108 > Pathos > ♀
Aquolina > 2004 > Arancia e Vaniglia > ♀
Aquolina > 2004 > Bignè Orchidea e Cioccolato Bianco > ♀
Aquolina > 2004 > Cioccolato Bianco > ♀
Aquolina > 2004 > Cocco > ♀
Aquolina > 2004 > Crema alla Violetta > ♀
Aquolina > 2004 > Fragolina di Bosco > ♀
Aquolina > 2004 > Latte di Mandorla > ♀
Aquolina > 2004 > Liquirizia e Mora > ♀
Aquolina > 2004 > Mango Fresco > ♀
Aquolina > 2004 > More e Musk > ♀
Aquolina > 2004 > Mousse ai Fiori di Vaniglia > ♀
Aquolina > 2004 > Pesca e Albicocca > ♀
Aquolina > 2004 > Pink Sugar > ♀
Aquolina > 2004 > Sfogliatella alla Mimosa > ♀
Aquolina > 2004 > Succo di Lampone > ♀
Aquolina > 2004 > The Verde > ♀
Aquolina > 2004 > Vaniglia > ♀
Aquolina > 2004 > Vaniglia e Anice > ♀
Aquolina > 2004 > Zucchero a Velo > ♀
Aquolina > 2006 > Blue Sugar > ♀
Aquolina > 2006 > Chocolovers > ♀
Aquolina > 2008 > Tweety > ♀
Aquolina > 2009 > Pink Sugar Luxury Extract > ♀
Aquolina > 2009 > Pink Sugar Sensual > ♀
Aquolina > 2012 > Pink Sugar Sparks > ♀
Aquolina > 2013 > Black Sugar > ♀
Aquolina > 2013 > Gold Sugar > ♀
Aquolina > 2013 > Simply Pink > ♀
Aquolina > 2013 > Steel Sugar > ♀
Aquolina > 2015 > Pasticcino alla Rosa glassata > ♀
Aquolina > 2015 > Pink Flower > ♀
Aquolina > 2017 > Luna Park > ♀
Aquolina > 2018 > Sweet Me > ♀
Araxi Parfum > 2019 > Araxi Parfum > ♀
Araxi Parfum > 2019 > Mora > ♀
Araxi Parfum > 2019 > Moro > ♀

Arrogance > 1981 > Arrogance pour Femme > ♀
Arrogance > 1982 > Arrogance pour Homme > ♂
Arrogance > 1983 > Arrogance Uomo > ♂
Arrogance > 2002 > Arrogance pour Elle > ♀
Arrogance > 2003 > Arrogance Man > ♂
Arrogance > 2004 > Glamour > ♀
Arrogance > 2005 > Arrogance Mix Lime, Zucchero > ♀
Arrogance > 2005 > Arrogance Mix Litchi, Mandorla > ♀
Arrogance > 2005 > Arrogance Mix Melograno, Vite > ♀
Arrogance > 2005 > Arrogance Mix Muschio Bianco, Mela > ♀
Arrogance > 2005 > Arrogance Mix Vaniglia, Papaya > ♀
Arrogance > 2006 > Gelsomino Jasmine > ♀
Arrogance > 2007 > Arrogance Poudre pour Femme > ♀
Arrogance > 2008 > Angelique Arrogance > ♀
Arrogance > 2010 > Arrogance Les Perfumes Absolute de Mate > ♀
Arrogance > 2010 > Arrogance Les Perfumes Fleur de Crystal > ♀
Arrogance > 2010 > Arrogance Les Perfumes Heliotrophine > ♀
Arrogance > 2011 > Blue Straps > ♂
Arrogance > 2015 > Arrogance Passion > ♀
Ars Mirabile > 2016 > Alma Bianca > ♀
Ars Mirabile > 2016 > Alma Nera > ♀
Ars Mirabile > 2016 > Canto dell'Angelo > ♀
Ars Mirabile > 2016 > Filtro d'Amore > ♀
Ars Mirabile > 2016 > Lato Oscuro > ♀
Ars Mirabile > 2016 > Oblio dei Sensi > ♀
Arshia Parfums > 2015 > Babel Bourbon > ♀
Arshia Parfums > 2015 > Kashan Rosé > ♀
Arshia Parfums > 2015 > Persepolis Ambré > ♀
Arshia Parfums > 2017 > Golden Taif > ♀
Art Landi Profumi > 2014 > Art 01 Acqua Mia > ♀
Art Landi Profumi > 2014 > Art 02 Voglie di Mare > ♀
Art Landi Profumi > 2014 > Art 03 Legni Dolci Bruciati > ♀
Art Landi Profumi > 2014 > Art 04 Il Solo e L'unico legno > ♀
Art Landi Profumi > 2014 > Art 05 Cocktail di Frutta Esotica >
Art Landi Profumi > 2014 > Art 06 Esotico Assoluto > ♀
Art Landi Profumi > 2014 > Art 07 Rosa del Deserto > ♀
Art Landi Profumi > 2017 > Art 08 Muschio di Liatride > ♀
Art Landi Profumi > 2017 > Art 09 Karo Karounde > ♀
Art Landi Profumi > 2019 > Art 10 Vetiver Weeds (Belin Che Cana) > ♀
Arte Profumi > 2013 > A'mare > ♀
Arte Profumi > 2013 > Bohèmien > ♀
Arte Profumi > 2013 > Ecclesiae > ♀
Arte Profumi > 2013 > Fumoir > ♀
Arte Profumi > 2013 > Harem Soirée > ♀
Arte Profumi > 2013 > Mitti > ♀
Arte Profumi > 2013 > O-Furo > ♀
Arte Profumi > 2013 > Pomelo > ♀
Arte Profumi > 2013 > Secret > ♀
Arte Profumi > 2013 > Sucre Noir > ♀
Arte Profumi > 2013 > Velvet Rouge > ♀
Arte Profumi > 2015 > Bois Sacre > ♀
Arte Profumi > 2015 > Jardin de Giverny > ♀
Arte Profumi > 2015 > Tribal > ♀
Arte Profumi > 2016 > Artissima > ♀
Arte Profumi > 2016 > Carpe Diem > ♀
Arte Profumi > 2016 > Giallo Riviera > ♀
Arte Profumi > 2016 > Racconti di Viaggio > ♀
Arte Profumi > 2017 > Figomoro > ♀
Arte Profumi > 2017 > Samharam > ♀
Arte Profumi > 2018 > Attar Davana > ♀
Arte Profumi > 2018 > Habanera > ♀
Arte Profumi > 2018 > Sine Tempore > ♀
Arteolfatto > 2013 > Black Hashish > ♀
Arteolfatto > 2013 > Bois Precious > ♀
Arteolfatto > 2013 > Brise Marine > ♀
Arteolfatto > 2013 > Habano Vanilla > ♀
Arteolfatto > 2013 > Vanesya > ♀
Arteolfatto > 2013 > Wild Orchid > ♀
Arteolfatto > 2015 > Oud Khasian > ♀
Arteolfatto > 2015 > Paropamiso > ♀
Arteolfatto > 2015 > Avenue Imperial > ♀
Arteolfatto > 2015 > Biancofiore > ♀
Arteolfatto > 2015 > Bois Tendre > ♀
Arteolfatto > 2015 > Eau Epices > ♀
Arteolfatto > 2015 > Giuggiola > ♀
Arteolfatto > 2015 > Gorgeous > ♀
Arteolfatto > 2015 > Jardin Afghan > ♀
Arteolfatto > 2015 > La Savina > ♀
Arteolfatto > 2015 > Oud > ♀
Arteolfatto > 2015 > Patchoulystan > ♀
Arteolfatto > 2015 > Purple Orchid > ♀
Arteolfatto > 2015 > Very Musk > ♀

Arteolfatto > 2017 > Ambre Delicieuse > ♀
Arteolfatto > 2017 > Sine More > ♀
Arteolfatto > 2018 > Tuberose Vanilla > ♀
Arteolfatto > 2019 > Vetiverve > ♀
Aulentissima > 2017 > Amande > ♀
Aulentissima > 2017 > Jardin de Marrakesh > ♀
Aulentissima > 2017 > The Queen of all Waters > ♀
Aulentissima > 2017 > Tupinambà > ♀
Automobili Lamborghini > 2014 > L1 > ♂
Automobili Lamborghini > 2015 > L2 > ♂
Automobili Lamborghini > 2015 > L3 > ♂
Automobili Lamborghini > 2015 > L4 > ♂
Automobili Lamborghini > 2018 > Urus > ♀
Avery > 2017 > A > ♀
Avery > 2017 > E > ♀
Avery > 2017 > R > ♀
Avery > 2017 > V > ♀
Avery > 2017 > Y > ♀
Avery > 2018 > Amour Bakhoor > ♀
Avery > 2018 > Chypre Elixir > ♀
Avery > 2018 > Cuir Touch > ♀
Avery > 2018 > Musk Melange > ♀
Avery > 2018 > Noisy Noisette > ♀
Avery > 2018 > Twist de Bois > ♀
Avery > 2018 > Why Not > ♀
Avery > 2019 > Peep pour Toi > ♀
Avery > 2019 > Sunday Sorbet > ♀
Avery > 2019 > Vanille Bakery > ♀
Baldi > 2013 > Ametista > ♀
Baldi > 2013 > Lapislazzuli > ♀
Baldi > 2013 > Malachite > ♀
Baldi > 2013 > Occhio di Tigre > ♀
Baldinini > 2008 > Baldinini > ♀
Baldinini > 2008 > Baldinini Man > ♂
Baldinini > 2009 > Baldinini de Nuit > ♀
Baldinini > 2009 > Baldinini Parfum Glace > ♀
Baldinini > 2010 > Gimmy > ♀
Baldinini > 2010 > Or Noir > ♀
Baldinini > 2014 > Baldinini for Man > ♂
Baldinini > 2014 > Baldinini for Woman > ♀
Baldinini > 2015 > Or Pur > ♀
Baldinini > 2017 > Amber Straps > ♀
Baldinini > 2017 > Blue Straps > ♀
Baldinini > 2017 > Emerald Straps > ♀
Baldinini > 2017 > Pink Straps > ♀
Baldinini > 2017 > Yellow Straps > ♀
Bamotte > 2014 > Deliziare > ♀
Bamotte > 2014 > Frizzante > ♀
Bamotte > 2014 > Incantare > ♀
Bamotte > 2014 > Sentimento > ♀
Bamotte > 2014 > Tentazione > ♀
Bamotte > 2014 > Tesoro > ♀
Baratti > 2007 > Want a Summer Cocktail? > ♀
Basile > 1986 > Basile > ♀
Basile > 1987 > Basile Uomo > ♂
Basile > 1989 > Uomo Forte >
Basile > 2000 > Basile Young > ♀
Basile > 2000 > Basile Young Uomo > ♂
Basile > 2003 > Femme > ♀
Basile > 2003 > Homme > ♂
Basile > 2010 > Basile Style Femme > ♀
Basile > 2010 > Basile Style Homme > ♂
Basile > 2016 > Basile Donna Red Woman > ♀
Basile > 2016 > Basile Uomo Blue Square > ♂
Basile > 2016 > Basile Uomo Green Square > ♂
Battistoni > 1986 > Marta > ♀
Battistoni > 1986 > Marte > ♂
Battistoni > 1990 > Classico > ♂
Battistoni > 1990 > Marte Concentrée > ♂
Battistoni > 1994 > Etherea > ♀
Battistoni > 1996 > Idea > ♀
Battistoni > 1997 > Marte 61 > ♂
Battistoni > 2000 > Black Tie > ♂
Battistoni > 2000 > Creation Donna > ♀
Battistoni > 2000 > Creation Uomo > ♂
Battistoni > 2010 > Marte Ii > ♀
Battistoni > 2010 > Marterosso > ♂
Battistoni > 2011 > Fantasy Flower in Pink > ♀
Battistoni > 2011 > Fantasy Flower in Yellow > ♀
Battistoni > 2012 > Marte Evolution > ♀
Battistoni > 2015 > Le Gemme Rubino > ♀
Battistoni > 2015 > Le Gemme Smeraldo > ♀

Battistoni > 2015 > Le Gemme Zaffiro > ♀
Battistoni > 2015 > Marte Collezione Privata Arancio & Vaniglia > ♂
Battistoni > 2015 > Marte Collezione Privata Bergamotto & Legno di Cedro > ♂
Battistoni > 2015 > Marte Collezione Privata Cuoio & Patchouly > ♂
Battistoni > 2015 > Marte Collezione Privata Pepe & Vetiver > ♂
Battistoni > 2015 > Marte Collezione Privata Zenzero & Sandalo > ♂
Battistoni > 2015 > Mighty > ♂
Battistoni > 2016 > Marte Red Planet > ♂
B&B Cosmetics > 2018 > Delirivm > ♀
B&B Cosmetics > 2019 > 909 Nine o Nine Woman > ♀
Benetton > 1987 > Colors de Benetton > ♂
Benetton > 1988 > Colors de Benetton Man > ♂
Benetton > 1993 > Tribù > ♀
Benetton > 1995 > Tribù Acqua Fresca > ♀
Benetton > 1997 > Benetton Cold > ♀
Benetton > 1997 > Benetton Hot > ♂
Benetton > 1997 > Cold > ♀
Benetton > 1997 > Hot > ♂
Benetton > 1999 > Benetton Pure Sport Men > ♂
Benetton > 1999 > Benetton Pure Sport Women > ♀
Benetton > 1999 > Pure Sport > ♂
Benetton > 1999 > Pure Sport > ♀
Benetton > 2000 > Benetton Sport Man > ♂
Benetton > 2000 > Benetton Sport Women > ♀
Benetton > 2000 > Funtastic Sweet Fruits for Girls > ♀
Benetton > 2000 > Funtastic Wild Citrus for Boys > ♂
Benetton > 2001 > Paradiso Inferno Blue > ♂
Benetton > 2001 > Paradiso Inferno Man > ♂
Benetton > 2001 > Paradiso Inferno Woman > ♀
Benetton > 2002 > B.clean Energy > ♂
Benetton > 2002 > B.clean Fresh > ♂
Benetton > 2002 > B.clean Relax > ♀
Benetton > 2002 > B.clean Soft > ♀
Benetton > 2003 > On Benny's Farm > ♀
Benetton > 2004 > B.united Man > ♂
Benetton > 2004 > B.united Woman > ♀
Benetton > 2004 > Paradiso Inferno Pink > ♀
Benetton > 2005 > Cumbia Colors Man > ♂
Benetton > 2005 > Cumbia Colors Woman > ♀
Benetton > 2005 > Stimulating Aqua > ♀
Benetton > 2006 > Gold > ♀
Benetton > 2006 > United Colors of Benetton Man > ♂
Benetton > 2006 > United Colors of Benetton Unisex > ♂
Benetton > 2006 > United Colors of Benetton Woman > ♀
Benetton > 2007 > B.united Jeans Man > ♂
Benetton > 2007 > B.united Jeans Woman > ♀
Benetton > 2008 > Benetton White Night Man > ♂
Benetton > 2008 > Benetton White Night Woman > ♀
Benetton > 2008 > Energy Games > ♂
Benetton > 2008 > Energy Man > ♂
Benetton > 2008 > Energy Pop > ♀
Benetton > 2008 > Energy Pop > ♂
Benetton > 2008 > Energy Woman > ♂
Benetton > 2008 > Essence of United Colors of Benetton Man > ♂
Benetton > 2008 > Essence of United Colors of Benetton Woman > ♀
Benetton > 2008 > Silver Man > ♂
Benetton > 2010 > Benetton Blu Man > ♂
Benetton > 2010 > Benetton Giallo Woman > ♀
Benetton > 2010 > Benetton Rosso Woman > ♀
Benetton > 2010 > Benetton Verde Man > ♂
Benetton > 2011 > Benetton Bianco > ♀
Benetton > 2011 > Benetton Nero > ♂
Benetton > 2011 > Nero > ♂
Benetton > 2012 > Cold Silver > ♂
Benetton > 2012 > Hot Gold > ♀
Benetton > 2012 > Let's Love > ♀
Benetton > 2012 > Let's Move > ♂
Benetton > 2013 > Appealing Lily > ♀
Benetton > 2013 > Let's Fly > ♀
Benetton > 2014 > United Dreams: Live Free > ♀
Benetton > 2014 > United Dreams: Love Yourself > ♀
Benetton > 2014 > United Dreams: Stay Positive > ♀
Benetton > 2015 > United Dreams: Aim High > ♂
Benetton > 2015 > United Dreams: Be Strong > ♂
Benetton > 2015 > United Dreams: Go Far > ♂
Benetton > 2015 > United Dreams: Open your Mind > ♀
Benetton > 2016 > Colors de Benetton Blue > ♂
Benetton > 2016 > Colors de Benetton Pink > ♀
Benetton > 2016 > United Dreams: Dream Big > ♂
Benetton > 2016 > United Dreams: Dream Big > ♀
Benetton > 2016 > United Dreams: Just United > ♀

Benetton > 2016 > United Dreams: Just United > ♂
Benetton > 2017 > Colors de Benetton Purple > ♂
Benetton > 2017 > United Dreams: Love Yourself > ♀
Benetton > 2017 > United Dreams: One Love > ♂
Benetton > 2017 > United Dreams: One Summer > ♀
Benetton > 2018 > Colors de Benetton Green > ♂
Benetton > 2019 > Colors de Benetton Black > ♂
Benetton > 2019 > Colors de Benetton Rose > ♀
Benetton > 2019 > Colors Man Black > ♂
Benetton > 2019 > United Dreams: Together for Her > ♀
Benetton > 2019 > United Dreams: Together for Him > ♂
Best Company > 1990 > Donna > ♀
Best Company > 1999 > Uomo > ♂
BK Perfume > 2018 > BK pour Femme > ♀
BK Perfume > 2018 > BK pour Homme > ♂
Blancheide > 2016 > Au Jour d'hui > ♂
Blancheide > 2016 > Bois Sauvage > ♂
Blancheide > 2016 > Cacao > ♂
Blancheide > 2016 > Ebano > ♂
Blancheide > 2016 > Jamboree > ♂
Blancheide > 2016 > Joa > ♂
Blancheide > 2016 > Le Supreme Patchouly > ♂
Blancheide > 2016 > Mae > ♂
Blancheide > 2016 > Makali > ♂
Blancheide > 2016 > Musc > ♂
Blancheide > 2016 > Rose > ♂
Blancheide > 2016 > Vanille > ♂
Blauer > 2018 > Uni1t3d Man > ♂
Blauer > 2018 > Uni1t3d Woman > ♀
Blauer > 2019 > Blauer Uni1t3d States Man > ♂
Blauer > 2019 > Blauer Uni1t3d States Woman > ♀
Blood Concept > 2011 > 0 > ♂
Blood Concept > 2011 > A > ♂
Blood Concept > 2011 > AB > ♂
Blood Concept > 2011 > B > ♂
Blood Concept > 2012 > +Ma > ♂
Blood Concept > 2012 > Red+Ma > ♂
Blood Concept > 2013 > Black Collection 0 > ♂
Blood Concept > 2013 > Black Collection A > ♂
Blood Concept > 2013 > Black Collection AB > ♂
Blood Concept > 2013 > Black Collection B > ♂
Blood Concept > 2015 > O Absolute Suede > ♂
Blood Concept > 2015 > O Cruel Incense > ♂
Blood Concept > 2015 > A Green Cachemire > ♂
Blood Concept > 2015 > A Killer Vanilla > ♂
Blood Concept > 2015 > AB Liquid Spice > ♂
Blood Concept > 2015 > AB Tokyo Musk > ♂
Blood Concept > 2015 > B Magic Amber > ♂
Blood Concept > 2015 > B Wonder Tonka > ♂
Blood Concept > 2015 > PH Bright Oud > ♂
Blood Concept > 2015 > XI Oxygen Vert > ♂
Blood Concept > 2016 > XX Metro Velvet > ♂
Blood Concept > 2016 > XY Nude Wood > ♂
Blumarine > 1988 > Blumarine > ♀
Blumarine > 1996 > Blu > ♀
Blumarine > 2000 > Blumarine II > ♀
Blumarine > 2004 > Vintage > ♀
Blumarine > 2009 > Bellissima > ♀
Blumarine > 2010 > Bellissima Parfum Intense > ♀
Blumarine > 2010 > Jus N. 1 Blugirl > ♀
Blumarine > 2011 > Bellissima Acqua di Primavera > ♀
Blumarine > 2011 > Blugirl Jus de Fleurs > ♀
Blumarine > 2012 > Innamorata > ♀
Blumarine > 2013 > Innamorata Lovely Rose > ♀
Blumarine > 2014 > Anna > ♀
Blumarine > 2015 > Ninfea > ♀
Blumarine > 2016 > Blumarine Rosa > ♀
Blumarine > 2017 > Dange-Rose > ♀
Blumarine > 2019 > B. Blumarine > ♀
Boellis > 2010 > Panama 1924: Millesimé > ♂
Boellis > 2010 > Panama 1924: Millesimé 150 Italia > ♂
Boellis > 2011 > Amaryllis Bianco > ♂
Boellis > 2011 > Panama 1924: Femme > ♀
Boellis > 2012 > Sport of Panama > ♂
Boellis > 2013 > Panama 1924: Daytona > ♂
Boellis > 2014 > Chiaia 9 > ♂
Boellis > 2014 > Condotti > ♂
Boellis > 2014 > Spiga > ♂
Boellis > 2015 > Panama 1924: Fefé (Dandy Napoletano) > ♂
Boellis > 2015 > Women of Panama > ♀
Boellis > 2017 > Panama 1924: Sport > ♂
Boellis > 2018 > Espresso Napoletano > ♂

Boellis > 2018 > Fiore di Mandorlo di Sicilia > ⚥
Boellis > 2018 > Iris di Capri > ⚥
Boellis > 2018 > Mandorlo e Cedro di Calabria > ⚥
Boellis > 2018 > Panama 1924: 2.0 > ♂
Boellis > 2020 > Panama 1924: Rosso > ♀
Bogue > 2012 > Castello > ⚥
Bogue > 2012 > Eau D'E > ⚥
Bogue > 2012 > Piazza Arnaldo > ⚥
Bogue > 2012 > Piazza Duomo > ⚥
Bogue > 2012 > Piazza Garibaldi > ⚥
Bogue > 2012 > Piazza Mercato > ⚥
Bogue > 2013 > Cologne Reloaded > ⚥
Bogue > 2014 > Ker > ⚥
Bogue > 2014 > Maai > ⚥
Bogue > 2015 > Oe > ⚥
Bogue > 2016 > Cadavre Exquis > ⚥
Bogue > 2016 > Gardelia > ⚥
Bogue > 2017 > Mem > ⚥
Bogue > 2018 > Noun > ⚥
Bogue > 2019 > 7738 > ⚥
Bogue > 2019 > Doleur > ⚥
Bogue > 2019 > I Love YV > ⚥
Bogue > 2019 > Il Dieci X > ⚥
Bois 1920 > 2004 > Verde di Mare > ⚥
Bois 1920 > 2005 > 1920 Extreme > ⚥
Bois 1920 > 2005 > Agrumi Amari di Sicilia > ⚥
Bois 1920 > 2005 > Classic 1920 > ⚥
Bois 1920 > 2005 > Rael Patchouly > ⚥
Bois 1920 > 2005 > Sandalo e Thé > ⚥
Bois 1920 > 2005 > Sushi Imperiale > ⚥
Bois 1920 > 2005 > Sutra Ylang > ⚥
Bois 1920 > 2005 > Vetiver Ambrato > ⚥
Bois 1920 > 2008 > Come la Luna > ♀
Bois 1920 > 2008 > Vento di Fiori > ♀
Bois 1920 > 2010 > Le Voluttuose Kimono Rosé > ♀
Bois 1920 > 2010 > Le Voluttuose La Vaniglia > ♀
Bois 1920 > 2010 > Le Voluttuose Notturno Fiorentino > ♀
Bois 1920 > 2011 > Come L'amore > ♀
Bois 1920 > 2011 > Oltremare > ⚥
Bois 1920 > 2012 > Le Voluttuose Rosa di Filare > ♀
Bois 1920 > 2013 > Dolce di Giorno > ⚥
Bois 1920 > 2013 > Oro 1920 > ♀
Bois 1920 > 2013 > Relativamente Rosso > ⚥
Bois 1920 > 2013 > Sensual Tuberose > ⚥
Bois 1920 > 2013 > Vento nel Vento > ⚥
Bois 1920 > 2014 > Aethereus > ⚥
Bois 1920 > 2014 > Spigo 1920 > ⚥
Bois 1920 > 2015 > Come Il Sole > ⚥
Bois 1920 > 2015 > Itruk > ⚥
Bois 1920 > 2015 > Nagud > ⚥
Bois 1920 > 2016 > Ancora Amore > ⚥
Bois 1920 > 2016 > Magia > ⚥
Bois 1920 > 2016 > Rosa 23 > ♀
Bois 1920 > 2016 > Virtù > ⚥
Bois 1920 > 2017 > Oro Nero > ⚥
Bois 1920 > 2018 > Parana > ⚥
Bois 1920 > 2018 > Sopra Il Mare > ⚥
Bois 1920 > 2019 > Cannabis > ⚥
Bois 1920 > 2019 > Cannabis Fruttata > ⚥
Bois 1920 > 2019 > Elite I > ⚥
Bois 1920 > 2019 > Elite II > ⚥
Bois 1920 > 2019 > Elite III > ⚥
Bois 1920 > 2019 > Elite V > ⚥
Bois 1920 > 2019 > Insieme > ⚥
Bois 1920 > 2019 > Oro Bianco > ⚥
Bois 1920 > 2019 > Oro Rosso > ⚥
Borbonese > 1993 > Borbonese > ♀
Borghese > 1978 > Di Borghese > ♀
Borghese > 1993 > Il Bacio > ♀
Borghese > 2001 > La Carezza d'amore > ♀
Borotalco > 2008 > Acqua di Borotalco > ⚥
Borsalino > 1984 > Borsalino > ♂
Borsalino > 1994 > L'altro > ♀
Borsalino > 1995 > Donna > ♀
Borsalino > 1997 > Chapeau > ⚥
Borsalino > 2007 > Panama > ♂
Borsalino > 2008 > Borsalino pour Elle > ♀
Borsalino > 2009 > Borsalino pour Elle Fleurie > ♀
Borsalino > 2009 > Cologne Intense > ♂
Borsalino > 2011 > La Vie en Blue > ♂
Borsalino > 2011 > La Vie en Rose > ♀
Borsari > 1970 > Violetta di Parma > ♀

Borsari > 1980 > Bouquet di Violette > ♀
Borsari > 1996 > Acqua Azzurra dei Fiori Bianchi > ⚥
Borsari > 1996 > Acqua delle Terre Rosse > ⚥
Borsari > 1997 > Acqua della Macchia Mediterranea > ⚥
Borsari > 1997 > Finestrella > ♀
Borsari > 2010 > Assenzio > ♂
Borsari > 2010 > Black Calla > ⚥
Borsari > 2010 > Boccioli d'Arancio e Zenzero > ⚥
Borsari > 2010 > Lampone, Fior di Melo e Semi di Cacao > ♀
Borsari > 2010 > Lemongrass e Cassis > ♀
Borsari > 2010 > Mirra E Anice Stellato > ♂
Borsari > 2010 > Neroli, Bamboo e Fior di Loto > ⚥
Borsari > 2010 > Rosa e Pepe > ♀
Bottega del Profumo > 2010 > Piazza delle Cinque Lune > ⚥
Bottega del Profumo > 2010 > Piazza Esedra > ⚥
Bottega del Profumo > 2010 > Via degli Avignonesi > ⚥
Bottega del Profumo > 2010 > Via dei Condotti > ⚥
Bottega del Profumo > 2010 > Via del Corso > ⚥
Bottega del Profumo > 2010 > Via di Campo Marzio > ⚥
Bottega del Profumo > 2010 > Via Frattina > ♀
Bottega del Profumo > 2010 > Via Margutta > ♀
Bottega Profumiera > 2013 > Galantuomo > ♂
Bottega Profumiera > 2013 > Gourmand > ⚥
Bottega Profumiera > 2013 > Mon Jardin > ♀
Bottega Profumiera > 2013 > Polianthes > ♀
Bottega Profumiera > 2013 > Rose Poudre > ♀
Bottega Profumiera > 2013 > Shardana > ⚥
Bottega Profumiera > 2016 > Inflora > ♀
Bottega Veneta > 2011 > Bottega Veneta > ♀
Bottega Veneta > 2013 > Bottega Veneta Eau Légère > ♀
Bottega Veneta > 2013 > Bottega Veneta pour Homme > ♂
Bottega Veneta > 2014 > Bottega Veneta Essence Aromatique > ♀
Bottega Veneta > 2014 > Knot > ♀
Bottega Veneta > 2015 > Bottega Veneta pour Homme Extreme > ♂
Bottega Veneta > 2015 > Knot Eau Florale > ♀
Bottega Veneta > 2016 > Bottega Veneta pour Homme Essence Aromatique > ♂
Bottega Veneta > 2016 > Eau Sensuelle > ♀
Bottega Veneta > 2016 > Parco Palladiano I: Magnolia > ⚥
Bottega Veneta > 2016 > Parco Palladiano II: Cipresso > ⚥
Bottega Veneta > 2016 > Parco Palladiano III: Pera > ⚥
Bottega Veneta > 2016 > Parco Palladiano IV: Azalea > ⚥
Bottega Veneta > 2016 > Parco Palladiano V: Lauro > ⚥
Bottega Veneta > 2016 > Parco Palladiano VI: Rosa > ⚥
Bottega Veneta > 2017 > Bottega Veneta Eau de Velours > ♀
Bottega Veneta > 2017 > Bottega Veneta pour Homme Parfum > ♂
Bottega Veneta > 2017 > Parco Palladiano VII: Lillà > ⚥
Bottega Veneta > 2017 > Parco Palladiano VIII: Neroli > ⚥
Bottega Veneta > 2017 > Parco Palladiano IX: Violetta > ⚥
Bottega Veneta > 2018 > Bottega Veneta L'absolu > ♀
Bottega Veneta > 2018 > Knot Eau Absolue > ♀
Bottega Veneta > 2018 > Parco Palladiano X: Olivo > ⚥
Bottega Veneta > 2018 > Parco Palladiano XI: Castagno > ⚥
Bottega Veneta > 2018 > Parco Palladiano XII: Quercia > ⚥
Bottega Veneta > 2018 > Parco Palladiano XIII: Quadrifoglio > ⚥
Bottega Veneta > 2018 > Parco Palladiano XIV: Melagrana > ⚥
Bottega Veneta > 2018 > Parco Palladiano XV: Salvia Blu > ⚥
Bottega Veneta > 2019 > Illusione for Her > ♀
Bottega Veneta > 2019 > Illusione for Him > ♂
Bottega Verde > 2000 > Abete Argentato > ♂
Bottega Verde > 2000 > Acqua di Bottega Verde N. 1 > ⚥
Bottega Verde > 2000 > Acqua di Bottega Verde N. 2 > ⚥
Bottega Verde > 2000 > Acqua di Bottega Verde N. 3 > ⚥
Bottega Verde > 2000 > Acqua di Bottega Verde N. 4 > ⚥
Bottega Verde > 2000 > Armonia Vellutata > ♀
Bottega Verde > 2000 > Bacio d'Estate > ♀
Bottega Verde > 2000 > Brazilian Soul > ♀
Bottega Verde > 2000 > BV Amour > ♀
Bottega Verde > 2000 > BV Feel > ♀
Bottega Verde > 2000 > BV Girl > ♀
Bottega Verde > 2000 > BV Secret > ♀
Bottega Verde > 2000 > BV Style > ♂
Bottega Verde > 2000 > Cioccolato > ♀
Bottega Verde > 2000 > Dream Collection > ♀
Bottega Verde > 2000 > Eau de Parfum Bijoux > ♀
Bottega Verde > 2000 > Essenza di Sogni > ♀
Bottega Verde > 2000 > Fiori di Ciliegio > ♀
Bottega Verde > 2000 > Iris > ♀
Bottega Verde > 2000 > Lady > ♀
Bottega Verde > 2000 > Lady Noire > ♀
Bottega Verde > 2000 > Le Zuccherose > ♀
Bottega Verde > 2000 > Love > ♂

Bottega Verde > 2000 > Man Original > ♂
Bottega Verde > 2000 > Melodia Esotica > ♀
Bottega Verde > 2000 > Mylla > ♀
Bottega Verde > 2000 > Natural Charme > ♀
Bottega Verde > 2000 > Naturalmente Tu > ♀
Bottega Verde > 2000 > Note per Due > ♂
Bottega Verde > 2000 > Passione Dolce > ♀
Bottega Verde > 2000 > Pepe Nero > ♂
Bottega Verde > 2000 > Rosa Romantica > ♀
Bottega Verde > 2000 > The Verde > ♀
Bottega Verde > 2000 > Uomo – Ambra e Tabacco > ♂
Bottega Verde > 2000 > Uomo – Blu di Spezie > ♂
Bottega Verde > 2000 > Uomo – Legni e Cachemire > ♂
Bottega Verde > 2000 > Uomo – Legno Marino > ♂
Bottega Verde > 2000 > Uomo – The Rosso > ♂
Bottega Verde > 2000 > Vaniglia > ♀
Bottega Verde > 2000 > Vaniglia e Cardamomo > ♀
Bottega Verde > 2000 > Vaniglia e Mirra > ♀
Bottega Verde > 2000 > Vaniglia Nera > ♀
Bottega Verde > 2000 > Violetta della Sera > ♀
Bottega Verde > 2000 > Argan > ♂
Bottega Verde > 2000 > Camelia d'Inverno > ♀
Bottega Verde > 2000 > Cocco > ♀
Bottega Verde > 2000 > Cuore di Fiaba > ♀
Bottega Verde > 2000 > Dahlia Imperiale > ♀
Bottega Verde > 2000 > Iris Bianco > ♀
Bottega Verde > 2000 > Iris dell'Aurora > ♀
Bottega Verde > 2000 > Lady Flower > ♀
Bottega Verde > 2000 > Muschio di BV > ♀
Bottega Verde > 2000 > Note per due energy > ♂
Bottega Verde > 2000 > Orchidea > ♀
Bottega Verde > 2002 > Fashion > ♀
Bottega Verde > 2008 > Momenti di Bottega Verde > ♀
Bottega Verde > 2008 > Man Sport > ♂
Bottega Verde > 2008 > Man Style > ♂
Bottega Verde > 2009 > Bijoux Nuit > ♀
Bottega Verde > 2009 > Dream > ♀
Bottega Verde > 2011 > Lei by Bottega Verde > ♀
Bottega Verde > 2011 > Violetta > ♀
Bottega Verde > 2012 > Summer Chic > ♀
Bottega Verde > 2012 > Giardini Toscani – Fontana delle Muse > ♀
Bottega Verde > 2012 > Giardini Toscani – Frutteto del Sole > ♀
Bottega Verde > 2012 > Giardini Toscani – Passeggiata delle Rose > ♀
Bottega Verde > 2012 > Giardini Toscani – Prato dei Baci > ♀
Bottega Verde > 2012 > Giardini Toscani – Sentiero dei Fiori > ♀
Bottega Verde > 2012 > Giardini Toscani – Vialetto delle Delizie > ♀
Bottega Verde > 2012 > Lei Glam > ♀
Bottega Verde > 2012 > Lei Rouge > ♀
Bottega Verde > 2014 > Ethno Flower > ♀
Bottega Verde > 2014 > Ethno Fruit > ♂
Bottega Verde > 2015 > Giglio Dorato > ♀
Bottega Verde > 2015 > Gioiosa > ♀
Bottega Verde > 2015 > Via del Bacio > ♀
Bottega Verde > 2015 > Via dell'amore > ♀
Bottega Verde > 2015 > Gardenia Reale > ♀
Bottega Verde > 2015 > Gelsomino > ♀
Bottega Verde > 2015 > Magnolia Nera > ♀
Bottega Verde > 2015 > Mughetto > ♀
Bottega Verde > 2015 > Peonia Splendida > ♀
Bottega Verde > 2015 > Pepe Rosa > ♀
Bottega Verde > 2016 > Incanto Marino > ♀
Bottega Verde > 2016 > Petali di Vaniglia > ♀
Bottega Verde > 2016 > Tentazione Marina > ♀
Bottega Verde > 2017 > Gelsomino Notturno > ♀
Bottega Verde > 2017 > Per Lei Eau de Toilette > ♀
Bottega Verde > 2017 > Per Lui Eau de Toilette > ♂
Bottega Verde > 2019 > Tiarè > ♀
Bozzini > 1980 > Bozzini > ♂
Bozzini > 1980 > Lady > ♀
Braccialini > 2008 > Braccialini Women > ♀
Braccialini > 2015 > Braccialini Eau de Parfum pour Femme > ♀
Braccialini > 2016 > Blue Casual > ♀
Braccialini > 2016 > Braccialini Fashion > ♀
Braccialini > 2016 > Cherry Chic > ♀
Braccialini > 2016 > Purple > ♀
Braccialini > 2017 > Glossy Green > ♀
Braccialini > 2018 > Decò > ♀
Breil Milano > 2007 > Breil Milano Fragrance for Man > ♂
Breil Milano > 2007 > Breil Milano Fragrance for Woman > ♀
Breil Milano > 2008 > My Breil > ♀
Breil Milano > 2009 > Complicity for Her > ♀
Breil Milano > 2009 > Complicity for Him > ♂

Brera6 Perfumes > 2008 > Foyer > ♀
Brera6 Perfumes > 2018 > 1848! > ♀
Brera6 Perfumes > 2018 > 60mph Club > ♂
Brera6 Perfumes > 2018 > Hesperia > ♀
Brera6 Perfumes > 2018 > Liberty > ♀
Brera6 Perfumes > 2018 > No-Name > ♂
Brioni > 2009 > Brioni > ♂
Brioni > 2014 > Brioni Eau de Toilette > ♂
Brioni > 2015 > Brioni Extrait > ♂
Brooksfield > 1993 > Brooksfield Men > ♂
Brooksfield > 1996 > Nuance > ♀
Brooksfield > 1998 > Royal Blue > ♂
Brooksfield > 2001 > B. Green > ♂
Brooksfield > 2003 > B5 Woman > ♀
Brooksfield > 2003 > B5 Woman > ♀
Bruno Acampora > 1974 > Blu Perfume Oil > ♀
Bruno Acampora > 1975 > Iranzol Perfume Oil > ♀
Bruno Acampora > 1975 > Musc Perfume Oil > ♀
Bruno Acampora > 1977 > Prima T Perfume Oil > ♀
Bruno Acampora > 1977 > Sballo Perfume Oil > ♀
Bruno Acampora > 1978 > Jasmine Perfume Oil > ♀
Bruno Acampora > 1980 > Seplasia Perfume Oil > ♀
Bruno Acampora > 2011 > Bianco > ♀
Bruno Acampora > 2011 > Nero > ♀
Bruno Acampora > 2012 > Blue Casual > ♀
Bruno Acampora > 2012 > Iranzol > ♀
Bruno Acampora > 2012 > Jasmin T > ♀
Bruno Acampora > 2012 > Musc > ♂
Bruno Acampora > 2012 > Prima T > ♀
Bruno Acampora > 2012 > Sballo > ♀
Bruno Acampora > 2012 > Seplasia > ♀
Bruno Acampora > 2013 > Volubilis > ♀
Bruno Acampora > 2015 > Musc Gold Perfume Oil > ♂
Bruno Acampora > 2016 > Azzurro di Capri > ♀
Bruno Acampora > 2016 > Collie Colonia > ♀
Bruno Acampora > 2016 > Courses Cuir > ♂
Bruno Acampora > 2016 > Egoi Patchouli > ♀
Bruno Acampora > 2016 > Où Oud > ♀
Bruno Acampora > 2016 > Sandan Sandalo > ♂
Bruno Acampora > 2016 > Vanyl Vaniglia > ♀
Bruno Acampora > 2016 > Vert Vetiver > ♀
Bruno Acampora > 2018 > Ruby > ♀
Bruno Acampora > 2019 > Citrea Prochyta > ♂
Bruno Acampora > 2019 > Freak Chic > ♀
Bruno Acampora > 2019 > Keep on Dancing > ♀
Bruno Acampora > 2019 > L'essence Bruno Perfume Oil > ♂
Bruno Acampora > 2019 > Malum > ♀
Bruno Acampora > 2019 > Mentuccia Romana > ♀
Bruno Acampora > 2019 > Read my Mind > ♂
Bruno Acampora > 2019 > Relight my Fire > ♀
Bruno Acampora > 2019 > Robin > ♀
Bruno Acampora > 2019 > Young Hearts > ♀
BSX > 2018 > BSX > ♂
Bugatti > 1999 > Design & Motion > ♂
Bugatti > 2006 > Home > ♀
Bugatti > 2010 > Pureblack > ♂
Bullfrog > 2016 > Secret Potion N. 1 > ♂
Bullfrog > 2016 > Secret Potion N. 2 > ♂
Bullfrog > 2017 > Secret Potion N. 3 > ♂
Bvlgari > 1992 > Eau Parfumée au Thé Vert > ♀
Bvlgari > 1994 > Bvlgari pour Femme > ♀
Bvlgari > 1996 > Bvlgari pour Homme > ♂
Bvlgari > 1996 > Eau Parfumée au Thé Vert Extreme > ♂
Bvlgari > 1997 > Eau Fraiche > ♀
Bvlgari > 1997 > Petits et Mamans > ♀
Bvlgari > 1998 > Black > ♀
Bvlgari > 1999 > Bvlgari Extreme > ♀
Bvlgari > 2000 > BLV > ♀
Bvlgari > 2001 > BLV pour Homme > ♂
Bvlgari > 2002 > BLV Absolute > ♀
Bvlgari > 2003 > Eau Parfumée au Thé Blanc > ♂
Bvlgari > 2003 > Omnia > ♀
Bvlgari > 2004 > BLV Notte pour Femme > ♀
Bvlgari > 2004 > BLV Notte pour Homme > ♀
Bvlgari > 2005 > Aqva pour Homme > ♂
Bvlgari > 2005 > Omnia Crystalline > ♀
Bvlgari > 2006 > Bvlgari pour Homme Soir > ♂
Bvlgari > 2006 > Eau Parfumée au Thé Rouge > ♂
Bvlgari > 2006 > Omnia Amethyste > ♀
Bvlgari > 2006 > Rose Essentiele > ♀
Bvlgari > 2006 > Voile de Jasmin > ♀
Bvlgari > 2007 > Aqva pour Homme Edition Limitée > ♂

Bvlgari > 2007 > Bvlgari Rose Essentielle Edt Rosée > ♀
Bvlgari > 2008 > Aqva pour Homme Marine > ♂
Bvlgari > 2008 > Jasmin Noir > ♀
Bvlgari > 2009 > BLV Eau de Parfum II > ♀
Bvlgari > 2009 > Jasmin Noir Edt > ♀
Bvlgari > 2009 > Omnia Green Jade > ♀
Bvlgari > 2010 > BLV Eau d'Été > ♀
Bvlgari > 2010 > Bvlgari Man > ♂
Bvlgari > 2011 > Aqva pour Homme Marine Toniq > ♂
Bvlgari > 2011 > Aqva pour Homme Toniq > ♂
Bvlgari > 2011 > Bvlgari Man The Silver Limited Edition > ♂
Bvlgari > 2011 > Jasmin Noir L'essence > ♀
Bvlgari > 2011 > Mon Jasmin Noir > ♀
Bvlgari > 2012 > Jasmin Noir L'elixir Edp > ♀
Bvlgari > 2012 > Mon Jasmin Noir L'eau Exquise > ♀
Bvlgari > 2012 > Mon Jasmin Noir L'Elixir Edp > ♀
Bvlgari > 2012 > Omnia Coral > ♀
Bvlgari > 2013 > Bvlgari Man Extreme > ♂
Bvlgari > 2013 > Omnia Crystalline Edp > ♀
Bvlgari > 2014 > Aqva Amara > ♂
Bvlgari > 2014 > Bvlgari Man in Black > ♂
Bvlgari > 2014 > Le Gemme: Amarena > ♀
Bvlgari > 2014 > Le Gemme: Ashlemah > ♀
Bvlgari > 2014 > Le Gemme: Calaluna > ♀
Bvlgari > 2014 > Le Gemme: Lilaia > ♀
Bvlgari > 2014 > Le Gemme: Maravilla > ♀
Bvlgari > 2014 > Le Gemme: Noorah > ♀
Bvlgari > 2014 > Omnia Indian Garnet > ♀
Bvlgari > 2014 > Opera Prima > ♀
Bvlgari > 2015 > Aqva Divina > ♀
Bvlgari > 2015 > Bvlgari Man Extreme All Blacks Limite Edition > ♂
Bvlgari > 2015 > Bvlgari Man in Black All Blacks Limited Edition > ♂
Bvlgari > 2015 > Eau Parfumee au Thé Bleu > ♀
Bvlgari > 2015 > Eau Parfumée au Thé Noir > ⚥
Bvlgari > 2015 > Goldea > ♀
Bvlgari > 2015 > Le Gemme Orientali: Lazulia > ♀
Bvlgari > 2015 > Le Gemme Orientali: Selima > ♀
Bvlgari > 2015 > Le Gemme Orientali: Zahira > ♀
Bvlgari > 2015 > Omnia Paraiba > ♀
Bvlgari > 2016 > Bvlgari Man Black Cologne > ♂
Bvlgari > 2016 > Bvlgari Man Black Orient > ♂
Bvlgari > 2016 > Le Gemme Imperiali: Desiria > ♀
Bvlgari > 2016 > Le Gemme Imperiali: Irina > ♀
Bvlgari > 2016 > Le Gemme Imperiali: Splendia > ♀
Bvlgari > 2016 > Le Gemme Men: Ambero > ♂
Bvlgari > 2016 > Le Gemme Men: Garanat > ♂
Bvlgari > 2016 > Le Gemme Men: Gyan > ♂
Bvlgari > 2016 > Le Gemme Men: Malakeos > ♂
Bvlgari > 2016 > Le Gemme Men: Onekh > ♂
Bvlgari > 2016 > Le Gemme Men: Tygar > ♂
Bvlgari > 2016 > Rose Goldea > ♀
Bvlgari > 2017 > Aqva pour Homme Atlantiqve > ♂
Bvlgari > 2017 > Bvlgari Man in Black Essence > ♂
Bvlgari > 2017 > Goldea the Roman Night > ♀
Bvlgari > 2017 > Splendida Iris d'Or > ♀
Bvlgari > 2017 > Splendida Jasmin Noir > ♀
Bvlgari > 2017 > Splendida Rose Rose > ♀
Bvlgari > 2018 > Bvlgari Man Wood Essence > ♂
Bvlgari > 2018 > Eau Parfumée au Thé Noir Intense > ⚥
Bvlgari > 2018 > Goldea The Roman Night Absolute > ♀
Bvlgari > 2018 > Le Gemme Collezione Murano: Calaluna > ♀
Bvlgari > 2018 > Le Gemme Collezione Murano: Lazulia > ♀
Bvlgari > 2018 > Le Gemme Collezione Murano: Noorah > ♀
Bvlgari > 2018 > Le Gemme Collezione Murano: Noorah > ♀
Bvlgari > 2018 > Le Gemme Collezione Murano: Selima > ♀
Bvlgari > 2018 > Le Gemme Collezione Murano: Zahira > ♀
Bvlgari > 2018 > Le Gemme Reali: Nylaia > ♀
Bvlgari > 2018 > Le Gemme Reali: Rubinia > ♀
Bvlgari > 2018 > Le Gemme Reali: Veridia > ♀
Bvlgari > 2018 > Omnia Pink Sapphire > ♀
Bvlgari > 2018 > Rose Goldea Jacky Tsai Edition > ♀
Bvlgari > 2018 > Splendida Magnolia Sensuel > ♀
Bvlgari > 2019 > Bvlgari Man Wood Neroli > ♂
Bvlgari > 2019 > Le Gemme Men: Falkar > ♂
Bvlgari > 2019 > Le Gemme Men: Opalon > ♂
Bvlgari > 2019 > Le Gemme Men: Yasep > ♂
Bvlgari > 2019 > Le Gemme: Coralia > ♀
Bvlgari > 2019 > Rose Goldea Blossom Delight > ♀
Bvlgari > 2019 > Splendida Tubereuse Mystique > ♀
Bvlgari > 2020 > Omnia Golden Citrine > ♀
Byblos > 1990 > Byblos > ♀
Byblos > 1993 > Byblos Uomo > ♂

Byblos > 1997 > Cielo > ♀
Byblos > 1997 > Fuoco > ♀
Byblos > 1997 > Mare > ♀
Byblos > 1997 > Terra > ♀
Byblos > 1998 > Ghiaccio > ♀
Byblos > 2000 > Brezza > ♀
Byblos > 2000 > Uragano > ♀
Byblos > 2001 > Byblos Uomo 2001 > ♂
Byblos > 2002 > Musk > ♀
Byblos > 2002 > Patchouly > ⚥
Byblos > 2002 > Sandalo > ♀
Byblos > 2003 > Feel Pink > ♀
Byblos > 2004 > Bamboo > ♀
Byblos > 2005 > Blu Man Energy > ♂
Byblos > 2005 > Blu Men Cool > ♂
Byblos > 2005 > Blu Men Enjoy > ♂
Byblos > 2005 > Byblos Woman > ♀
Byblos > 2006 > Blu Happy Hour > ♀
Byblos > 2006 > Blu Light Fever > ♀
Byblos > 2006 > Blu Love Affair > ♀
Byblos > 2006 > Blu Wake Up! > ♀
Byblos > 2006 > Byblos Man > ♂
Byblos > 2007 > Byblos Eater Flower for Women > ♀
Byblos > 2008 > Essence > ♀
Byblos > 2010 > Byblos Passion > ♀
Byblos > 2011 > In Black > ♀
Byblos > 2012 > Miss Byblos > ♀
Byblos > 2013 > Byblos Fusion > ♂
Byblos > 2013 > Miss Byblos Special Edition > ♀
Byblos > 2014 > Butterfly > ♀
Byblos > 2014 > Byblos Luna > ♀
Byblos > 2014 > Byblos Sole > ♀
Byblos > 2017 > Leather Sensation > ♂
Byblos > 2017 > Metal Sensation > ♂
Byblos > 2017 > September Morn > ♀
Calé Fragranze d'Autore > 2008 > Allegro con Brio > ⚥
Calé Fragranze d'Autore > 2008 > Assolo > ⚥
Calé Fragranze d'Autore > 2008 > Brezza di Seta > ♀
Calé Fragranze d'Autore > 2008 > Dolce Riso > ⚥
Calé Fragranze d'Autore > 2008 > Mistero > ⚥
Calé Fragranze d'Autore > 2008 > Ozio > ⚥
Calé Fragranze d'Autore > 2008 > Tepidarium > ⚥
Calé Fragranze d'Autore > 2011 > Fulgor > ⚥
Calé Fragranze d'Autore > 2011 > Roboris > ⚥
Calé Fragranze d'Autore> 2018 > Sottosopra > ⚥
Calé Fragranze d'Autore > 2019 > Libera Mente > ⚥
Calzedonia > 2014 > Fabulous > ♀
Calzedonia > 2014 > In Love > ♀
Calzedonia > 2014 > Lady Rock > ♀
Canali > 2005 > Canali Men > ♂
Canali > 2005 > Summer Night > ♂
Canali > 2007 > Black Diamond > ♂
Canali > 2008 > Canali Men Prestige > ♂
Canali > 2008 > Canali Style > ♂
Canali > 2009 > Canali dal 1934 > ♂
Canali > 2009 > Winter Tale Special Edition > ♂
Carla Fracci > 2003 > Carla Fracci > ♀
Carla Fracci > 2004 > Giselle > ♀
Carla Fracci > 2006 > Medea > ♀
Carla Fracci > 2007 > Salomè > ♀
Carla Fracci > 2008 > Odette > ♀
Carla Fracci > 2009 > Hamlet > ♀
Carla Fracci > 2012 > Aurora > ♀
Carla Fracci > 2014 > Giulietta > ♀
Carlo Colucci > 2002 > Carlo Colucci Uomo > ♂
Carlo Colucci > 2008 > Emozione Uomo > ♂
Carlo Colucci > 2018 > DCCLIIII per L'uomo > ♂
Carlo Colucci > 2018 > DCCLIIII per La Donna > ♀
Carrera > 1988 > Carrera (Original) > ♂
Carrera > 1988 > Carrera Femme > ♀
Carrera > 2000 > Carrera Emotion > ♂
Carrera > 2002 > Carrera Emotion pour Femme > ♀
Carrera > 2005 > Carrera Master > ♂
Carrera Jeans Parfums > 2016 > Carrera Jeans 700 Original Uomo > ♂
Carrera Jeans Parfums > 2016 > Carrera Jeans 770 Original Donna > ♀
Carrera Jeans Parfums > 2019 > Carrera Jeans 707 Camouflage Uomo > ♂
Carrera Jeans Parfums > 2019 > Carrera Jeans 767 Camouflage Donna > ♀
Carthusia – I Profumi di Capri > 1990 > Fiori di Capri > ⚥
Carthusia – I Profumi di Capri > 2000 > Io Capri > ♂
Carthusia – I Profumi di Capri > 2000 > Ligea (La Sirena) > ⚥
Carthusia – I Profumi di Capri > 2003 > Aria di Capri > ♀
Carthusia – I Profumi di Capri > 2003 > Mediterraneo > ⚥

Carthusia – I Profumi di Capri > 2004 > Carthusia Uomo > ♂
Carthusia – I Profumi di Capri > 2006 > Via Camerelle > ♀
Carthusia – I Profumi di Capri > 2007 > Numero Uno > ♀
Carthusia – I Profumi di Capri > 2009 > Caprissimo > ♀
Carthusia – I Profumi di Capri > 2009 > Gelsomini di Capri > ♀
Carthusia – I Profumi di Capri > 2010 > 1681 > ♂
Carthusia – I Profumi di Capri > 2010 > Corallium > ♀
Carthusia – I Profumi di Capri > 2011 > Carthusia Lady > ♀
Carthusia – I Profumi di Capri > 2012 > Capri Forget Me Not > ♀
Carthusia – I Profumi di Capri > 2013 > Prima del Teatro di San Carlo > ♀
Carthusia – I Profumi di Capri > 2014 > Acqua di Carthusia Aloe > ♂
Carthusia – I Profumi di Capri > 2014 > Acqua di Carthusia Bergamotto > ♀
Carthusia – I Profumi di Capri > 2014 > Acqua di Carthusia Geranio > ♀
Carthusia – I Profumi di Capri > 2014 > Acqua di Carthusia Zagara > ♂
Carthusia – I Profumi di Capri > 2015 > Essence of the Park > ♀
Carthusia – I Profumi di Capri > 2017 > Gelsomini di Capri 2017 > ♀
Carthusia – I Profumi di Capri > 2017 > Terra Mia > ♂
Carthusia – I Profumi di Capri > 2019 > Tuberosa > ♀
Castello di Ama > 2014 > Iris Mater > ♀
Castello di Ama > 2019 > Nomen Rosae Absolue > ♀
Cerchi nell'acqua > 2000 > Ambr'ero > ♂
Cerchi nell'acqua > 2000 > Piccolo Amor > ♂
Cerchi nell'acqua > 2000 > Waves > ♂
Cerchi nell'acqua > 2000 > White Out > ♀
Cerchi nell'acqua > 2000 > Armonia > ♂
Cerchi nell'acqua > 2005 > E5 > ♂
Cerchi nell'acqua > 2011 > Isotta > ♀
Cerchi nell'acqua > 2012 > Ipazia > ♀
Cerchi nell'acqua > 2012 > L'Exotique > ♀
Cerchi nell'acqua > 2013 > Emilie > ♀
Cerchi nell'acqua > 2014 > Atelier Marrakech > ♂
Cerchi nell'acqua > 2014 > Peau d'Ange > ♂
Cerchi nell'acqua > 2014 > Raysuli > ♂
Cerchi nell'acqua > 2014 > Usmar Venezia > ♂
Cerchi nell'acqua > 2014 > Visir > ♂
Cerchi nell'acqua > 2014 > Yubris > ♂
Cerchi nell'acqua > 2017 > L'amour Fleuri > ♀
Cerchi nell'acqua > 2017 > Le Bain de Minuit > ♀
Cerchi nell'acqua > 2017 > Syconia > ♂
Cerchi nell'acqua > 2018 > Jolie > ♂
Cerruti > 1979 > Nino Cerruti pour Homme > ♂
Cerruti > 1985 > Fair Play > ♂
Cerruti > 1987 > Nino Cerruti pour Femme > ♀
Cerruti > 1990 > 1881 Men > ♂
Cerruti > 1995 > 1881 > ♀
Cerruti > 1998 > Image > ♂
Cerruti > 2000 > Image Harmony > ♂
Cerruti > 2000 > Image Woman > ♀
Cerruti > 2002 > 1881 Amber pour Homme > ♂
Cerruti > 2003 > Cerruti 1881 Eau d'Été > ♀
Cerruti > 2003 > Cerrutisì > ♂
Cerruti > 2004 > 1881 Cerruti Eau d'Été 2004 > ♀
Cerruti > 2004 > Cerruti 1881 Summer Fragrance pour Homme > ♂
Cerruti > 2005 > Cerruti 1881 Collection > ♀
Cerruti > 2006 > Cerruti 1881 Black > ♀
Cerruti > 2006 > Cerruti 1881 Blanc > ♀
Cerruti > 2007 > Cerruti 1881 Lumieres d'Été > ♀
Cerruti > 2007 > Cerruti pour Homme > ♂
Cerruti > 2008 > Cerruti 1881 en Fleurs > ♀
Cerruti > 2008 > Cerruti 1881 Intense pour Homme > ♂
Cerruti > 2008 > Image Fresh Energy > ♂
Cerruti > 2008 > Cerruti pour Homme Couture Edition > ♂
Cerruti > 2009 > Cerruti 1881 Fraicheur d'Été > ♀
Cerruti > 2009 > L'essence de Cerruti > ♂
Cerruti > 2011 > 1881 Fairplay > ♂
Cerruti > 2012 > Cerruti 1881 Serie Limitée > ♂
Cerruti > 2013 > 1881 Acqua Forte > ♂
Cerruti > 2014 > 1881 Bella Notte Man > ♂
Cerruti > 2014 > 1881 Bella Notte Woman > ♀
Cerruti > 2015 > 1881 Edition Blanche > ♀
Cerruti > 2015 > 1881 Edition Blanche pour Homme > ♂
Cerruti > 2016 > Cerruti 1881 Sport > ♂
Cerruti > 2017 > 1881 Signature > ♂
Cerruti > 2018 > 1881 Essentiel > ♂
Cesare Paciotti > 2011 > Cesare Paciotti for Her > ♀
Cesare Paciotti > 2011 > Cesare Paciotti for Him > ♂
Cesare Paciotti > 2013 > Oriental Supreme for Her > ♀
Cesare Paciotti > 2013 > Oriental Supreme for Him > ♂
Chiara Boni > 1990 > Chiara Boni > ♀
Chiara Boni > 1992 > Vanilla > ♀
Chiara Boni > 1997 > Light > ♀
Chiara Boni > 1997/2001 > Chiara Boni L'uomo > ♂

Chiara Boni > 1998 > Sunshine > ♀
Chiara Boni > 1999 > Fleurs de Chiara Boni > ♀
Chiara Boni > 2001 > Chiara Boni Eau Fleurie > ♀
Chiara Boni > 2002 > White Musk > ♀
Chiara Boni > 2006 > Sensitivity > ♀
Chiara Boni > 2008 > Tango > ♀
Choix > 2018 > Lumière du Désert > ♂
Choix > 2018 > Mon Ami > ♀
Choix > 2018 > Rêve d'Or > ♀
Choix > 2018 > Une Nuit > ♂
Choix > 2018 > Matin d'Été > ♂
Ciatu – Soul of Sicily > 2014 > Ortughia > ♂
Ciatu – Soul of Sicily > 2014 > Taormina Eau de Parfum > ♂
Ciatu – Soul of Sicily > 2014 > Taormina Eau de Toilette > ♂
Ciatu – Soul of Sicily > 2018 > Catania > ♂
Cioccolato Mon Amour > 2007 > Bianco Classico > ♀
Cioccolato Mon Amour > 2007 > Fondente Extra > ♀
Claudia Scattolini > 2016 > Agrums > ♂
Claudia Scattolini > 2016 > Amber > ♂
Claudia Scattolini > 2016 > Marine > ♂
Claudia Scattolini > 2016 > Rose > ♀
Claudia Scattolini > 2016 > Vanilla > ♀
Claudia Scattolini > 2016 > Wild Fig > ♂
Claudia Scattolini > 2016 > Wood & Skin > ♂
Cliven > 2016 > Bengal Tea > ♂
Cliven > 2016 > Mimosa > ♀
Cliven > 2016 > Sicilian Citrus Fruit > ♂
Cliven > 2016 > Tibetan White Moss > ♂
Cliven > 2016 > Violetta > ♀
Cliven > 2018 > Ceylon Cinnamon > ♂
Cliven > 2018 > Japanese Lotus Flowers > ♂
Cliven > 2018 > Lily of The Valley > ♂
Cliven > 2019 > Madagascar Sweet Vanilla > ♂
Collistar > 2001 > Acqua Attiva Assoluta > ♂
Collistar > 2007 > Benessere > ♀
Collistar > 2008 > Benessere dei Sensi > ♀
Collistar > 2009 > Acqua Attiva > ♂
Collistar > 2009 > Benessere Notte > ♀
Collistar > 2011 > Profumo di Felicità > ♀
Collistar > 2012 > Acqua Attiva Ice > ♂
Collistar > 2013 > Acqua Attiva Green > ♂
Collistar > 2014 > Profumo di Armonia > ♀
Collistar > 2015 > Acqua Wood > ♂
Collistar > 2015 > L'Oud > ♂
Collistar > 2016 > L'ambra > ♂
Collistar > 2016 > Profumo dell'amore > ♀
Collistar > 2016 > Vetiver Forte > ♂
Collistar > 2017 > L'incenso > ♂
Collistar > 2017 > La Rosa > ♀
Collistar > 2017 > Profumo dei Sogni > ♀
Collistar > 2018 > La Vaniglia > ♀
Collistar > 2018 > Profumo di Energia > ♂
Como Lake > 2018 > Bacio nella Pioggia > ♀
Como Lake > 2018 > Note d'Amore > ♂
Como Lake > 2018 > Notturno > ♂
Como Lake > 2018 > Silenzio > ♂
Como Lake > 2018 > Un'altra Estate > ♀
Compagnia delle Indie > 2000 > Colonia > ♂
Compagnia delle Indie > 2000 > Donna > ♀
Compagnia delle Indie > 2000 > Uomo > ♂
Compagnia delle Indie > 2000 > Patchouly > ♂
Compagnia delle Indie > 2000 > Sandalo > ♂
Compagnia delle Indie > 2000 > Vetiver > ♂
Compagnia delle Indie > 2009 > Africa Desert Tobacco > ♂
Compagnia delle Indie > 2009 > Asia Ginger Dust > ♂
Compagnia delle Indie > 2009 > Europe Mediterranean Breeze > ♂
Compagnia delle Indie > 2009 > Le Americhe: Caribbean Fruits > ♂
Compagnia delle Indie > 2009 > Oceania: Tiare Blossom > ♀
Compagnia delle Indie > 2012 > Cannella dello Sri Lanka > ♂
Compagnia delle Indie > 2012 > Corallo dell'atollo di Ari > ♂
Compagnia delle Indie > 2012 > Giada della Birmania > ♂
Compagnia delle Indie > 2012 > Indaco di Persia > ♀
Compagnia delle Indie > 2012 > Muschi Bianchi del Tibet > ♀
Compagnia delle Indie > 2012 > Rosa del Deserto di Petra > ♀
Compagnia delle Indie > 2013 > Myrrha dello Yemen > ♂
Compagnia delle Indie > 2013 > Olibano del Siam > ♂
Compagnia delle Indie > 2013 > Topazio Imperiale Di Palmyra > ♂
Compagnia delle Indie > 2013 > Vaniglia del Kerala > ♂
Compagnia delle Indie > 2015 > Donna > ♀
Compagnia delle Indie > 2015 > Original Uomo > ♂
Compagnia delle Indie > 2015 > Wood Uomo > ♂
Compagnia delle Indie > 2017 > Blue Essence Parfum Intense > ♂

Compagnia delle Indie > 2017 > Green Spirit Parfum Intense > ⚥
Compagnia delle Indie > 2017 > Red Attraction Parfum Intense > ⚥
Compagnia delle Indie > 2017 > Yellow Secret Parfum Intense > ⚥
Coreterno > 2019 > Catharsis > ⚥
Coreterno > 2019 > Punk Motel > ⚥
Coreterno > 2019 > Rose and Me > ♀
Coreterno > 2019 > Yerba Nera > ⚥
Cortina 1224 > 2009 > Madame > ♀
Cortina 1224 > 2009 > Monsieur > ♂
Costume National > 2002 > Scent > ♀
Costume National > 2002 > Scent Intense > ⚥
Costume National > 2003 > Scent Sheer > ♀
Costume National > 2004 > Scent Gloss > ♀
Costume National > 2004 > Scent Intense Parfum > ⚥
Costume National > 2005 > Scent Cool Gloss > ♀
Costume National > 2006 > Scent Intense Parfum Limited Edition > ⚥
Costume National > 2007 > 21 > ⚥
Costume National > 2009 > Costume National Homme > ♂
Costume National > 2011 > Pop Collection > ♀
Costume National > 2012 > So Nude > ♀
Costume National > 2013 > Cyber Garden > ♂
Costume National > 2013 > So Nude Eau de toilette > ♀
Costume National > 2015 > Soul > ⚥
Costume National > 2018 > Scent Intense Parfum Red Edition > ⚥
Costume National > 2019 > Costume National 1 > ⚥
Costume National > 2019 > Costume National J > ⚥
Creso > 2016 > Babel > ⚥
Creso > 2016 > Logos > ⚥
Creso > 2016 > Panta Rei > ⚥
Creso > 2016 > Quarto Vuoto > ⚥
Creso > 2016 > Sappho > ⚥
Cristiana Bellodi > 2016 > B > ⚥
Cristiana Bellodi > 2016 > C > ⚥
Cristiana Bellodi > 2016 > E > ⚥
Cristiana Bellodi > 2016 > I > ⚥
Cristiana Bellodi > 2016 > L > ⚥
Cristiana Bellodi > 2016 > R > ⚥
Cristiano Fissore > 2007 > Cashmere for Men > ♂
Cristiano Fissore > 2007 > Cashmere for Women > ♀
Cristiano Fissore > 2007 > Rapsodia in Blu > ⚥
Culti > 2009 > Acqua Attiva > ⚥
Culti > 2009 > Acqua Tessuta > ⚥
Culti > 2009 > Anym'ale > ⚥
Culti > 2009 > Infinito > ⚥
Culti > 2009 > Mediterranea > ⚥
Culti > 2009 > Ode Rosae > ⚥
Culti > 2009 > Terraforte > ⚥
Culti > 2009 > Thessenza > ⚥
Dasa Concept Store > 2015 > Ambre Rouge > ⚥
Dasa Concept Store > 2015 > Blanche Patcholy > ⚥
Dasa Concept Store > 2015 > Deep Sea > ⚥
Dasa Concept Store > 2015 > Douce Chateau > ⚥
Dasa Concept Store > 2015 > Green Santal Wood > ⚥
Dasa Concept Store > 2015 > Mandarin Mousse > ⚥
Dasa Concept Store > 2015 > Oriental Dream > ⚥
Dasa Concept Store > 2015 > Touberouse Noir > ⚥
Dasa Concept Store > 2015 > Vert Musc > ⚥
Deborah > 1991 > Grand Prix > ⚥
Deborah > 1994 > Grand Prix Extreme > ♂
Deborah > 2000 > Frutti Rossi > ♀
Deborah > 2000 > Mandorla > ⚥
Deborah > 2000 > Vaniglia > ⚥
Deborah > 2005 > Fantasy Flowers Green > ♀
Deborah > 2005 > Fantasy Flowers Sky Blue > ♀
Deborah > 2005 > Funny Flowers Dark Blue > ♀
Deborah > 2005 > Funny Flowers Red > ♀
Deborah > 2005 > Funny Flowers White > ♀
Deborah > 2006 > Be Gourmand – Bon Bon > ⚥
Deborah > 2006 > Fisichella > ♂
Deborah > 2006 > Vee is around for Her > ♀
Deborah > 2006 > Vee Is around for Him > ♂
Deborah > 2007 > Be Gourmand – Be Mandy > ♀
Deborah > 2007 > Be Gourmand – Candy Fruit > ♀
Deborah > 2007 > Be Gourmand – Lovely Cream > ♀
Deborah > 2007 > Be Gourmand – Soft Sugar > ♀
Deborah > 2016 > Accordo di Fior di Patchouli > ♀
Deborah > 2016 > Accordo di Fresca Fresia > ♀
Deborah > 2016 > Accordo di Mandorlo Ambrato > ♀
Deborah > 2016 > Accordo di Papavero Nero > ♀
Deborah > 2016 > Accordo di Rosa Vellutata > ♀
Deborah > 2016 > Accordo di Rosa Violetta > ♀
Decotto di Neve > 2017 > Boulevard al Mare > ⚥

Decotto di Neve > 2017 > Felicità per la madre > ♀
Decotto di Neve > 2017 > Forza nella comprensione > ⚥
Decotto di Neve > 2017 > Gravità dentro di noi > ⚥
Decotto di Neve > 2017 > Gravità intorno a noi > ⚥
Decotto di Neve > 2017 > Gravità tra noi > ♀
Decotto di Neve > 2017 > Scopritore di Marmellata > ⚥
Decotto di Neve > 2018 > Fiore di Felce > ⚥
Decotto di Neve > 2018 > Glicosidi Cardiaci > ⚥
Decotto di Neve > 2018 > Orizzonte degli Eventi > ⚥
Decotto di Neve > 2018 > Rosso Ortodosso > ⚥
Decotto di Neve > 2018 > 6 e 5 > ⚥
Decotto di Neve > 2018 > Umanamente > ♂
Decotto di Neve > 2018 > Vecchia Aiuola > ⚥
Denim > 1976 > Denim 1976 > ♂
Denim > 1976 > Original > ♂
Denim > 1982 > Musk > ♂
Denim > 1982 > Aqua > ♂
Denim > 1982 > Azure > ♂
Denim > 1982 > Black > ♂
Denim > 1982 > Chill > ♂
Denim > 1982 > Heat > ♂
Denim > 1982 > Illusion > ♂
Denim > 1982 > Raw Passion > ♂
Denim > 1982 > River > ♂
Denim > 1982 > Sync > ♂
Denim > 1982 > Temptation > ♂
Denim > 1982 > Vibe > ♂
Denim > 1982 > Wild > ♂
Derbe-Speziali Fiorentini > 2000 > Acqua degli Speziali > ⚥
Derbe-Speziali Fiorentini > 2000 > Acqua del Benessere > ⚥
Derbe-Speziali Fiorentini > 2000 > Baby Profumo > ⚥
Derbe-Speziali Fiorentini > 2000 > Boy Profumo > ⚥
Derbe-Speziali Fiorentini > 2000 > Camelia e Coriandolo > ⚥
Derbe-Speziali Fiorentini > 2000 > Canapa e Mirto > ⚥
Derbe-Speziali Fiorentini > 2000 > Caramel > ⚥
Derbe-Speziali Fiorentini > 2000 > Cedro e Pepe Rosa > ⚥
Derbe-Speziali Fiorentini > 2000 > Fiori Bianchi e Foglie Verdi > ⚥
Derbe-Speziali Fiorentini > 2000 > Fiori del Chianti > ⚥
Derbe-Speziali Fiorentini > 2000 > Frangipani > ⚥
Derbe-Speziali Fiorentini > 2000 > Ginger e Jasmin > ⚥
Derbe-Speziali Fiorentini > 2000 > Girl Profumo > ⚥
Derbe-Speziali Fiorentini > 2000 > Lavanda > ⚥
Derbe-Speziali Fiorentini > 2000 > Liquirizia e Mandarino > ⚥
Derbe-Speziali Fiorentini > 2000 > Mela e Tulipani > ⚥
Derbe-Speziali Fiorentini > 2000 > Nontiscordardime > ⚥
Derbe-Speziali Fiorentini > 2000 > Olivo e Girasole > ⚥
Derbe-Speziali Fiorentini > 2000 > Papavero e Fico > ⚥
Derbe-Speziali Fiorentini > 2000 > Peonia e Lime > ⚥
Derbe-Speziali Fiorentini > 2000 > Pepe e Pompelmo > ⚥
Derbe-Speziali Fiorentini > 2000 > Rosa e Mora > ⚥
Derbe-Speziali Fiorentini > 2000 > Spezie e Patchouli > ⚥
Derbe-Speziali Fiorentini > 2000 > Tè Bianco > ⚥
Derbe-Speziali Fiorentini > 2000 > Tè Nero > ⚥
Derbe-Speziali Fiorentini > 2000 > Terre di Amerigo > ⚥
Derbe-Speziali Fiorentini > 2000 > Young > ⚥
DFG 1924 > 2017 > Aroma Arancio Verde > ⚥
DFG 1924 > 2017 > Aroma Blu > ⚥
DFG 1924 > 2017 > Aroma Caldo > ⚥
DFG 1924 > 2017 > Aroma d'Inverno > ⚥
DFG 1924 > 2017 > Aroma Frutta d'Estate > ♀
DFG 1924 > 2017 > Aroma Fruttato > ⚥
DFG 1924 > 2017 > Aroma Intenso > ⚥
DFG 1924 > 2017 > Aroma Vivienne > ⚥
DFG 1924 > 2017 > Cento Orizzonti > ⚥
DFG 1924 > 2017 > Ghiaccio Bollente > ♂
DFG 1924 > 2017 > Il Giardino di Freya > ♀
DFG 1924 > 2017 > Il Mercante di Spezie > ⚥
DFG 1924 > 2017 > Il Risveglio delle Esperidi > ⚥
DFG 1924 > 2017 > La Fontana di Titti > ⚥
DFG 1924 > 2017 > La Sorgente di Ninfee > ⚥
DFG 1924 > 2017 > Narciso > ⚥
DFG 1924 > 2017 > Noor > ⚥
DFG 1924 > 2019 > Il Sentiero degli Dei > ⚥
DFG 1924 > 2019 > La Baia di Jasmine > ⚥
DFG 1924 > 2019 > Non dire No > ⚥
Diadema Exclusif > 2016 > Absolu Gelsomino > ⚥
Diadema Exclusif > 2016 > Absolu Neroli > ⚥
Diadema Exclusif > 2016 > Absolu Rosa di Maggio > ⚥
Diadema Exclusif > 2016 > Absolu Vaniglia > ⚥
Diadema Exclusif > 2016 > Anuar > ⚥
Diadema Exclusif > 2016 > Armonie della Sera > ♀
Diadema Exclusif > 2016 > Milonga > ♀

Dr. Taffi > 2012 > I Macchiaioli – Rilassante > ♀
Dr. Taffi > 2012 > Jazz Mulberry > ♀
Dr. Taffi > 2012 > Lino – Tè Bianco > ♀
Dr. Taffi > 2014 > Seta Fior di Loto > ♀
Dr. Taffi > 2014 > Velluto Vaniglia > ♀
Dr. Taffi > 2014 > Yuta Zenzero > ♀
Dr. Taffi > 2014 > Batik Maracuja Fiori > ♀
Dr. Taffi > 2014 > Cady Ambra > ♀
Dr. Taffi > 2014 > Camelia Chic > ♀
Dr. Taffi > 2014 > Camelia Gold > ♀
Dr. Taffi > 2014 > Canapa Pepe Nero > ♀
Dr. Taffi > 2014 > Cashmere Iris > ♀
Dr. Taffi > 2014 > Cotone – Muschio Bianco > ♀
Dr. Taffi > 2014 > Jeans Pepe Bianco > ♀
Dr. Taffi > 2014 > Kenaf Karkadè > ♀
Dr. Taffi > 2014 > Ramiè > ♀
Dr. Taffi > 2014 > Tulle e Papaveri > ♀
Dr. Taffi > 2015 > Merlot & Rovere > ♂
Dr. Taffi > 2015 > Sangiovese e Bacche Blu > ♂
Dr. Taffi > 2015 > Satin – Perla > ♀
Dr. Taffi > 2015 > Taffetà Note di Mandorla > ♀
Dr. Taffi > 2015 > Macramè Agrumi e Spezie > ♀
Dr. Taffi > 2015 > Peperoncino > ♀
Dr. Taffi > 2018 > Sauvignon & Tabacco > ♂
Dr. Taffi > 2019 > Sangria e Dragoncello > ♂
Dr. Vranjes Firenze > 2010 > Ambra e Iris > ♀
Dr. Vranjes Firenze > 2010 > Bergamotto Mirto > ♀
Dr. Vranjes Firenze > 2010 > Gingember Estragone > ♂
Dr. Vranjes Firenze > 2010 > Rosa Cassis > ♀
Dr. Vranjes Firenze > 2010 > Vetiver Poivre > ♂
Dr. Vranjes Firenze > 2010 > Zagara Patchouli > ♂
Dr. Vranjes Firenze > 2016 > 17 Agosto – L'enfleurage > ⚥
Dr. Vranjes Firenze > 2016 > 19 Settembre – Ego > ⚥
Dr. Vranjes Firenze > 2016 > 28 Gennaio – Il Cuore > ⚥
Dr. Vranjes Firenze > 2016 > 7 Settembre – L'unione > ⚥
Dr. Vranjes Firenze > 2016 > 9 Febbraio – L'origine > ⚥
Dsquared2 > 2007 > He Wood > ♂
Dsquared2 > 2008 > She Wood > ♀
Dsquared2 > 2009 > He Wood Rocky Mountainn > ♂
Dsquared2 > 2009 > She Wood Velvet Forest > ♀
Dsquared2 > 2010 > He Wood Ocean Wet > ♂
Dsquared2 > 2010 > She Wood Crystal Creek > ♀
Dsquared2 > 2011 > He Wood Silver Wind > ♂
Dsquared2 > 2011 > Potion > ♀
Dsquared2 > 2011 > She Wood Golden Light > ♀
Dsquared2 > 2012 > Potion for Women > ♀
Dsquared2 > 2013 > Potion Blue Cadet > ♂
Dsquared2 > 2014 > Intense He Wood > ♂
Dsquared2 > 2014 > Wild > ♂
Dsquared2 > 2015 > Want > ♀
Dsquared2 > 2016 > Want Pink Ginger > ♀
Dsquared2 > 2017 > He Wood Cologne > ♂
Dsquared2 > 2018 > Wood for Her > ♀
Dsquared2 > 2018 > Wood for Him > ♂
Dsquared2 > 2019 > Green Wood > ♂
Dsquared2 > 2019 > Red Wood > ♀
Ducati > 2010 > Ducati > ♂
Ducati > 2011 > Fight for Me > ♂
Ducati > 2012 > Fight for me Extreme > ♂
Ducati > 2013 > Trace Me > ♂
Ducati > 2017 > Ducati 1926 > ♂
Ducati > 2018 > Ducati Sport > ♂
Ducati > 2019 > Ducati Ice > ♂
Eau d'Italie > 2005 > Eau d'Italie > ⚥
Eau d'Italie > 2006 > Bois d'Ombrie > ⚥
Eau d'Italie > 2006 > Paestum Rose > ⚥
Eau d'Italie > 2006 > Sienne L'hiver > ⚥
Eau d'Italie > 2008 > Baume du Doge > ⚥
Eau d'Italie > 2008 > Magnolia Romana > ⚥
Eau d'Italie > 2010 > Au Lac > ♀
Eau d'Italie > 2011 > Jardin du Poete > ⚥
Eau d'Italie > 2012 > Un Bateau pour Capri > ⚥
Eau d'Italie > 2013 > Acqua Decima > ⚥
Eau d'Italie > 2014 > Graine de Joie > ⚥
Eau d'Italie > 2015 > Morn to Dusk > ⚥
Eau d'Italie > 2017 > Rosa Greta > ⚥
Eau d'Italie > 2018 > Fior Fiore > ⚥
Eau d'Italie > 2019 > Easy to Love > ⚥
El Charro > 1991 > El Charro for Woman > ♀
E. Marinella > 1997/2012 > E. Marinella Napoli (The Original) > ♂
E. Marinella > 2000/2012 > Seta > ♀
E. Marinella > 2002/2012 > 287 > ♂

E. Marinella > 2006 > Chiaja > ♀
E. Marinella > 2006 > Muscade > ♀
E. Marinella > 2007 > Ambra Royale > ♀
E. Marinella > 2008 > Costa Nera > ♂
E. Marinella > 2010 > Frenesia > ♀
E. Marinella > 2012 > Capodimonte > ♂
E. Marinella > 2012 > Posillipo > ♂
E. Marinella > 2014 > 100 – 1914-2014 > ♂
E. Marinella > 2015 > Tabacco Imperiale > ♂
E. Marinella > 2016 > Malia > ♀
E. Marinella > 2017 > 4.0 Collection – Cyber Cuir > ⚥
E. Marinella > 2017 > 4.0 Collection – Hyper Wood > ⚥
E. Marinella > 2017 > 4.0 Collection – Spicy Lab > ⚥
E. Marinella > 2019 > Suite > ⚥
Emilio Pucci > 1965/2007 > Vivara > ♀
Emilio Pucci > 1970 > Eau de Zadig > ♀
Emilio Pucci > 1970 > Signor Vivara > ♂
Emilio Pucci > 1970 > Stra-Vivara > ♀
Emilio Pucci > 1971 > Monsieur Zadig > ♂
Emilio Pucci > 1971 > Zadig > ♀
Emilio Pucci > 1973 > Miss Zadig > ♀
Emilio Pucci > 1977 > Miss Zadig Eau Fraiche > ♀
Emilio Pucci > 1981 > Pucci > ♀
Emilio Pucci > 1982 > Pucci Eau Fraiche > ♀
Emilio Pucci > 2008 > Vivara Silver Edition > ♀
Emilio Pucci > 2009 > Vivara – Acqua 330 > ♀
Emilio Pucci > 2009 > Vivara – Sabbia 167 > ♀
Emilio Pucci > 2009 > Vivara – Sole 149 > ♀
Emilio Pucci > 2009 > Vivara Black Edition > ♀
Emilio Pucci > 2010 > Miss Pucci > ♀
Emilio Pucci > 2010 > Vivara Turquoise Edition > ♀
Emilio Pucci > 2011 > Miss Pucci Intense > ♀
Emilio Pucci > 2011 > Vivara – Verde 072 > ♀
Enrico Coveri > 1983 > Dollars > ♂
Enrico Coveri > 1983 > Paillettes > ♀
Enrico Coveri > 1984 > Enrico Coveri pour Homme > ♂
Enrico Coveri > 1986 > Enrico Coveri pour Homme L'eau > ♂
Enrico Coveri > 1987 > Enrico Coveri pour Femme > ♀
Enrico Coveri > 1993 > Firenze > ♀
Enrico Coveri > 2002 > Kinky you Young Femme > ♀
Enrico Coveri > 2002 > Kinky you Young Homme > ♂
Enrico Coveri > 2003 > Paillettes (Ried.) > ♀
Enrico Coveri > 2006 > Enrico Coveri MiO6 Man > ♂
Enrico Coveri > 2006 > Enrico Coveri MiO6 Woman > ♀
Enrico Coveri > 2010 > Paillettes 3 > ♀
Enrico Coveri > 2011 > Pop Heart for Her > ♀
Enrico Coveri > 2011 > Pop Heart for Him > ♂
Enrico Coveri > 2014 > Paillettes Nuit > ♀
Enrico Coveri > 2015 > Firenze Primo Amore > ♀
Enrico Coveri > 2016 > Coveri pour Elle > ♀
Enrico Coveri > 2017 > La Rose > ♀
Enrico Coveri > 2018 > Enrico Coveri Nouvel Homme > ♂
Enrico Coveri > 2018 > Le Nouvel Homme > ♂
Enrico Coveri > 2018 > Paillettes Pearl > ♀
Eolie Parfums > 2014 > Ericusa > ♀
Eolie Parfums > 2014 > Hierà > ♀
Eolie Parfums > 2014 > Ikesia > ♀
Eolie Parfums > 2014 > La Sciara > ♀
Eolie Parfums > 2014 > Le Saline > ♂
Eolie Parfums > 2014 > Meligunis > ♂
Eolie Parfums > 2014 > Phoenicus > ♂
Eolie Parfums > 2015 > Ventus > ♂
Eolie Parfums > 2015 > Zephyrus > ♂
Eolie Parfums > 2017 > Abraxas > ♀
Erbario Toscano > 2012 > Cuore di Pepe Nero > ♂
Erbario Toscano > 2012 > Vaniglia Piccante > ♀
Erbario Toscano > 2013 > Gocce di Resina > ♂
Erbario Toscano > 2013 > Legno di Rosa > ♂
Erbario Toscano > 2013 > Polvere di Siena > ♂
Erbario Toscano > 2014 > Primavera Toscana > ♀
Erbario Toscano > 2014 > Violetta Nobile > ♀
Erbario Toscano > 2015 > Agrumato di Costa > ♀
Erbario Toscano > 2015 > Bacche di Tuscia > ♀
Erbario Toscano > 2015 > Fico d'Elba > ♀
Erbario Toscano > 2015 > Fumo di Oppio > ♂
Erbario Toscano > 2015 > Noble Flowers > ♀
Erbario Toscano > 2016 > Cuoio Bianco > ♂
Erbariso Toscano > 2016 > Elicriso Marino > ♂
Erbario Toscano > 2016 > Fior Gentile > ♀
Erbario Toscano > 2016 > Foglia Ghiacciata > ♀
Erbario Toscano > 2016 > Iris Muschiato > ♂
Erbario Toscano > 2016 > Legno Patchoulli > ♀

Erbario Toscano > 2016 > Rabarbaro Esperidato > ♂
Erbario Toscano > 2016 > Speziato Nero > ♂
Erbario Toscano > 2016 > Sugar Spicy > ♂
Erbario Toscano > 2016 > Tabacco Dolce > ♂
Erbario Toscano > 2016 > Terra > ♀
Erbario Toscano > 2016 > Tuberosa Ambrata > ♀
Erbario Toscano > 2016 > Wild Musk > ♂
Erbario Toscano > 2017 > Salis > ♂
Erboristeria Magentina > 2018 > Profumo degli Angeli > ♀
Erboristeria Magentina > 2018 > Profumo degli Elfi > ♀
Erboristeria Magentina > 2018 > Profumo degli Esseni > ♀
Erboristeria Magentina > 2019 > Profumo delle Fate > ♀
Ermanno Scervino > 2019 > Ermanno Scervino Eau de Parfum > ♀
Ermenegildo Zegna > 1992 > Zegna pour Homme > ♂
Ermenegildo Zegna > 2003 > Essenza di Zegna > ♂
Ermenegildo Zegna > 2004 > Essenza di Zegna Intense > ♂
Ermenegildo Zegna > 2005 > Acqua d'Estate Essenza > ♂
Ermenegildo Zegna > 2005 > Z Zegna > ♂
Ermenegildo Zegna > 2007 > Acqua d'Estate Essenza 2007 > ♂
Ermenegildo Zegna > 2007 > Zegna Intenso > ♂
Ermenegildo Zegna > 2008 > Acqua d'Estate Essenza di Zegna > ♂
Ermenegildo Zegna > 2008 > Z Zegna Extreme > ♂
Ermenegildo Zegna > 2008 > Z Zegna Fresh > ♂
Ermenegildo Zegna > 2008 > Zegna Intenso Limited Edition > ♂
Ermenegildo Zegna > 2009 > Essenza di Zegna Acqua d'Estate > ♂
Ermenegildo Zegna > 2009 > Zegna Colonia > ♂
Ermenegildo Zegna > 2010 > Zegna Forte > ♂
Ermenegildo Zegna > 2012 > Florentine Iris > ♂
Ermenegildo Zegna > 2012 > Indonesian Oud > ♂
Ermenegildo Zegna > 2012 > Italian Bergamot > ♂
Ermenegildo Zegna > 2012 > Javanese Patchouli > ♂
Ermenegildo Zegna > 2012 > Sicilian Mandarin > ♂
Ermenegildo Zegna > 2013 > Uomo > ♂
Ermenegildo Zegna > 2014 > Haitian Vetiver > ♂
Ermenegildo Zegna > 2014 > Peruvian Ambrette > ♂
Ermenegildo Zegna > 2014 > Uomo Absolute > ♂
Ermenegildo Zegna > 2015 > Acqua di Bergamotto > ♂
Ermenegildo Zegna > 2015 > Mediterranean Neroli > ♂
Ermenegildo Zegna > 2015 > Z Zegna Energy > ♂
Ermenegildo Zegna > 2016 > Amber Gold > ♂
Ermenegildo Zegna > 2016 > Incense Gold > ♂
Ermenegildo Zegna > 2016 > Musk Gold > ♂
Ermenegildo Zegna > 2016 > Z Zegna Milan > ♂
Ermenegildo Zegna > 2016 > Z Zegna New York > ♂
Ermenegildo Zegna > 2016 > Z Zegna Shanghai > ♂
Ermenegildo Zegna > 2017 > Acqua di Iris > ♂
Ermenegildo Zegna > 2017 > Bourbon Vanilla > ♂
Ermenegildo Zegna > 2017 > Elements of Man: Integrity > ♂
Ermenegildo Zegna > 2017 > Elements of Man: Passion > ♂
Ermenegildo Zegna > 2017 > Elements of Man: Strength > ♂
Ermenegildo Zegna > 2017 > Elements of Man: Talent > ♂
Ermenegildo Zegna > 2017 > Elements of Man: Wisdom > ♂
Ermenegildo Zegna > 2017 > Indian Spice > ♂
Ermenegildo Zegna > 2017 > Persian Saffron > ♂
Ermenegildo Zegna > 2018 > Acqua di Neroli > ♂
Ermenegildo Zegna > 2019 > Madras Cardamom > ♂
Ermenegildo Zegna > 2020 > Roman Wood > ♂
Erreuno > 1995 > Erreuno > ♀
Erreuno > 1996 > Miss Erreuno > ♀
Essenza > 2018 > Ambra & Vaniglia > ♀
Essenza > 2018 > Muschio Bianco > ♀
Essenza > 2018 > Patchouli > ♀
Essenza > 2018 > Vetiver > ♀
Essenzialmente Laura > 2017 > Achab > ♀
Essenzialmente Laura > 2017 > Acqua Barocca > ♀
Essenzialmente Laura > 2017 > Alcor > ♀
Essenzialmente Laura > 2017 > Alioth > ♀
Essenzialmente Laura > 2017 > Ambra Antica > ♀
Essenzialmente Laura > 2017 > Avorio > ♀
Essenzialmente Laura > 2017 > Bellatrix > ♀
Essenzialmente Laura > 2017 > Bosco > ♀
Essenzialmente Laura > 2017 > Calabash > ♀
Essenzialmente Laura > 2017 > Core 'Ngrato > ♀
Essenzialmente Laura > 2017 > Coronari 57 > ♀
Essenzialmente Laura > 2017 > Cuoio Imperiale > ♀
Essenzialmente Laura > 2017 > Ebano > ♀
Essenzialmente Laura > 2017 > Flora > ♀
Essenzialmente Laura > 2017 > Il Cortile delle Zagare > ♀
Essenzialmente Laura > 2017 > Indaco > ♀
Essenzialmente Laura > 2017 > Kismet > ♀
Essenzialmente Laura > 2017 > La Corte > ♀
Essenzialmente Laura > 2017 > La Fuga > ♀

Essenzialmente Laura > 2017 > La Lavanda > ♂
Essenzialmente Laura > 2017 > La Lavanda di Leonardo > ♂
Essenzialmente Laura > 2017 > La Regina di Taif > ♀
Essenzialmente Laura > 2017 > Lavambra > ♂
Essenzialmente Laura > 2017 > Le Rose di Afrodite > ♀
Essenzialmente Laura > 2017 > Lilibet > ♀
Essenzialmente Laura > 2017 > Madeleine > ♀
Essenzialmente Laura > 2017 > Majorelle > ♀
Essenzialmente Laura > 2017 > Manto Rosso > ♂
Essenzialmente Laura > 2017 > Mare > ♂
Essenzialmente Laura > 2017 > Megrez > ♀
Essenzialmente Laura > 2017 > Merak > ♀
Essenzialmente Laura > 2017 > Mizar > ♀
Essenzialmente Laura > 2017 > Notturno > ♂
Essenzialmente Laura > 2017 > Ombra > ♂
Essenzialmente Laura > 2017 > Orens > ♂
Essenzialmente Laura > 2017 > Oxo > ♂
Essenzialmente Laura > 2017 > Pepe > ♂
Essenzialmente Laura > 2017 > Talitha > ♀
Essenzialmente Laura > 2017 > Tangerino > ♂
Essenzialmente Laura > 2017 > The Scents of the Bible – Incenso delle Chiese di Roma > ♂
Essenzialmente Laura > 2017 > The Scents of the Bible – Mystic Rose > ♀
Essenzialmente Laura > 2017 > The Scents of the Bible – Nardo Della Maddalena > ♀
Essenzialmente Laura > 2017 > Vermiglio > ♂
Essenzialmente Laura > 2017 > Vi > ♂
Essenzialmente Laura > 2017 > Viola > ♀
Essenzialmente Laura > 2017 > Voi Sapete ch'io V'amo > ♀
Essenzialmente Laura > 2018 > Gli Essenziali – Assai > ♂
Essenzialmente Laura > 2018 > Gli Essenziali – Fimmina > ♀
Essenzialmente Laura > 2018 > Gli Essenziali – Fior d'Ambra > ♂
Essenzialmente Laura > 2018 > Gli Essenziali – Fior di Pero > ♂
Essenzialmente Laura > 2018 > Gli Essenziali – Fior di Pesco > ♂
Essenzialmente Laura > 2018 > Gli Essenziali – Fiore Nero > ♂
Essenzialmente Laura > 2018 > Gli Essenziali – Fiore Stellare > ♂
Essenzialmente Laura > 2018 > Gli Essenziali – Focu Meo > ♂
Essenzialmente Laura > 2018 > Gli Essenziali – Italia > ♂
Esse Strikes the Notes > 2018 > Anita > ♀
Esse Strikes the Notes > 2018 > Donatella > ♀
Esse Strikes the Notes > 2018 > Miranda > ♀
Esse Strikes the Notes > 2018 > Priscilla > ♀
Esse Strikes the Notes > 2019 > Vittoria > ♀
E – Suitcase > 2018 > Ciao Stronzo > ♂
E – Suitcase > 2018 > Giramondo > ♂
E – Suitcase > 2018 > Oca Giuliva > ♀
E – Suitcase > 2018 > Party Amo > ♂
E – Suitcase > 2019 > Arco – Balena > ♂
E – Suitcase > 2019 > J-Eva > ♀
E – Suitcase > 2019 > My Airbag > ♂
E – Suitcase > 2019 > Tempo Perso > ♂
Etro > 1989 > Ambra > ♂
Etro > 1989 > Gomma > ♀
Etro > 1989 > Heliotrope > ♀
Etro > 1989 > Jacquard > ♀
Etro > 1989 > Magot > ♂
Etro > 1989 > Palais Jamais > ♀
Etro > 1989 > Patchouly > ♀
Etro > 1989 > Royal Pavillion > ♂
Etro > 1989 > Sandalo > ♂
Etro > 1989 > Vetiver > ♂
Etro > 1994 > Messe de Minuit > ♀
Etro > 1996 > Vicolo Fiori > ♀
Etro > 1997 > Shaal Nur > ♂
Etro > 1999 > Etra Etro > ♀
Etro > 2001 > Benetroessere Raving > ♀
Etro > 2001 > Benetroessere Relent > ♀
Etro > 2001 > Benetroessere Resort > ♀
Etro > 2002 > New Tradition > ♀
Etro > 2004 > Anice > ♂
Etro > 2004 > Mahogany > ♂
Etro > 2004 > Musk > ♂
Etro > 2006 > Dianthus > ♀
Etro > 2008 > Via Verri Vintage Limited Edition > ♀
Etro > 2009 > Pegaso > ♀
Etro > 2010 > Relent > ♂
Etro > 2011 > Paisley > ♂
Etro > 2011 > Vicolo Fiori Edp > ♀
Etro > 2012 > Greene Street > ♂
Etro > 2013 > Rajasthan > ♂
Etro > 2014 > Lemon Sorbet > ♀
Etro > 2015 > Io Myself > ♂

Etro > 2015 > Marquetry > ⚥
Etro > 2016 > Patchouly Edp > ⚥
Etro > 2016 > Shantung > ⚥
Etro > 2017 > Manrose > ♂
Etro > 2018 > Musk Edp > ⚥
Etro > 2018 > Udaipur > ⚥
Ex Floribus Vinis > 2009 > N. 1 Anans Sativa > ♀
Ex Floribus Vinis > 2009 > N. 2 Armenica Vulgaris > ♀
Ex Floribus Vinis > 2009 > N. 3 Ribes Rubrum > ♀
Ex Floribus Vinis > 2009 > N. 4 Rubus Idaeus > ♀
Ex Floribus Vinis > 2009 > N. 5 Anthemis Nobilis > ⚥
Ex Floribus Vinis > 2009 > N. 6 Piper Officinarum > ⚥
Exò Fragranze > 2011 > Amore > ⚥
Exò Fragranze > 2011 > Benessere > ⚥
Exò Fragranze > 2011 > Concentrazione > ⚥
Exò Fragranze > 2011 > Potere > ⚥
Exò Fragranze > 2011 > Sicurezza > ⚥
Exò Fragranze > 2011 > Tranquillità > ⚥
Extè > 2005 > J'S Extè Woman > ♀
Extè > 2006 > J'S Extè Man > ♂
Extè > 2007 > J'S Extè Pop > ⚥
Extrait d'Atelier > 2016 > Maître Chausseur > ⚥
Extrait d'Atelier > 2016 > Maître Couturier > ⚥
Extrait d'Atelier > 2016 > Maître Joallier > ⚥
Extrait d'Atelier > 2018 > Maître Céramiste > ⚥
Extrait d'Atelier > 2019 > Maître Jardinier > ⚥
Fabi > 2008 > Fabi per Lei > ♀
Fabi > 2008 > Fabi per Lui > ♂
Fabio lo Coco Fragrance > 2015 > Moorish > ⚥
Fabio lo Coco Fragrance > 2015 > Oud Narang > ⚥
Falconeri > 2014 > Ambra > ♀
Falconeri > 2014 > Elicriso > ⚥
Falconeri > 2014 > Fico > ⚥
Familia Familia > 2018 > Deal > ⚥
Familia Familia > 2018 > Enjoy the Weekend > ⚥
Familia Familia > 2018 > Family in Love > ⚥
Familia Familia > 2018 > Family in Love Baby > ⚥
Familia Familia > 2018 > Wake Me Up > ⚥
Familia Familia > 2018 > Wake Me Up Baby > ⚥
Farmacia del Castello (Strega del Castello) > > >
Farmacia SS. Annunziata > 2011 > 450 > ⚥
Farmacia SS. Annunziata > 2011 > Agrumi > ⚥
Farmacia SS. Annunziata > 2011 > Ambra Nera > ♀
Farmacia SS. Annunziata > 2011 > Arabico > ⚥
Farmacia SS. Annunziata > 2011 > Aromadite > ⚥
Farmacia SS. Annunziata > 2011 > Aurora > ♀
Farmacia SS. Annunziata > 2011 > Cara > ♀
Farmacia SS. Annunziata > 2011 > Chia > ♀
Farmacia SS. Annunziata > 2011 > Fiore di Riso > ⚥
Farmacia SS. Annunziata > 2011 > Gelsorosa > ♀
Farmacia SS. Annunziata > 2011 > Kama > ♀
Farmacia SS. Annunziata > 2011 > Ker > ♀
Farmacia SS. Annunziata > 2011 > Nero > ⚥
Farmacia SS. Annunziata > 2011 > Patchouly Indonesiano > ⚥
Farmacia SS. Annunziata > 2011 > Perla > ♀
Farmacia SS. Annunziata > 2011 > Regina > ♀
Farmacia SS. Annunziata > 2011 > Sofron > ⚥
Farmacia SS. Annunziata > 2011 > Ybris > ⚥
Farmacia SS. Annunziata > 2012 > Sweet Musk > ♀
Farmacia SS. Annunziata > 2012 > Takis > ⚥
Farmacia SS. Annunziata > 2012 > Talc Gourmand > ♀
Farmacia SS. Annunziata > 2012 > Vetiver Incenso > ⚥
Farmacia SS. Annunziata > 2014 > Hyle > ♂
Farmacia SS. Annunziata > 2014 > Isos > ⚥
Farmacia SS. Annunziata > 2014 > Nero Incenso > ⚥
Farmacia SS. Annunziata > 2015 > Tabacco d'Autore > ⚥
Farmacia SS. Annunziata > 2016 > Cuoio Fiorentino > ⚥
Farmacia SS. Annunziata > 2016 > Vaniglia del Madagascar > ⚥
Farmacia SS. Annunziata > 2016 > Verde di Persia > ⚥
Farmacia SS. Annunziata > 2017 > Eden > ⚥
Farmacia SS. Annunziata > 2018 > Giardini di Firenze > ⚥
Farmacia SS. Annunziata > 2018 > Whisky Oud > ⚥
Farmacia SS. Annunziata > 2019 > Tahiti Vanilla > ⚥
Fendi > 1985 > Fendi > ♀
Fendi > 1988 > Fendi Uomo > ♂
Fendi > 1988 > Touch of Fendi > ♀
Fendi > 1992 > Asja > ♀
Fendi > 1996 > Fantasia Fendi > ♀
Fendi > 1996 > Life Essence > ♂
Fendi > 1998 > Theorema > ♀
Fendi > 1999 > Theorema Esprit d'Été > ♀
Fendi > 2002 > Theorema Leggero > ♀

Fendi > 2003 > Theorema Leggero for Summer > ♀
Fendi > 2004 > Celebration > ♀
Fendi > 2004 > Fendi > ♀
Fendi > 2004 > Fendi for Men > ♂
Fendi > 2007 > Palazzo > ♀
Fendi > 2008 > Palazzo Edt > ♀
Fendi > 2010 > Fan di Fendi > ♀
Fendi > 2011 > Fan di Fendi Edt > ♀
Fendi > 2011 > Theorema Uomo > ♂
Fendi > 2012 > Fan di Fendi Extreme > ♀
Fendi > 2012 > Fan di Fendi pour Homme > ♂
Fendi > 2013 > Fan di Fendi pour Homme Acqua > ♂
Fendi > 2013 > Fan di Fendi Eau Fraiche > ♀
Fendi > 2013 > Fan di Fendi pour Homme Acqua > ♂
Fendi > 2013 > L'acquarossa > ♀
Fendi > 2014 > Fan di Fendi Blossom > ♀
Fendi > 2014 > Fan di Fendi Leather Essence > ♀
Fendi > 2014 > Fan di Fendi pour Homme Assoluto > ♂
Fendi > 2014 > Furiosa > ♀
Fendi > 2014 > L'acquarossa Edt > ♀
Fendi > 2015 > L'acquarossa Elixir > ♀
Ferrari > 1995 > Donna > ♀
Ferrari > 1997 > Yellow > ♀
Ferrari > 1999 > Ferrari Black > ♂
Ferrari > 2001 > Ferrari N. 1 > ♂
Ferrari > 2003 > Racing > ♂
Ferrari > 2005 > Ferrari Passion Unlimited > ♂
Ferrari > 2006 > Ferrari Extreme > ♂
Ferrari > 2009 > Ferrari Uomo > ♂
Ferrari > 2010 > Scuderia Ferrari > ♂
Ferrari > 2010 > Scuderia Ferrari Red > ♂
Ferrari > 2011 > Scuderia Ferrari Black Shine > ♂
Ferrari > 2012 > Essence Oud > ♂
Ferrari > 2012 > Ferrari Silver Essence > ♂
Ferrari > 2012 > Red Power > ♂
Ferrari > 2012 > Scuderia Ferrari Light Essence Bright > ⚥
Ferrari > 2013 > Essence Musk > ♂
Ferrari > 2013 > Leather Essence > ♂
Ferrari > 2013 > Scuderia Ferrari Black > ♂
Ferrari > 2013 > Scuderia Ferrari Black Signature > ♂
Ferrari > 2013 > Scuderia Ferrari Racing Red > ♂
Ferrari > 2013 > Scuderia Ferrari Scuderia Club > ♂
Ferrari > 2014 > Cedar Essence > ♂
Ferrari > 2014 > Red Power Intense > ♂
Ferrari > 2014 > Scuderia Ferrari Black Limited Edition > ♂
Ferrari > 2014 > Scuderia Ferrari Light Essence Acqua > ⚥
Ferrari > 2014 > Vetiver Essence > ♂
Ferrari > 2015 > Amber Essence > ♂
Ferrari > 2015 > Bright Neroli > ⚥
Ferrari > 2015 > Man in Red > ♂
Ferrari > 2015 > Noble Fig > ⚥
Ferrari > 2015 > Pure Lavender > ⚥
Ferrari > 2015 > Red Power Ice 3 > ♂
Ferrari > 2016 > Amber Essence 2016 > ♂
Ferrari > 2016 > Radiant Bergamot > ⚥
Ferrari > 2017 > Ferrari Light Essence > ♂
Ferrari > 2017 > Scuderia Ferrari Forte > ♂
Ferrari > 2018 > Scuderia Ferrari Extreme > ♂
Fiat 500 > 2018 > Fiat 500 for Her > ♀
Fiat 500 > 2018 > Fiat 500 for Him > ♂
Fila > 2016 > Fila for Men > ♂
Fila > 2016 > Fila for Women > ♂
Fila > 2018 > Citrus Sundae > ⚥
Fila > 2018 > Loose Savon > ⚥
Fila > 2018 > Sweet Coaster > ⚥
Filippo Sorcinelli > 2014 > Unum Collection: Lavs > ⚥
Filippo Sorcinelli > 2015 > Unum Collection: Rosa Nigra > ⚥
Filippo Sorcinelli > 2016 > Sauf Collection – Contre Bombarde 32 > ⚥
Filippo Sorcinelli > 2016 > Sauf Collection – Plein Jeu II – V > ⚥
Filippo Sorcinelli > 2016 > Sauf Collection – Voix Humaine 8 > ⚥
Filippo Sorcinelli > 2016 > Unum Collection: Ennui-Noir > ⚥
Filippo Sorcinelli > 2016 > Unum Collection: Symphonie-Passion > ⚥
Filippo Sorcinelli > 2017 > Nebbia Densa > ⚥
Filippo Sorcinelli > 2017 > Nebbia Fitta > ⚥
Filippo Sorcinelli > 2017 > Nebbia Spessa > ⚥
Filippo Sorcinelli > 2017 > Unum Collection: Io non ho mani che mi accarezzino il volto > ⚥
Filippo Sorcinelli > 2018 > Sauf Collection – Unda Maris 8 > ⚥
Filippo Sorcinelli > 2018 > Sauf Collection – Violon Basse 16 > ⚥
Filippo Sorcinelli > 2018 > Unum Collection: But not Today > ⚥
Filippo Sorcinelli > 2019 > Epicentro > ⚥
Filippo Sorcinelli > 2019 > Unum Collection: Quando Rapita in Estasi > ⚥

Fiorucci > 1971 > Vanilla Scent > ⚥
Fiorucci > 2000 > Buffalo > ♀
Fiorucci > 2000 > Danger > ♂
Fiorucci > 2000 > Extreme Black > ♂
Fiorucci > 2000 > Extreme Sport > ♂
Fiorucci > 2000 > Fiorucci > ⚥
Fiorucci > 2000 > Fiorucci Loves You Forever > ♀
Fiorucci > 2000 > I Love London > ♀
Fiorucci > 2000 > I Love New York > ♀
Fiorucci > 2000 > I Love Paris > ♀
Fiorucci > 2000 > Monsieur > ♂
Fiorucci > 2000 > Musk > ⚥
Fiorucci > 2000 > Rock with Style > ♀
Fiorucci > 2000 > Touch > ♀
Fiorucci > 2000 > Dolce Amore > ♀
Fiorucci > 2001 > Fiorucci Loves You > ♀
Fiorucci > 2002 > Acqua degli Angeli > ♀
Fiorucci > 2005 > Miss Fiorucci Only Love > ♀
Fiorucci > 2005 > Miss Fiorucci so Sexy > ♀
Fiorucci > 2005 > So Sexy! > ♀
Fiorucci > 2006 > Glittery > ♀
Fiorucci > 2007 > Pin Up I'm Funny > ♀
Fiorucci > 2007 > Pin Up I'm Juicy > ♀
Fiorucci > 2007 > Pin Up I'm Sensual > ♀
Fiorucci > 2007 > Pin Up I'm Spicy > ♀
Fiorucci > 2009 > Amore 14 Red > ♀
Fiorucci > 2009 > Amore 14 White > ♀
Fiorucci > 2011 > Kisses of Fire > ♀
Fiorucci > 2011 > Western Girl > ⚥
Fiorucci > 2012 > Delicious > ♀
Fiorucci > 2012 > Donna > ♀
Fiorucci > 2012 > Golden > ♀
Fiorucci > 2012 > Icy Fantasy > ♀
Fiorucci > 2012 > Uomo > ♂
Fiorucci > 2013 > Pink Diamond > ♀
Fiorucci > 2014 > Passione > ♀
Fiorucci > 2014 > Star > ♀
Fiorucci > 2015 > Black Lions > ♂
Fiorucci > 2015 > Majestic > ♀
Fiorucci > 2015 > Maximus > ♂
Fiorucci > 2015 > Mr. Grey > ♂
Fiorucci > 2015 > Nuit Rose > ♀
Fiorucci > 2015 > Paris > ♀
Fiorucci > 2015 > Paris La Nuit > ♀
Fiorucci > 2015 > Pegasus > ♂
Fiorucci > 2015 > Provence > ♀
Fiorucci > 2015 > Red Lions > ♂
Fiorucci > 2015 > Touch > ♀
Fiorucci > 2015 > Wall Street > ♂
Fiorucci > 2016 > Chrome > ♂
Fiorucci > 2016 > Fiorucci Gold Lions > ♂
Fiorucci > 2017 > L'amour > ♀
Fiorucci > 2017 > Lumière > ♀
Fiorucci > 2018 > Miss Grey > ♀
Fiorucci > 2019 > Majestic Esmeralda > ♀
Fiorucci > 2019 > Paris Eau de Parfum > ♀
Florian > 2018 > Aqua Admirabilis > ♂
Florian > 2018 > Aqua Moresca > ♂
Flumen Profumi > 2015 > Accento d'Amore > ⚥
Flumen Profumi > 2015 > Adagio > ⚥
Flumen Profumi > 2015 > Ancora una volta soltanto > ⚥
Flumen Profumi > 2015 > Armonia > ⚥
Flumen Profumi > 2015 > Bramato Coraggio > ⚥
Flumen Profumi > 2015 > Caldo Abbraccio > ⚥
Flumen Profumi > 2015 > Dama > ⚥
Flumen Profumi > 2015 > Fugace Silenzio > ⚥
Flumen Profumi > 2015 > Incanto > ⚥
Flumen Profumi > 2015 > Inedito Ricordo > ⚥
Flumen Profumi > 2015 > Leggera Follia > ⚥
Flumen Profumi > 2015 > Melodico Stupore > ⚥
Flumen Profumi > 2015 > Meraviglioso Istante > ⚥
Flumen Profumi > 2015 > Nettare d'Aurora > ⚥
Flumen Profumi > 2015 > Rintocchi di Gioia > ⚥
Flumen Profumi > 2015 > Ritratto Notturno > ⚥
Flumen Profumi > 2015 > Ritrovarsi Ancora > ⚥
Flumen Profumi > 2015 > Sorso di Quiete > ⚥
Flumen Profumi > 2015 > Tocco di Ghiaccio > ⚥
Flumen Profumi > 2015 > Utopia > ⚥
Flumen Profumi > 2018 > Adagio > ⚥
Frais Monde > 2000-2015 > Alizé > ⚥
Frais Monde > 2000-2015 > Alloro Bianco e Fico > ⚥
Frais Monde > 2000-2015 > Ambra Argan > ⚥

Frais Monde > 2000-2015 > Ambra Grigia > ⚥
Frais Monde > 2000-2015 > Ambra Mediterranea > ⚥
Frais Monde > 2000-2015 > Anice e Vaniglia > ⚥
Frais Monde > 2000-2015 > Bacche > ⚥
Frais Monde > 2000-2015 > Bergamotto > ⚥
Frais Monde > 2000-2015 > Black Musk > ⚥
Frais Monde > 2000-2015 > Cassis e Muschio Bianco > ⚥
Frais Monde > 2000-2015 > Castagno e Cisto > ⚥
Frais Monde > 2000-2015 > Cedro Bianco e Muschio > ⚥
Frais Monde > 2000-2015 > Ciliegio > ⚥
Frais Monde > 2000-2015 > Corteccia di Mango > ⚥
Frais Monde > 2000-2015 > Dalia Nera > ⚥
Frais Monde > 2000-2015 > Etesian > ⚥
Frais Monde > 2000-2015 > Fiori > ⚥
Frais Monde > 2000-2015 > Fiori di Albizia > ⚥
Frais Monde > 2000-2015 > Fiori di Melograno > ⚥
Frais Monde > 2000-2015 > Foglie > ⚥
Frais Monde > 2000-2015 > Frutti > ⚥
Frais Monde > 2000-2015 > Gelsomino > ⚥
Frais Monde > 2000-2015 > Giglio > ⚥
Frais Monde > 2000-2015 > Iris Grigio > ⚥
Frais Monde > 2000-2015 > Magnolia e Cashmere > ⚥
Frais Monde > 2000-2015 > Malva e Bacche di Biancospino > ⚥
Frais Monde > 2000-2015 > Mandarino Nero > ⚥
Frais Monde > 2000-2015 > Mandorla > ⚥
Frais Monde > 2000-2015 > Mare, Arancio e Bacche > ⚥
Frais Monde > 2000-2015 > Mare, Limone e Mimosa > ⚥
Frais Monde > 2000-2015 > Mughetto > ⚥
Frais Monde – Brambles & Moor > 1990-2000 > Cocco > ⚥
Frais Monde – Brambles & Moor > 1990-2000 > Cocco e Abete > ⚥
Frais Monde – Brambles & Moor > 1990-2000 > Cocco e Muschio Bianco > ⚥
Frais Monde – Brambles & Moor > 1990-2000 > Cotone e Guayava > ⚥
Frais Monde – Brambles & Moor > 1990-2000 > Legno di Oud e Macis > ⚥
Frais Monde – Brambles & Moor > 1990-2000 > Macchia Marina > ⚥
Frais Monde – Brambles & Moor > 1990-2000 > Mandorla e Gardenia > ⚥
Frais Monde – Brambles & Moor > 1990-2000 > Muschio Selvatico > ⚥
Frais Monde – Brambles & Moor > 1990-2000 > Muschio Veneziano > ⚥
Frais Monde – Brambles & Moor > 1990-2000 > Oceano > ⚥
Frais Monde – Brambles & Moor > 1990-2000 > Palissandro e Henné > ⚥
Frais Monde – Brambles & Moor > 1990-2000 > Riso e Muschio Bianco > ⚥
Frais Monde – Brambles & Moor > 1990-2000 > Sandalo > ⚥
Frais Monde – Brambles & Moor > 1990-2000 > Tè Verde e Bergamotto > ⚥
Frais Monde – Brambles & Moor > 1990-2000 > Vaniglia e Mate Colombiano > ⚥
Frais Monde – Brambles & Moor > 1990-2000 > Vaniglia e Muschio Bianco > ⚥
Frais Monde – Brambles & Moor > 1990-2000 > Vetiver > ⚥
Francesca Dell'Oro > 2013 > Ambrosine > ⚥
Francesca Dell'Oro > 2013 > Lullaby > ♀
Francesca Dell'Oro > 2013 > Unsaid > ♀
Francesca Dell'Oro > 2013 > Very Tight > ♂
Francesca Dell'Oro > 2013 > White Plumage > ♀
Francesca Dell'Oro > 2014 > Francine > ♀
Francesca Dell'Oro > 2015 > Anvoutant > ♀
Francesca Dell'Oro > 2015 > Fleurdenya > ♀
Francesca Dell'Oro > 2015 > Page 29 > ♀
Francesca Dell'Oro > 2017 > Ice Yasmill > ♀
Francesca Dell'Oro > 2017 > Irupe > ♀
Francesca Dell'Oro > 2017 > Rosmenthe > ♀
Francesca Dell'Oro > 2017 > Rubia Sucrée > ♀
Francesca Dell'Oro > 2017 > Voile Confit > ♀
Francesca Dell'Oro > 2018 > Bihaku > ♀
Francesca Dell'Oro > 2018 > Onemore > ♀
Francesca Dell'Oro > 2019 > There's a Place > ♀
François Deli > 2012 > Bois Aromatique > ♂
François Deli > 2012 > Citrus Leather > ♂
François Deli > 2012 > Fleurs de la Soirée > ♀
François Deli > 2012 > Fumée Toxique > ♂
François Deli > 2012 > Habitude de l'Est > ♂
François Deli > 2012 > Herbe et Jasmin > ♂
François Deli > 2012 > Moghul Garden > ♀
François Deli > 2012 > Mure et Orange > ♀
François Deli > 2012 > Neroli Nobile > ♂
François Deli > 2012 > Spicy Agarwood > ♂
François Deli > 2013 > Bouquet de Roses > ♀
François Deli > 2013 > Sweet Tobacco > ♂
François Deli > 2013 > Zone Blanche > ♀
Frankie Garage > 2017 > She > ♀
Frankie Garage > 2017 > Sporty Fragrance > ♂
Frankie Garage > 2017 > 1st Avenue > ♀

Frankie Garage > 2017 > Evo > ♂
Frankie Garage > 2017 > Frankie Garage > ♂
Frankie Garage > 2017 > Sporty Fragrance Blackout > ♂
Frankie Garage > 2017 > Street > ♂
Frankie Morello > 2010 > Collection > ♀
Frankie Morello > 2010 > Milan > ♀
Frankie Morello > 2010 > Women's Collection > ♀
Frankie Morello > 2017 > Man > ♂
Frankie Morello > 2017 > Woman > ♀
Gabriella Chieffo > 2014 > Camaheu > ♂
Gabriella Chieffo > 2014 > Hystera > ♀
Gabriella Chieffo > 2014 > Lye > ♂
Gabriella Chieffo > 2014 > Ragù > ♂
Gabriella Chieffo > 2015 > Acquasala > ♂
Gabriella Chieffo > 2015 > Variazione di Ragù > ♂
Gabriella Chieffo > 2016 > Maisia > ♂
Gabriella Chieffo > 2016 > Taersia > ♂
Gabriella Chieffo > 2017 > Quasicielo > ♂
Gabriella Chieffo > 2018 > Lattedoro > ♂
Gabriella Chieffo > 2019 > 1,2,3 Stella! > ♂
Gai Mattiolo > 1997 > Gai Mattiolo > ♀
Gai Mattiolo > 1998 > Gai Mattiolo Uomo > ♂
Gai Mattiolo > 2000 > That's Amore! Lei > ♀
Gai Mattiolo > 2000 > That's Amore! Lui > ♂
Gai Mattiolo > 2002 > That's Amore! Kisses XXX > ♀
Gai Mattiolo > 2002 > That's Amore! Kisses XXX > ♂
Gai Mattiolo > 2003 > Gai Mattiolo Man's > ♂
Gai Mattiolo > 2003 > Gai Mattiolo Woman's > ♀
Gai Mattiolo > 2005 > That's Amore! Tattoo Lei > ♀
Gai Mattiolo > 2005 > That's Amore! Tattoo Lui > ♂
Gai Mattiolo > 2006 > Be Sparkling > ♀
Gai Mattiolo > 2007 > That's Amore! Dance Lei > ♀
Gai Mattiolo > 2007 > That's Amore! Dance Lui > ♂
Gai Mattiolo > 2009 > That's Amore! Exotic Paradise Hawaiian Vanilla > ♀
Gai Mattiolo > 2009 > That's Amore! Exotic Paradise Hawaiian Water > ♂
Gandini 1896 > 2003 > Muschio Bianco > ♀
Gandini 1896 > 2003 > Tè Bianco > ♀
Gandini 1896 > 2005 > Mora & Muschio > ♀
Gandini 1896 > 2010 > Foglia e Fiori d'arancio > ♂
Gandini 1896 > 2010 > Lavanda ed Ambra d'Oro > ♂
Gandini 1896 > 2010 > Legno di Teak > ♂
Gandini 1896 > 2010 > Lime e Basilico > ♂
Gandini 1896 > 2010 > Melograno e Incenso > ♂
Gandini 1896 > 2010 > Muschio Blu > ♂
Gandini 1896 > 2010 > Pompelmo ed Agrumi > ♂
Gandini 1896 > 2010 > Rosa Rossa e Fiori di Pesco > ♀
Gandini 1896 > 2010 > Tabacco > ♂
Gandini 1896 > 2012 > Patchouli Irresistibile > ♂
Gandini 1896 > 2012 > Pioggia d'Estate > ♂
Gandini 1896 > 2012 > Vaniglia Essenziale > ♂
Gandini 1896 > 2012 > Violetta di Provenza > ♀
Gandini 1896 > 2014 > Peonia Rosa > ♀
Gas > 2005 > Gas > ♀
Gas > 2005 > Gas for Your Soul > ♂
Gattinoni > 2003 > Gattinoni Couture > ♀
Gattinoni > 2004 > Neo Man > ♂
Gattinoni > 2004 > Neo Woman > ♀
Gattinoni > 2007 > Prêt à Porter > ♀
Gattinoni > 2018 > Armonia > ♀
Genny > 1987 > Genny > ♀
Genny > 1992 > Genny Shine > ♀
Genny > 2003 > Caress > ♀
Genny > 2003 > Eau de Genny > ♀
Genny > 2014 > Eterea > ♀
Genny > 2016 > Genny Noir > ♀
Genny > 2017 > Eau de Genny Edp > ♀
Genny > 2017 > Genny Caress > ♀
Genny > 2017 > Genny Edp > ♀
Genny > 2017 > My Genny > ♀
Genny > 2018 > Platinum Genny > ♀
Gerani > 1999 > Gerani > ♀
Gerani > 1999 > Gerani pour Homme > ♂
Ghost Nose Parfums > 2016 > Arthemisia > ♂
Ghost Nose Parfums > 2016 > Estrosa > ♂
Ghost Nose Parfums > 2016 > My Oud > ♂
Ghost Nose Parfums > 2016 > Scent of Bali > ♂
Ghost Nose Parfums > 2017 > Arsenico > ♂
Ghost Nose Parfums > 2017 > Etherno > ♂
Ghost Nose Parfums > 2017 > Follja > ♂
Ghost Nose Parfums > 2018 > Ribelle > ♂
Ghost Nose Parfums > 2019 > Overdose > ♂
Gianfranco Ferré > 1984 > Eau du Matin > ♀

Gianfranco Ferré > 1984 > Ferré > ♀
Gianfranco Ferré > 1984 > Gianfranco Ferré > ♀
Gianfranco Ferré > 1986 > Gianfranco Ferré for Man > ♂
Gianfranco Ferré > 1991 > Ferré by Ferré > ♀
Gianfranco Ferré > 1995 > Gieffeffe > ♀
Gianfranco Ferré > 1998 > 20 for Woman > ♀
Gianfranco Ferré > 1998 > Gff Donna > ♀
Gianfranco Ferré > 1998 > Gff Uomo > ♂
Gianfranco Ferré > 2000 > Pontaccio 21 > ♀
Gianfranco Ferré > 2003 > Essence d'Eau > ♀
Gianfranco Ferré > 2004 > Fgf Ferré Lui-Him > ♂
Gianfranco Ferré > 2004 > Gf Ferré Lei-Her > ♀
Gianfranco Ferré > 2005 > Ferré Edp > ♀
Gianfranco Ferré > 2005 > Gianfranco Ferré Bergamotto Marino > ♂
Gianfranco Ferré > 2006 > Ferré for Men > ♂
Gianfranco Ferré > 2007 > Ferré Rose > ♀
Gianfranco Ferré > 2007 > Gf Ferré Bluemusk > ♀
Gianfranco Ferré > 2008 > Ferré Acqua Azzurra > ♂
Gianfranco Ferré > 2008 > Ferré Rose Diamond Limited Edition > ♀
Gianfranco Ferré > 2008 > Ferré Rose Princesse > ♀
Gianfranco Ferré > 2009 > In the Mood for Love > ♀
Gianfranco Ferré > 2010 > In the Mood for Love Pure > ♀
Gianfranco Ferré > 2011 > In the Mood for Love Man > ♂
Gianfranco Ferré > 2011 > In the Mood for Love Tender > ♀
Gianfranco Ferré > 2015 > Camicia 113 > ♀
Gianfranco Ferré > 2015 > Ferré Black > ♂
Gianfranco Ferré > 2016 > Camicia 113 Edt > ♀
Gianfranco Ferré > 2016 > L'uomo > ♂
Gianfranco Ferré > 2019 > Blooming Rose > ♀
Gianluca Bulega Couture > 2008 > Amami Alfredo > ♀
Gianluca Bulega Couture > 2010 > Amado Mio > ♀
Gianluca Bulega Couture > 2010 > Amami per Sempre > ♀
Gianluca Bulega Couture > 2011 > Makeda > ♀
Gianluca Bulega Couture > 2011 > Marghelove > ♀
Gianluca Bulega Couture > 2012 > Parnassus > ♀
Gian Marco Venturi > 1985 > Gian Marco Venturi > ♀
Gian Marco Venturi > 1991 > Donna > ♀
Gian Marco Venturi > 1997 > GMV Uomo > ♂
Gian Marco Venturi > 1998 > GMV Uomo Energy > ♂
Gian Marco Venturi > 1999 > GMV Donna > ♀
Gian Marco Venturi > 2000 > GMV Uomo Hot > ♂
Gian Marco Venturi > 2001 > GMV 2001 > ♂
Gian Marco Venturi > 2001 > Woman > ♀
Gian Marco Venturi > 2003 > Girl > ♀
Gian Marco Venturi > 2004 > Trybe > ♂
Gian Marco Venturi > 2006 > Girl 2 > ♀
Gian Marco Venturi > 2008 > Gian Marco Venturi Women > ♀
Gian Marco Venturi > 2010 > Frames Essence > ♀
Gian Marco Venturi > 2010 > GMV Essence for Men > ♂
Gian Marco Venturi > 2014 > Frames Homme Sport > ♂
Gian Marco Venturi > 2015 > Gian Marco Venturi Femme > ♀
Gian Marco Venturi > 2017 > Frames Oud > ♂
Gian Marco Venturi > 2018 > Aqua > ♂
Gianni Campagna > 2006 > Bespoke > ♂
Gianni Campagna > 2006 > Ciuri Ciuri > ♀
Gianni Campagna > 2006 > Gelsomino > ♀
Giardino Benessere > 2015 > Amber > ♂
Giardino Benessere > 2015 > Cotton Flower > ♂
Giardino Benessere > 2015 > Sandalo e Mirra > ♂
Giardino Benessere > 2015 > The Bianco > ♂
Giardino Benessere > 2015 > Tuberose > ♂
Giardino Benessere > 2015 > White Musk > ♂
Giardino Benessere > 2016 > Pompei Garden > ♂
Giardino Benessere > 2016 > Rosa Dorotea > ♂
Giardino Benessere > 2017 > Aurelia > ♂
Giardino Benessere > 2017 > Salaria > ♂
Giardino Benessere > 2018 > Crio > ♂
Giardino Benessere > 2018 > Febe > ♂
Giardino Benessere > 2018 > Kronos > ♂
Giardino Benessere > 2018 > Tethys > ♂
Giardino Benessere > 2019 > Oceania > ♂
Giardino Benessere > 2019 > Rea > ♂
Giardino dei Sensi > 2017 > Bacche di Goji > ♂
Giardino dei Sensi > 2018 > Fior di Loto Candido > ♀
Giardino dei Sensi > 2018 > Fiordaliso Vivace > ♀
Giardino dei Sensi > 2018 > Giglio Gentile > ♀
Giardino dei Sensi > 2018 > Legni Mediterranei for Men > ♂
Giardino dei Sensi > 2018 > Orchidea Romantica > ♀
Giardino dei Sensi > 2018 > Tiare Esotico > ♀
Giardino dei Sensi > 2018 > Iris Poetico > ♀
Giardino dei Sensi > 2018 > Segreto Narciso > ♀
Giardino dei Sensi > 2018 > Sublime Peonia > ♀

Giardino dei Sensi > 2019 > Essenziale Vaniglia > ♀
Giardino dei Sensi > 2019 > Avena > ♂
Giardino dei Sensi > 2019 > Legni Esotici > ♂
Giardino dei Sensi > 2019 > Soave Magnolia > ♀
Giglio – Elisir Toscano > 2018 > Giglio Assoluto > ♂
Giorgio Armani > 1982 > Armani > ♀
Giorgio Armani > 1984 > Armani Eau pour Homme > ♂
Giorgio Armani > 1992 > Giò > ♀
Giorgio Armani > 1995 > Acqua di Giò > ♀
Giorgio Armani > 1996 > Acqua di Giò > ♂
Giorgio Armani > 1998 > Emporio Armani Lei > ♀
Giorgio Armani > 1998 > Emporio Armani Lui > ♂
Giorgio Armani > 2000 > Mania > ♀
Giorgio Armani > 2001 > Emporio Armani White for Her > ♀
Giorgio Armani > 2001 > Emporio Armani White for Him > ♂
Giorgio Armani > 2002 > Armani Mania > ♂
Giorgio Armani > 2002 > Sensi > ♀
Giorgio Armani > 2003 > Emporio Armani Night > ♀
Giorgio Armani > 2004 > Armani Code > ♂
Giorgio Armani > 2004 > Armani Mania > ♀
Giorgio Armani > 2004 > Armani Privé Ambre Soie > ♂
Giorgio Armani > 2004 > Armani Privé Bois d'Encens > ♂
Giorgio Armani > 2004 > Armani Privé Pierre de Lune > ♂
Giorgio Armani > 2004 > Ermani Privé Eau de Jade > ♂
Giorgio Armani > 2004 > Sensi Jewel > ♀
Giorgio Armani > 2004 > Sensi White Notes > ♀
Giorgio Armani > 2005 > Armani Privé Cuir Amethyste > ♂
Giorgio Armani > 2005 > City Glam for Her > ♀
Giorgio Armani > 2005 > City Glam for Him > ♂
Giorgio Armani > 2006 > Armani Code Elixir > ♀
Giorgio Armani > 2006 > Emporio Remix for Her > ♀
Giorgio Armani > 2006 > Emporio Remix for Him > ♂
Giorgio Armani > 2006 > Summer Mania Femme > ♀
Giorgio Armani > 2006 > Summer Mania Homme > ♂
Giorgio Armani > 2007 > Armani Code Sheer > ♀
Giorgio Armani > 2007 > Armani Privé Eclat de Jasmin > ♂
Giorgio Armani > 2007 > Attitude > ♂
Giorgio Armani > 2007 > Emporio Armani Diamonds > ♀
Giorgio Armani > 2007 > Emporio Armani Red pour Elle > ♀
Giorgio Armani > 2007 > Emporio Armani Red pour Lui > ♂
Giorgio Armani > 2007 > Summer Mania Eau Fraiche pour Femme > ♀
Giorgio Armani > 2007 > Summer Mania Eau Fraiche pour Homme > ♂
Giorgio Armani > 2008 > Armani Code Casino Limited Edition 2008 > ♂
Giorgio Armani > 2008 > Armani Code Le Parfum > ♂
Giorgio Armani > 2008 > Armani Code Mirror Edition > ♂
Giorgio Armani > 2008 > Armani Privé Les Eaux: Oranger Alhambra > ♂
Giorgio Armani > 2008 > Armani Privé Les Eaux: Rose Alexandrie > ♀
Giorgio Armani > 2008 > Armani Privé Les Eaux: Vetiver d'Hiver (Vetiver Babylonie) > ♂
Giorgio Armani > 2008 > Emporio Armani Diamonds for Men > ♂
Giorgio Armani > 2008 > Emporio Armani for Her 2008 > ♀
Giorgio Armani > 2008 > Emporio Armani for Him 2008 > ♂
Giorgio Armani > 2008 > Emporio Armani diamonds Intense > ♀
Giorgio Armani > 2008 > Onde Collection: Onde Extase > ♀
Giorgio Armani > 2008 > Onde Collection: Onde Mystere > ♀
Giorgio Armani > 2008 > Onde Collection: Onde Vertige > ♀
Giorgio Armani > 2009 > Armani Code Summer pour Femme > ♀
Giorgio Armani > 2009 > Armani Code Summer pour Homme > ♂
Giorgio Armani > 2009 > Armani Privé Les Eaux: Cedre Olympe > ♂
Giorgio Armani > 2009 > Attitude Extreme > ♂
Giorgio Armani > 2009 > Emporio Armani Diamonds Edt > ♀
Giorgio Armani > 2009 > Emporio Armani Diamonds He Limite Edition > ♂
Giorgio Armani > 2009 > Idole d'Armani > ♀
Giorgio Armani > 2010 > Acqua di Gioia > ♀
Giorgio Armani > 2010 > Armani Code Summer pour Femme 2010 > ♀
Giorgio Armani > 2010 > Armani Code Summer pour Homme 2010 > ♂
Giorgio Armani > 2010 > Armani Privé Ambre Orient > ♂
Giorgio Armani > 2010 > Armani Privé Oud Royal > ♂
Giorgio Armani > 2010 > Armani Privé Rose d'Arabie > ♂
Giorgio Armani > 2010 > Emporio Armani Diamonds for Men Summer Edition > ♂
Giorgio Armani > 2010 > Emporio Armani Diamonds for Women Summer Edition > ♀
Giorgio Armani > 2010 > Idole d'Armani Edt > ♀
Giorgio Armani > 2011 > Acqua di Giò – Acqua di Life Edition > ♂
Giorgio Armani > 2011 > Acqua di Gioia Essenza > ♀
Giorgio Armani > 2011 > Armani Code Sport > ♂
Giorgio Armani > 2011 > Armani Code Summer pour Femme 2011 > ♀
Giorgio Armani > 2011 > Armani Code Summer pour Homme 2011 > ♂
Giorgio Armani > 2011 > Armani Privé Cuir Noir > ♂
Giorgio Armani > 2011 > Armani Privé Les Editions Couture: Le Femme Bleue > ♀

Giorgio Armani > 2011 > Emporio Armani Diamonds Black Carat for Her > ♀
Giorgio Armani > 2011 > Emporio Armani Diamonds Black Carat for Him > ♂
Giorgio Armani > 2012 > Acqua di Giò Essenza > ♂
Giorgio Armani > 2012 > Acqua di Gioia Edp Satinée > ♀
Giorgio Armani > 2012 > Armani Code Couture Edition > ♀
Giorgio Armani > 2012 > Armani Code Luna > ♀
Giorgio Armani > 2012 > Armani Code Sport Athlete > ♂
Giorgio Armani > 2012 > Armani Code Ultimate > ♂
Giorgio Armani > 2012 > Armani Privé Les Eaux: Figuier Eden > ♂
Giorgio Armani > 2012 > Armani Privé Les Editions Couture: La Femme Nacre > ♀
Giorgio Armani > 2012 > Emporio Armani Diamonds Summer Fraiche for Men > ♂
Giorgio Armani > 2012 > Emporio Armani Diamonds Summer Fraiche for Women > ♀
Giorgio Armani > 2013 > Acqua di Gioia Eau Fraiche > ♀
Giorgio Armani > 2013 > Armani Code Golden Edition > ♂
Giorgio Armani > 2013 > Armani Eau de Nuit > ♂
Giorgio Armani > 2013 > Armani Eau pour Homme > ♂
Giorgio Armani > 2013 > Armani Privé Les Editions Couture: Nuances > ♀
Giorgio Armani > 2013 > Armani Privé Myrrhe Imperiale > ♀
Giorgio Armani > 2013 > Armani Privé Rose d'Arabie L'or du Desert > ♂
Giorgio Armani > 2013 > Emporio Armani Diamonds Rose > ♀
Giorgio Armani > 2013 > Sì > ♀
Giorgio Armani > 2014 > Acqua di Giò Blue Edition pour Homme > ♂
Giorgio Armani > 2014 > Acqua di Gioia Edt > ♀
Giorgio Armani > 2014 > Armani Code Ice > ♂
Giorgio Armani > 2014 > Armani Eau d'Aromes > ♂
Giorgio Armani > 2014 > Armani Privé Encens Satin > ♀
Giorgio Armani > 2014 > Armani Privé Les Eaux: Pivoine Suzhou > ♀
Giorgio Armani > 2014 > Armani Privé Les Editions Couture: Ombre & Lumière > ♀
Giorgio Armani > 2014 > Armani Privé Rose d'Arabie Limited Edition Swarovski > ♀
Giorgio Armani > 2014 > Emporio Armani Diamonds Rocks > ♂
Giorgio Armani > 2014 > Sì Intense > ♀
Giorgio Armani > 2014 > Sì White > ♀
Giorgio Armani > 2015 > Acqua di Giò Profumo > ♂
Giorgio Armani > 2015 > Acqua di Gioia Jasmine > ♀
Giorgio Armani > 2015 > Armani Code Satin > ♀
Giorgio Armani > 2015 > Armani Code Special Blend > ♂
Giorgio Armani > 2015 > Armani Code Turquoise for Men > ♂
Giorgio Armani > 2015 > Armani Code Turquoise for Women > ♀
Giorgio Armani > 2015 > Armani Eau de Cedre > ♂
Giorgio Armani > 2015 > Armani Privé Ambre Eccentrico > ♂
Giorgio Armani > 2015 > Armani Privé Sable Fume > ♀
Giorgio Armani > 2015 > Armani Privé Sable Or > ♀
Giorgio Armani > 2015 > Emporio Armani Diamonds Violet > ♀
Giorgio Armani > 2015 > Sì Edt > ♀
Giorgio Armani > 2015 > Sì Golden Bow > ♀
Giorgio Armani > 2015 > Sì Huile de Parfum > ♀
Giorgio Armani > 2016 > Air di Gioia > ♀
Giorgio Armani > 2016 > Armani Code Profumo > ♂
Giorgio Armani > 2016 > Armani Code Sport Edition 2016 > ♂
Giorgio Armani > 2016 > Armani Eau de Nuit Oud > ♂
Giorgio Armani > 2016 > Armani Privé Cuir Majeste > ♀
Giorgio Armani > 2016 > Armani Privé Les Eaux: Pivoine Suzhou Soie de Nacre > ♀
Giorgio Armani > 2016 > Armani Privé Les Editions Couture: Fil Rouge > ♀
Giorgio Armani > 2016 > Armani Privé Rose Malachite > ♀
Giorgio Armani > 2016 > Armani Privé Vert Malachite > ♀
Giorgio Armani > 2016 > Emporio Armani Diamonds Club > ♀
Giorgio Armani > 2016 > Emporio Armani Diamonds Club for Him > ♂
Giorgio Armani > 2016 > Sì Intense Night Light > ♀
Giorgio Armani > 2016 > Sì Le Parfum > ♀
Giorgio Armani > 2016 > Sì Night Light > ♀
Giorgio Armani > 2016 > Sì Rose Signature > ♀
Giorgio Armani > 2016 > Sky di Gioia > ♀
Giorgio Armani > 2016 > Sun di Gioia > ♀
Giorgio Armani > 2017 > Acqua di Giò Profumo Special Blend > ♂
Giorgio Armani > 2017 > Armani Code Cashmere > ♀
Giorgio Armani > 2017 > Armani Code Colonia > ♂
Giorgio Armani > 2017 > Armani Privé Iris Celadon > ♀
Giorgio Armani > 2017 > Armani Privé Les Editions Couture: Charm' > ♀
Giorgio Armani > 2017 > Armani Privé New York > ♂
Giorgio Armani > 2017 > Armani Privé Rouge Malachite Limited Edition l'Or de Russie > ♂
Giorgio Armani > 2017 > Because It's You > ♀
Giorgio Armani > 2017 > Emporio Armani Stronger With You > ♂
Giorgio Armani > 2017 > Sì Hair Mist > ♀
Giorgio Armani > 2017 > Sì Passione > ♀
Giorgio Armani > 2017 > Sì Rose Signature II Edp > ♀

Giorgio Armani > 2017 > Sì Sono Io > ♀
Giorgio Armani > 2018 > Acqua di Giò Absolu > ♂
Giorgio Armani > 2018 > Acqua di Gioia Hair & Body Mist > ♀
Giorgio Armani > 2018 > Armani Code A-List > ♂
Giorgio Armani > 2018 > Armani Privé Bleu Lazuli > ♂
Giorgio Armani > 2018 > Armani Privé Bleu Turquoise > ♂
Giorgio Armani > 2018 > Armani Privé Les Editions Couture: Rose d'Artiste > ♀
Giorgio Armani > 2018 > Armani Privé Rose d'Arabie Limited Edition 2018 > ♂
Giorgio Armani > 2018 > Sì Nacre Edition > ♀
Giorgio Armani > 2018 > Sì Passione Limited Edition > ♀
Giorgio Armani > 2019 > Acqua di Giò Absolu Instinct > ♂
Giorgio Armani > 2019 > Armani Code Absolu > ♂
Giorgio Armani > 2019 > Armani Code Absolu Femme > ♀
Giorgio Armani > 2019 > Armani Privé Les Eaux: Orangerie Venise > ♂
Giorgio Armani > 2019 > Armani Privé Les Editions Couture: Laque > ♂
Giorgio Armani > 2019 > Armani Privé Musc Shamal > ♂
Giorgio Armani > 2019 > Emporio Armani Stronger With You Intensely > ♂
Giorgio Armani > 2019 > In Love With You > ♀
Giorgio Armani > 2019 > Light di Gioia > ♀
Giorgio Armani > 2019 > Sì Fiori > ♀
Giorgio Armani > 2019 > Sì Nacre Edition 2019 > ♀
Giorgio Armani > 2019 > Sì Passione Limited Edition 2019 > ♀
Giorgio Armani > 2019 > Sì Passione Red Maestro > ♀
Giorgio Armani > 2020 > Armani Code Absolu Gold > ♂
Giorgio Armani > 2020 > Armani Privé Les Eaux: Gardenia Antigua > ♂
Giorgio Armani > 2020 > Armani Privé Les Eaux: Jasmin Kusamono > ♀
Giorgio Armani > 2020 > Armani Privé Les Eaux: Rose Milano > ♀
Giorgio Armani > 2020 > Armani Privé Les Eaux: The Yulong > ♀
Giorgio Armani > 2020 > Emporio Armani in Love with you Freeze > ♀
Giorgio Armani > 2020 > Emporio Armani Stronger with you Freeze > ♂
Giorgio Armani > 2020 > Sì Passione Intense > ♀
Giulietta Capuleti > 2011 > Soul Drops > ♀
Giulietta Capuleti > 2014 > Ballo in Maschera > ♀
Giulietta Capuleti > 2014 > Bugia Bianca > ♂
Giulietta Capuleti > 2014 > Ritorno Amaro > ♀
Giulietta Capuleti > 2015 > Far from Balcony > ♂
Gocce di Byron > 2015 > N. 1 > ♂
Gocce di Byron > 2015 > N. 2 > ♂
Gocce di Byron > 2015 > N. 3 > ♂
Gocce di Byron > 2015 > N. 4 > ♂
Gocce di Byron > 2015 > N. 5 > ♂
Gocce di Byron > 2015 > Portovenere > ♀
Gocce di Byron > 2015 > Vernazza > ♂
Goti > 2008 > Black > ♂
Goti > 2008 > Earth > ♂
Goti > 2008 > White > ♂
Goti > 2013 > Gray > ♂
Goti > 2013 > Smoke > ♂
Goti > 2016 > Alchemico: Visione 2 – Acqua > ♂
Goti > 2016 > Alchemico: Visione 2 – Aria > ♂
Goti > 2016 > Alchemico: Visione 2 – Terra > ♂
Goti > 2016 > Alchemico: Visione 3 – Fuoco > ♂
Greta Mastroianni > 2013 > Greta Mastroianni > ♀
Gritti > 2010 > Antalya > ♂
Gritti > 2012 > Aqua Incanta > ♀
Gritti > 2012 > Damascus > ♀
Gritti > 2013 > White Edition Black Currant > ♂
Gritti > 2013 > White Edition Light Powdery > ♂
Gritti > 2013 > White Edition Sweet Vanilla > ♂
Gritti > 2013 > White Edition White Almond > ♂
Gritti > 2014 > Doped Tuberose > ♀
Gritti > 2014 > Fanos > ♂
Gritti > 2014 > Noctem Arabs > ♂
Gritti > 2015 > Collection Privé: Arete > ♂
Gritti > 2015 > Collection Privé: Ephesus > ♂
Gritti > 2015 > Collection Privé: Loody > ♂
Gritti > 2015 > Collection Privé: Mathi > ♂
Gritti > 2015 > Saraj > ♂
Gritti > 2016 > Collection Privé: Alexandra > ♀
Gritti > 2016 > Collection Privé: Lu > ♀
Gritti > 2016 > Decimo > ♂
Gritti > 2016 > Magnifica Lux > ♀
Gritti > 2016 > Delirium > ♂
Gritti > 2016 > Preludio > ♀
Gritti > 2017 > Arancia Ambrata > ♂
Gritti > 2017 > Costiera > ♀
Gritti > 2017 > Neroli Extreme > ♂
Gritti > 2017 > Pomelo Sorrento > ♂
Gritti > 2018 > Bra Series – Adele > ♀
Gritti > 2018 > Bra Series – Chantilly > ♀
Gritti > 2018 > Bra Series – Dame de L'Île > ♀

Gritti > 2018 > Bra Series – Macrame > ♀
Gritti > 2018 > Bra Series – Rebrode > ♀
Gritti > 2018 > Collection Privé: Fenice > ♂
Gritti > 2018 > Tangerina > ♂
Gritti > 2019 > 19-68 > ♂
Gritti > 2019 > Bra Series – Tutu > ♀
Gucci > 1974 > Gucci N. 1 > ♀
Gucci > 1976 > Gucci pour Homme > ♂
Gucci > 1982 > Eau de Gucci Concentrée > ♂
Gucci > 1985 > Gucci N. 3 > ♀
Gucci > 1988 > Gucci Nobile > ♂
Gucci > 1991 > L'arte di Gucci > ♀
Gucci > 1993 > Eau de Gucci > ♀
Gucci > 1995 > Gucci Accenti > ♀
Gucci > 1997 > Envy > ♀
Gucci > 1997 > Envy Edp > ♀
Gucci > 1998 > Envy for Men > ♂
Gucci > 1999 > Gucci Rush > ♀
Gucci > 2000 > Gucci Rush for Men > ♂
Gucci > 2001 > Gucci Rush 2 > ♀
Gucci > 2002 > Gucci Eau de Parfum > ♀
Gucci > 2003 > Gucci pour Homme > ♂
Gucci > 2003 > Gucci Rush Summer > ♀
Gucci > 2004 > Gucci Eau de Parfum II > ♀
Gucci > 2006 > Envy Me 2 > ♀
Gucci > 2007 > Gucci by Gucci Edp > ♀
Gucci > 2007 > Gucci pour Homme II > ♂
Gucci > 2008 > Gucci by Gucci Edt > ♀
Gucci > 2008 > Gucci by Gucci pour Homme > ♂
Gucci > 2009 > Flora by Gucci Edt > ♀
Gucci > 2010 > Flora by Gucci Edp > ♀
Gucci > 2010 > Gucci by Gucci Sport > ♂
Gucci > 2010 > Gucci Guilty > ♀
Gucci > 2011 > Flora by Gucci Eau Fraiche > ♀
Gucci > 2011 > Gucci Guilty Intense > ♀
Gucci > 2011 > Gucci Guilty Intense pour Homme > ♂
Gucci > 2011 > Gucci Guilty pour Homme > ♂
Gucci > 2012 > Flora Garden Collection: Generous Violet > ♀
Gucci > 2012 > Flora Garden Collection: Glamorous Magnolia > ♀
Gucci > 2012 > Flora Garden Collection: Glorius Mandarin > ♀
Gucci > 2012 > Flora Garden Collection: Gorgeous Gardenia > ♀
Gucci > 2012 > Gucci Première > ♀
Gucci > 2013 > Flora by Gucci 1966 > ♀
Gucci > 2013 > Gucci Guilty Black pour Femme > ♀
Gucci > 2013 > Gucci Guilty Black pour Homme > ♂
Gucci > 2013 > Gucci Guilty Studs pour Femme > ♀
Gucci > 2013 > Gucci Guilty Studs pour Homme > ♂
Gucci > 2013 > Gucci Museo: Forever Now > ♂
Gucci > 2013 > Made to Measure > ♂
Gucci > 2014 > Gucci Guilty Diamond > ♀
Gucci > 2014 > Gucci Guilty pour Homme Diamond > ♂
Gucci > 2014 > Gucci Oud > ♂
Gucci > 2014 > Gucci Premiere Edt > ♀
Gucci > 2015 > Gucci Bamboo > ♀
Gucci > 2015 > Gucci Guilty Eau > ♀
Gucci > 2015 > Gucci Guilty Eau pour Homme > ♂
Gucci > 2016 > Flora by Gucci Anniversary Edition > ♀
Gucci > 2016 > Gucci Bamboo Edt > ♀
Gucci > 2016 > Gucci Guilty Platinum > ♀
Gucci > 2016 > Intense Oud > ♂
Gucci > 2017 > Gucci Bloom > ♀
Gucci > 2017 > Gucci Guilty Absolute > ♂
Gucci > 2018 > Flora Gorgeous Gardenia Limited Edition > ♀
Gucci > 2018 > Flora Gorgeous Gardenia Limited Edition 2018 > ♀
Gucci > 2018 > Gucci Bloom Acqua di Fiori > ♀
Gucci > 2018 > Gucci Bloom Nettare di Fiori > ♀
Gucci > 2018 > Gucci Guilty Absolute pour Femme > ♀
Gucci > 2018 > Gucci Guilty Oud > ♂
Gucci > 2019 > Flora Emerald Gardenia > ♀
Gucci > 2019 > Gucci Bloom Ambrosia di Fiori > ♀
Gucci > 2019 > Gucci Bloom Gocce di Fiori > ♀
Gucci > 2019 > Gucci Bloom Hair Mist > ♀
Gucci > 2019 > Gucci Guilty Edp > ♀
Gucci > 2019 > Memoire d'une Odeur > ♂
Gucci > 2019 > The Alchemist Garden: A Forgotten Rose Perfume Oil > ♂
Gucci > 2019 > The Alchemist Garden: A Kiss from Violet Perfume Oil > ♂
Gucci > 2019 > The Alchemist Garden: A Nocturnal Whisper Perfume Oil > ♂
Gucci > 2019 > The Alchemist Garden: A Song for the Rose Edp > ♂
Gucci > 2019 > The Alchemist Garden: A Winter Melody Scented Water > ♂
Gucci > 2019 > The Alchemist Garden: Fading Autumn Scented Water > ♂
Gucci > 2019 > The Alchemist Garden: Moonlight Serenade Scented Water > ♂

Iceberg > 2000 > Fluid Man > ♂
Iceberg > 2000 > Fluid Woman > ♀
Iceberg > 2001 > Iceberg Effusion Man > ♂
Iceberg > 2001 > Iceberg Effusion Woman > ♀
Iceberg > 2004 > Light Fluid Iceberg Man > ♂
Iceberg > 2004 > Light Fluid Iceberg Woman > ♀
Iceberg > 2008 > The Iceberg Fragrance > ⚥
Iceberg > 2009 > The Iceberg Fragrance for Men > ♂
Iceberg > 2010 > Eau de Iceberg 74 pour Femme > ♀
Iceberg > 2010 > Eau de Iceberg 74 pour Homme > ♂
Iceberg > 2012 > Burning Ice > ♂
Iceberg > 2012 > Eau de Iceberg 74 Amber > ♂
Iceberg > 2012 > Eau de Iceberg 74 Cedar > ♂
Iceberg > 2012 > Eau de Iceberg 74 Jasmin > ♀
Iceberg > 2012 > Eau de Iceberg 74 Wild Rose > ♀
Iceberg > 2013 > Eau de Iceberg 74 Oud > ♂
Iceberg > 2013 > Eau de Iceberg 74 Sandalwood > ♂
Iceberg > 2013 > Eau de Iceberg 74 Sensual Musk > ♀
Iceberg > 2013 > Iceberg White > ⚥
Iceberg > 2014 > Tender White > ♀
Iceberg > 2015 > Iceberg Man > ♂
Iceberg > 2018 > Iceberg since 1974 for Her > ♀
Iceberg > 2018 > Iceberg since 1974 for Him > ♂
I Coloniali > 1994 > Acqua Tenera alla Peonia Cinese > ♀
I Coloniali > 1994 > Macerato Aromatico per Donna alla Cananga di Java > ♀
I Coloniali > 1994 > Macerato Aromatico per Uomo al Legno di Guajaco > ♂
I Coloniali > 1995 > Mirra & Mirra > ⚥
I Coloniali > 1995 > Tea & Tea > ⚥
I Coloniali > 1995 > Vaniglia & Vaniglia > ⚥
I Coloniali > 1995 > Woody & Spicy > ⚥
I Coloniali > 1999 > Ebano & Ebano > ♂
I Coloniali > 2012 > Seductive Elixir: Angel Musk > ♀
I Coloniali > 2012 > Seductive Elixir: Animal Oud > ♀
I Coloniali > 2012 > Seductive Elixir: Ardent Amber > ♀
I Coloniali > 2012 > Seductive Elixir: Luxurious Datura > ♀
I Coloniali > 2012 > Seductive Elixir: Mysterious Rose > ♀
I Coloniali > 2012 > Seductive Elixir: Playful Lychee > ♀
I Coloniali > 2012 > Seductive Elixir: Sensual Silk > ♀
I Coloniali > 2012 > Seductive Elixir: Sexy Vanilla > ♀
I Fiori del Male > 2018 > Rose Narcotique > ⚥
I Fiori del Male > 2018 > Tubereuse Malefique > ⚥
I Fiori del Male > 2018 > Violette Lysergique > ⚥
I Fiori del Male > 2019 > Gourmand 1 > ⚥
I Fiori del Male > 2019 > Gourmand 2 > ⚥
I Fiori del Male > 2019 > Gourmand 3 > ⚥
I Fiori del Male > 2019 > Iris Obscur > ⚥
I Fiori del Male > 2019 > Ylang Additif > ⚥
Il Profvmo > 1997 > Chocolat > ♀
Il Profvmo > 1998 > Amour > ♀
Il Profvmo > 1998 > Café Vert > ♀
Il Profvmo > 2000 > Chocolat Amère > ♂
Il Profvmo > 2002 > Aria di Mare > ⚥
Il Profvmo > 2003 > Touaregh > ⚥
Il Profvmo > 2004 > Ambre d'Or > ⚥
Il Profvmo > 2004 > Citron Sauvage > ⚥
Il Profvmo > 2004 > Encens Epicé > ♂
Il Profvmo > 2004 > Gardenia Royal > ♀
Il Profvmo > 2004 > Mandarine > ♀
Il Profvmo > 2004 > Musc Bleu > ♀
Il Profvmo > 2004 > Nymphea > ♀
Il Profvmo > 2004 > Palmerose > ⚥
Il Profvmo > 2004 > Vanille Bourbon > ♀
Il Profvmo > 2005 > Eclair de Tubereuse > ♀
Il Profvmo > 2005 > Musc Bleu Absolu > ♀
Il Profvmo > 2005 > Rose Secrete > ♀
Il Profvmo > 2005 > Vent de Jasmin > ♀
Il Profvmo > 2006 > Aventure > ♂
Il Profvmo > 2006 > Chocolat Frais > ♀
Il Profvmo > 2006 > G11 > ♂
Il Profvmo > 2006 > Patchouli Noir > ⚥
Il Profvmo > 2007 > Macadam > ♀
Il Profvmo > 2008 > Blanche Jacinthe > ♀
Il Profvmo > 2008 > Coquelicot > ♀
Il Profvmo > 2008 > Coquelicot > ♀
Il Profvmo > 2008 > Imprinting > ♂
Il Profvmo > 2008 > Songe de Tulipe > ♀
Il Profvmo > 2008 > Brise de Lavande > ⚥
Il Profvmo > 2008 > Vetiver de Java > ♂
Il Profvmo > 2009 > Pioggia Salata > ⚥
Il Profvmo > 2010 > Nuda > ♀
Il Profvmo > 2011 > Cannabis > ⚥
Il Profvmo > 2011 > Chocolat Bambola > ⚥
Il Profvmo > 2011 > Fleur de Bambu > ♀
Il Profvmo > 2011 > Ginger Osmo > ⚥
Il Profvmo > 2011 > Osé > ♀
Il Profvmo > 2011 > Profumo d'Italia > ⚥
Il Profvmo > 2011 > Santal Rouge > ♂
Il Profvmo > 2013 > Black Dianthus > ⚥
Il Profvmo > 2014 > Quai des Lices > ⚥
Il Profvmo > 2014 > Viole Blanche > ♀
Il Profvmo > 2015 > Cortigiana > ♀
Il Profvmo > 2016 > Caramella d'Amore > ♀
Il Profvmo > 2016 > Othello > ♂
Il Profvmo > 2017 > Lysander > ♂
Il Profvmo > 2017 > Silvana > ⚥
Il Profvmo > 2018 > Romeo > ♂
Il Profvmo > 2019 > Fleur de Cerisier > ♀
Imperial Fashion > 2015 > Magico Imperial #1 for Her > ♀
Imperial Fashion > 2015 > Magico Imperial #2 for Him > ♂
Inspiritv > 2015 > Fortitvdo > ⚥
Inspiritv > 2015 > Ivstitia > ⚥
Inspiritv > 2015 > Lvx > ⚥
Inspiritv > 2015 > Prvdentia > ⚥
Inspiritv > 2015 > Temperantia > ⚥
Inspiritv > 2016 > Solstitivm > ⚥
Intimissimi > 2008 > Intimissimi > ♀
Intimissimi > 2013 > Innocente > ♀
Intimissimi > 2013 > Romantica > ♀
Intimissimi > 2013 > Sensuale > ♀
Intimissimi > 2015 > Mia > ♀
Intimissimi > 2015 > Unica > ♀
IO-KO 1954 > 2017 > I.EGOCENTRIC > ⚥
IO-KO 1954 > 2017 > I.MIRAGE 11 > ⚥
IO-KO 1954 > 2017 > I.MIRAGE 23 > ⚥
IO-KO 1954 > 2017 > I.OUD > ⚥
IO-KO 1954 > 2017 > I.PATCHOULY > ⚥
IO-KO 1954 > 2017 > I.UTOPIA > ⚥
IO-KO 1954 > 2018 > I.IOKORO > ⚥
IO-KO 1954 > 2019 > I.METAPHOR > ⚥
I Profumi del Marmo > 2014 > Calacatta > ⚥
I Profumi del Marmo > 2014 > Statuario > ⚥
I Profumi del Marmo > 2016 > Bianco Carrara > ⚥
I Profumi del Marmo > 2016 > Portoro > ⚥
I Profumi del Marmo > 2017 > Arabescato > ⚥
I Profumi del Marmo > 2017 > Bardiglio > ⚥
I Profumi del Marmo > 2017 > Fantastico > ⚥
I Profumi del Marmo > 2018 > Art Collection: Bugia > ⚥
I Profumi del Marmo > 2018 > Eminentia > ⚥
I Profumi del Marmo > 2018 > Pinocchio Solid Perfume > ⚥
I Profumi del Marmo > 2018 > Rosso Verona > ⚥
I Profumi del Marmo > 2019 > Travertino > ⚥
I Profumi del Mastro Profumaio > 2018 > Fior di Panna > ♀
I Profumi del Mastro Profumaio > 2018 > Granverde > ⚥
I Profumi del Mastro Profumaio > 2018 > La Riserva > ⚥
I Profumi del Mastro Profumaio > 2018 > Mantra > ⚥
I Profumi di d'Annunzio > 2017 > Aqva Nvntia > ♀
I Profumi di d'Annunzio > 2017 > Diva Musa > ♀
I Profumi di d'Annunzio > 2017 > Ermione > ♀
I Profumi di d'Annunzio > 2017 > Il Piacere > ♀
I Profumi di d'Annunzio > 2018 > Il Fuoco > ⚥
I Profumi di d'Annunzio > 2018 > Notturno > ⚥
I Profumi di Firenze > 1990 > Agrumi di Sicilia > ⚥
I Profumi di Firenze > 1990 > Ambra del Nepal > ⚥
I Profumi di Firenze > 1994 > Caterina de' Medici > ♀
I Profumi di Firenze > 1998 > Acqua Mirabile Odorosa di Firenze > ⚥
I Profumi di Firenze > 1998 > Acqua Mirabile Odorosa di Firenze N. 1 > ⚥
I Profumi di Firenze > 2000 > Acqua Chiara > ♀
I Profumi di Firenze > 2000 > Limone di Sicilia > ⚥
I Profumi di Firenze > 2000 > Spezie de' Medici > ⚥
I Profumi di Firenze > 2000 > Talco Delicato > ⚥
I Profumi di Firenze > 2000 > Vaniglia del Madagascar > ♀
I Profumi di Firenze > 2000 > Vaniglia e Zenzero > ⚥
I Profumi di Firenze > 2000 > Zenzero > ⚥
I Profumi di Firenze > 2000 > Vaniglia e Zenzero > ⚥
I Profumi di Firenze > 2000 > Eternelle > ♀
I Profumi di Firenze > 2000 > Florentia 16 Dolci Fiori > ♀
I Profumi di Firenze > 2000 > Florentia 22 Pesca e Fiori > ♀
I Profumi di Firenze > 2000 > Florentia 24 > ♀
I Profumi di Firenze > 2000 > Florentia 24 Rosa e Fiori > ♀
I Profumi di Firenze > 2000 > Florentia 26 Frutti Esotici > ♀
I Profumi di Firenze > 2000 > Fresco di Vetiver > ⚥
I Profumi di Firenze > 2000 > Magnifico 1 Mirto Imperiale > ⚥

I Profumi di Firenze > 2000 > Magnolia Purpurea > ♀
I Profumi di Firenze > 2000 > Mela Verde > ♀
I Profumi di Firenze > 2000 > Melograno Selvatico > ♂
I Profumi di Firenze > 2000 > Mirto Imperiale > ♂
I Profumi di Firenze > 2000 > Senza Fine > ♀
I Profumi di Firenze > 2000 > Magnifico 13 Cedro e Ciclamino > ♂
I Profumi di Firenze > 2002 > Costa Mediterranea > ♂
I Profumi di Firenze > 2002 > Sapore di Mare (Brezza Di Mare) > ♂
I Profumi di Firenze > 2002 > Ancienne La Vecchia Spezieria > ♂
I Profumi di Firenze > 2002 > Arancio di Sicilia > ♂
I Profumi di Firenze > 2002 > Bergamotto Calabro > ♂
I Profumi di Firenze > 2002 > Caprifoglio Rupestre > ♀
I Profumi di Firenze > 2002 > Cashmere > ♀
I Profumi di Firenze > 2002 > Cedro > ♂
I Profumi di Firenze > 2002 > Cuoio di Russia > ♂
I Profumi di Firenze > 2002 > Dolce Patchouli > ♀
I Profumi di Firenze > 2002 > Dolceamaro > ♀
I Profumi di Firenze > 2002 > Fior di Loto > ♀
I Profumi di Firenze > 2002 > Frangipane > ♂
I Profumi di Firenze > 2002 > Frangipane e Cocco > ♀
I Profumi di Firenze > 2002 > Vaniglia e Fichi > ♀
I Profumi di Firenze > 2002 > Vetiver di Giava > ♂
I Profumi di Firenze > 2002 > Violetta di Bosco > ♀
I Profumi di Firenze > 2002 > Zagara Neroli Flor > ♂
I Profumi di Firenze > 2002 > Zefiro > ♂
I Profumi di Firenze > 2004 > Muschio e Giglio > ♀
I Profumi di Firenze > 2004 > Muschio Nero > ♂
I Profumi di Firenze > 2006 > I Fiori del Cielo > ♀
I Profumi di Firenze > 2006 > Miele Rosa > ♀
I Profumi di Firenze > 2006 > Mirra Elemi > ♂
I Profumi di Firenze > 2006 > Muschio e Ambra > ♂
I Profumi di Firenze > 2006 > Muschio e Spezie > ♂
I Profumi di Firenze > 2006 > Spigo Fiorentino Lavanda Oxford > ♂
I Profumi di Firenze > 2007 > Magnifico 9 Zenzero e Peperoncino > ♂
I Profumi di Firenze > 2007 > Muschio Bianco > ♂
I Profumi di Firenze > 2007 > Terra di Siena > ♀
I Profumi di Firenze > 2007 > Mimosa Sensitiva > ♀
I Profumi di Firenze > 2008 > Tuscania > ♂
I Profumi di Firenze > 2008 > Verde Bosco > ♂
I Profumi di Firenze > 2008 > Muschio dell'Himalaya > ♀
I Profumi di Firenze > 2008 > Tabacco > ♂
I Profumi di Firenze > 2008 > Thé Verde > ♂
I Profumi di Firenze > 2008 > Tuberosa d'Autunno > ♀
I Profumi di Firenze > 2008 > Vento di Eros > ♂
I Profumi di Firenze > 2009 > Lillà Serenella > ♀
I Profumi di Firenze > 2010 > Gelsomino del Deserto > ♀
I Profumi di Firenze > 2010 > Giacinto Selvatico > ♀
I Profumi di Firenze > 2010 > Giglio Fiorentino > ♀
I Profumi di Firenze > 2010 > Glicine Rosacea > ♀
I Profumi di Firenze > 2010 > Hayan > ♀
I Profumi di Firenze > 2010 > Hidalgo > ♂
I Profumi di Firenze > 2010 > Mughetto di Primavera > ♀
I Profumi di Firenze > 2010 > Muschio Bianco 3 > ♀
I Profumi di Firenze > 2010 > Oltrarno > ♂
I Profumi di Firenze > 2010 > Syko e Danae Fico e Fior di Pesco > ♀
I Profumi di Firenze > 2010 > Tulipano Nero > ♀
I Profumi di Firenze > 2011 > Manto di Rugiada Melograno Selvatico > ♀
I Profumi di Firenze > 2012 > Osmanto > ♀
I Profumi di Firenze > 2012 > Plenilunio Fragole e Mughetto > ♀
I Profumi di Firenze > 2012 > Primavera a Firenze > ♂
I Profumi di Firenze > 2012 > Elisir de' Medici > ♂
I Profumi di Firenze > 2012 > Il Giardino di Boboli > ♂
I Profumi di Firenze > 2012 > Il Giorno di Iris > ♂
I Profumi di Firenze > 2012 > Il Sale e Le Dune > ♂
I Profumi di Firenze > 2012 > Incanto > ♀
I Profumi di Firenze > 2012 > Incenso d'Oriente > ♂
I Profumi di Firenze > 2012 > Iris di Firenze N. 1 > ♀
I Profumi di Firenze > 2012 > Iris di Firenze N. 2 > ♀
I Profumi di Firenze > 2012 > Jeunesse Il Giorno e La Notte > ♀
I Profumi di Firenze > 2012 > Kataleya > ♂
I Profumi di Firenze > 2012 > Patchouly Rosso > ♀
I Profumi di Firenze > 2012 > Rosa Bulgara > ♀
I Profumi di Firenze > 2012 > Rosa di Damasco > ♀
I Profumi di Firenze > 2012 > Sandalo della Malesia > ♂
I Profumi di Firenze > 2012 > Sandalo Indiano > ♂
I Profumi di Firenze > 2013 > Il Bosco e La Riva > ♂
I Profumi di Firenze > 2014 > Kumi > ♀
I Profumi di Firenze > 2014 > Le Pleiadi > ♀
I Profumi di Firenze > 2014 > Neroli Flor > ♂
I Profumi di Firenze > 2014 > Verso Andromeda > ♀
I Profumi di Firenze > 2014-2016 > L'uomo di Pitti > ♂
I Profumi di Firenze > 2014-2016 > La Chiantigiana > ♂

I Profumi di Firenze > 2014-2016 > La Vecchia Spezieria > ♂
I Profumi di Firenze > 2014-2016 > Legno Amaro > ♂
I Profumi di Firenze > 2015 > Bora Bora Ciliegia e Pepe Bianco > ♀
I Profumi di Firenze > 2015 > Il Fiume e Il Salice: Angelica e Mughetto > ♂
I Profumi di Firenze > 2015 > Tenero Narciso > ♂
I Profumi di Firenze > 2016 > La Notte di Angelica > ♀
I Profumi di Firenze > 2019 > Cleide > ♀
I Profumi di Firenze > 2019 > Olimpia > ♀
I Profumi di Firenze > 2019 > Sandalo Misore > ♂
Isabella Rossellini > 2000 > Manifesto > ♀
Isabella Rossellini > 2002 > Isabella > ♀
Isabella Rossellini > 2003 > My Manifesto > ♀
Isabella Rossellini > 2004 > Daring > ♀
Isabella Rossellini > 2006 > Storia > ♀
I Santi > 1995 > Via Veneto > ♀
Isole Mediterranee > 2005 > Aria > ♂
Isole Mediterranee > 2005 > Cielo > ♀
Isole Mediterranee > 2005 > Mare > ♀
Isole Mediterranee > 2005 > Terra > ♀
Jewel's Joy > 2015 > Violetta di Parma > ♀
Jusbox > 2016 > 14hour Dream > ♀
Jusbox > 2016 > Beat Café > ♀
Jusbox > 2016 > Micro Love > ♀
Jusbox > 2016 > Use Abuse > ♀
Jusbox > 2017 > Black Powder > ♀
Jusbox > 2017 > Feather Supreme > ♀
Jusbox > 2017 > Feel 'N' Chill > ♀
Jusbox > 2017 > Live 'N' Loud > ♀
Jusbox > 2018 > Cheeky Smile > ♀
Jusbox > 2018 > Golden Serenade > ♀
Jusbox > 2018 > Green Bubble > ♀
Jusbox > 2018 > No Rules > ♀
Jusbox > 2019 > Siren & Sailor > ♂
Juventus > 2008 > 1897 Man > ♂
Juventus > 2008 > 1897 Woman > ♀
Kappa > 2010 > Accelerazione Man > ♂
Kappa > 2010 > Acqua Woman > ♀
Kappa > 2010 > Azzuro Man > ♂
Kappa > 2010 > Marino Man > ♂
Kappa > 2010 > Moda Woman > ♀
Kappa > 2010 > Nero Man > ♂
Kappa > 2010 > Perla Woman > ♀
Kappa > 2010 > Rosa Woman > ♀
Kappa > 2011 > Platino Man > ♂
Kappa > 2011 > Viola Woman > ♀
Kemi Blending Magic > 2014 > Attar Oil: Elixir > ♂
Kemi Blending Magic > 2014 > Hayat > ♂
Kemi Blending Magic > 2014 > Ilm > ♂
Kemi Blending Magic > 2014 > Jabir > ♂
Kemi Blending Magic > 2014 > Kemi > ♂
Kemi Blending Magic > 2014 > Layla > ♂
Kemi Blending Magic > 2014 > Luna > ♀
Kemi Blending Magic > 2014 > Attar Oil: Tempest > ♂
Kemi Blending Magic > 2016 > Aqua Regia > ♂
Kemi Blending Magic > 2016 > Aurum > ♂
Kemi Blending Magic > 2016 > Hermetic (Harrod's Exclusive) > ♂
Kemi Blending Magic > 2017 > Solis > ♂
Ken Scott > 1987 > KS > ♀
Ken Scott > 1987 > Ken Scott Uomo> ♂
Ken Scott > 1989 > Ken Scott 2 > ♀
Kiko Milano > 2016 > Oasis Sunset > ♀
Kiko Milano > 2016 > Sahara Sun > ♀
Kiko Milano > 2016 > Velvet Passion > ♀
Killer Loop > 2002 > Killer Loop for Men > ♂
Killer Loop > 2002 > Killer Loop for Women > ♀
Kiton > 1996 > Kiton Men > ♂
Kiton > 1997 > Donna > ♀
Kiton > 1998 > Napoli > ♂
Kiton > 2007 > Kiton Black > ♂
Krizia > 1982 > K de Krizia > ♀
Krizia > 1984 > Krizia Uomo > ♂
Krizia > 1985 > Teatro alla Scala > ♀
Krizia > 1989 > Moods by Krizia Donna > ♀
Krizia > 1989 > Moods by Krizia Uomo > ♂
Krizia > 1991 > Krazy Krizia > ♀
Krizia > 1996 > Fiori di Krizia > ♀
Krizia > 1997 > Spazio Krizia Donna > ♀
Krizia > 1997 > Spazio Krizia Uomo > ♂
Krizia > 1999 > Aesy Krizia > ♀
Krizia > 2001 > Krizia > ♀
Krizia > 2002 > Eau de Krizia > ♀
Krizia > 2003 > Time Uomo > ♂

Krizia > 2003 > Time Woman > ♀
Krizia > 2006 > Krizia Donna Istinto > ♀
Krizia > 2006 > Krizia Uomo Istinto > ♂
Krizia > 2006 > My Afrika > ♀
Krizia > 2014 > Krizia pour Femme > ♀
Krizia > 2014 > Krizia pour Homme > ♂
L'Amande > 2012 > Antalya > ♀
L'Amande > 2012 > Armonie > ♀
L'Amande > 2012 > Calla > ♀
L'Amande > 2012 > Coriandolo > ♂
L'Amande > 2012 > Fior d'Arancio Supremo > ♀
L'Amande > 2012 > Fiori di Ciliegio > ♀
L'Amande > 2012 > Fleur de Sel & Vanille > ♀
L'Amande > 2012 > Gelsomino Supremo > ♀
L'Amande > 2012 > Glicine > ♀
L'Amande > 2012 > Iris Supremo > ♀
L'Amande > 2012 > Lanterne > ♀
L'Amande > 2012 > Lili > ♀
L'Amande > 2012 > Neroli > ♀
L'Amande > 2012 > Papavero > ♀
L'Amande > 2012 > Petali di Sambuco Polvere d'Ambra > ♀
L'Amande > 2012 > Petali di Spezie > ♀
L'Amande > 2012 > Rosa Suprema > ♀
Laboratorio Olfattivo > 2010 > Alambar > ♀
Laboratorio Olfattivo > 2010 > Alkemi > ♀
Laboratorio Olfattivo > 2010 > Cozumel > ♂
Laboratorio Olfattivo > 2010 > Daimiris > ♀
Laboratorio Olfattivo > 2010 > Nirmal > ♀
Laboratorio Olfattivo > 2011 > Esvedra > ♂
Laboratorio Olfattivo > 2012 > Decou-Vert > ♂
Laboratorio Olfattivo > 2012 > Noblige > ♂
Laboratorio Olfattivo > 2012 > Rosamunda > ♀
Laboratorio Olfattivo > 2013 > Kashnoir > ♂
Laboratorio Olfattivo > 2013 > Salina > ♂
Laboratorio Olfattivo > 2014 > Patchouliful > ♂
Laboratorio Olfattivo > 2016 > Mylo > ♂
Laboratorio Olfattivo > 2016 > Nerotic > ♂
Laboratorio Olfattivo > 2016 > Nun > ♂
Laboratorio Olfattivo > 2017 > Vanhera > ♂
Laboratorio Olfattivo > 2018 > Need-U > ♂
Laboratorio Olfattivo > 2018 > Sacreste > ♂
Laboratorio Olfattivo > 2019 > Baliflora > ♂
Laboratorio Olfattivo > 2019 > Nerosa > ♂
Laboratorio Olfattivo > 2019 > Tantrico > ♂
Laboratorio Olfattivo > 2019 > Tuberosis > ♂
Laboratorio Olfattivo > 2019 > Vetyverso > ♂
Laboratorio Olfattivo > 2020 > Tonkade > ♂
La Collina Toscana > 2008 > Belvedere Holm Oak > ♂
La Collina Toscana > 2008 > Hillock Sunflower > ♀
La Collina Toscana > 2008 > Iris of the Signory > ♀
La Collina Toscana > 2008 > Maremma's Tobacco > ♂
La Collina Toscana > 2008 > Oblivion Absinth > ♀
La Collina Toscana > 2008 > Poppy of Cliffs > ♀
La Collina Toscana > 2011 > Borgo delle Stelle > ♂
La Collina Toscana > 2011 > Loggia dei Mercanti > ♂
La Collina Toscana > 2011 > Poggio in Fiore > ♀
La Collina Toscana > 2011 > Rocca della Signoria > ♂
La Collina Toscana > 2013 > Corte Belfiore > ♀
La Collina Toscana > 2013 > Vicolo del Sellaio > ♀
Lancetti > 1976 > Lancetti > ♀
Lancetti > 1985 > Via Condotti pour Femme > ♀
Lancetti > 1990 > Elle > ♀
Lancetti > 1990 > Il > ♂
Lancetti > 1993 > Suspense > ♀
Lancetti > 1995 > Madame > ♀
Lancetti > 1995 > Monsieur > ♂
Lancetti > 1997 > Eau de Joie > ♀
Lancetti > 1999 > Lancetti pour Homme > ♂
Lancetti > 2001 > Lancetti Femme > ♀
Lancetti > 2001 > Lancetti Homme > ♂
Lancetti > 2001 > Via Condotti Pour Homme > ♂
Lancetti > 2002 > Etre Femme > ♀
Lancetti > 2002 > Etre Homme > ♂
Lancetti > 2004 > Etre Special Edition > ♀
Lancetti > 2004 > Etre Special Edition II > ♀
Lancetti > 2005 > Etre Special Edition III > ♀
Lancetti > 2006 > Lancetti Mood Man > ♂
Lancetti > 2006 > Lancetti Mood Woman > ♀
Lancetti > 2011 > Yuzen pour Femme > ♀
Lancetti > 2011 > Yuzen pour Homme > ♂
Lancetti > 2012 > Celebration I > ♀
Lancetti > 2012 > Celebration II > ♀

Lancetti > 2012 > Celebration III > ♀
Lancetti > 2012 > Celebration IV > ♀
Lancetti > 2017 > Argento Blu Man > ♂
Lancetti > 2017 > Argento Man > ♂
La Perla > 1987/2013 > La Perla > ♀
La Perla > 1991 > Grigioperla > ♂
La Perla > 1995 > Blue > ♀
La Perla > 1995 > Io > ♀
La Perla > 1997 > Parfum Privé > ♀
La Perla > 2000 > Eclix > ♀
La Perla > 2000 > Touch Grigioperla > ♂
La Perla > 2002 > Creation > ♀
La Perla > 2003 > Shiny Creation > ♀
La Perla > 2006 > Charme > ♀
La Perla > 2006 > Grigioperla Attitude > ♂
La Perla > 2007 > Grigioperla Hedò > ♂
La Perla > 2007 > J'aime La Perla > ♀
La Perla > 2007 > Love Frills: Dark Extacy > ♀
La Perla > 2007 > Love Frills: Languid Vanilla > ♀
La Perla > 2007 > Love Frills: Ruby Perlage > ♀
La Perla > 2008 > Grigioperla Hedò White > ♂
La Perla > 2008 > J'aime La Nuit > ♀
La Perla > 2008 > J'aime Les Fleurs > ♀
La Perla > 2009 > Charme Lace Collection > ♀
La Perla > 2009 > Grigioperla Essence > ♂
La Perla > 2009 > J'aime Precious Edition > ♀
La Perla > 2011 > Divina > ♀
La Perla > 2012 > Divina Gold Edition > ♀
La Perla > 2012 > Divina Silver Edition > ♀
La Perla > 2012 > Grigioperla Nero > ♂
La Perla > 2012 > La Perla in Rosa > ♀
La Perla > 2013 > Divina Edp > ♀
La Perla > 2013 > Just Precious > ♀
La Perla > 2014 > Grigioperla Touch Sport > ♂
La Perla > 2014 > Grigioperla Uomo > ♂
La Perla > 2014 > J'aime Gold Edition > ♀
La Perla > 2014 > La Perla in Rosa Edp > ♀
La Perla > 2014 > Peony Blossom > ♀
La Perla > 2015 > J'aime Elixir > ♀
La Perla > 2015 > Private Collection: Contemporary Tuberose > ♀
La Perla > 2015 > Private Collection: Lotus Shadow > ♀
La Perla > 2015 > Private Collection: White Iris > ♀
La Perla > 2017 > La Mia Perla > ♀
La Perla > 2019 > La Mia Perla Nera > ♀
Laura Biagiotti > 1982 > Laura Biagiotti > ♀
Laura Biagiotti > 1985 > Night > ♀
Laura Biagiotti > 1988 > Roma > ♀
Laura Biagiotti > 1989 > Laura Biagiotti Uomo > ♂
Laura Biagiotti > 1991 > Fiori Bianchi > ♀
Laura Biagiotti > 1992 > Roma Uomo > ♂
Laura Biagiotti > 1992/2011 > Venezia > ♀
Laura Biagiotti > 1994 > Laura > ♀
Laura Biagiotti > 1995 > Venezia Pastello > ♀
Laura Biagiotti > 1995 > Venezia Uomo > ♂
Laura Biagiotti > 1996 > Sotto Voce > ♀
Laura Biagiotti > 1999 > Tempore Donna > ♀
Laura Biagiotti > 1999 > Tempore Uomo > ♂
Laura Biagiotti > 2001 > Emotion > ♀
Laura Biagiotti > 2004 > Acqua di Roma > ♀
Laura Biagiotti > 2004 > Acqua di Roma Uomo > ♂
Laura Biagiotti > 2006 > Biagiotti Due Donna > ♀
Laura Biagiotti > 2006 > Biagiotti Due Uomo > ♂
Laura Biagiotti > 2008 > Donna > ♀
Laura Biagiotti > 2009 > Laura Rose > ♀
Laura Biagiotti > 2010 > Mistero di Roma Donna > ♀
Laura Biagiotti > 2010 > Mistero di Roma Uomo > ♂
Laura Biagiotti > 2012 > Venezia Eau de Toilette > ♀
Laura Biagiotti > 2013 > Essenza di Roma > ♀
Laura Biagiotti > 2013 > Essenza di Roma Uomo > ♂
Laura Biagiotti > 2014 > Blu di Roma Donna > ♀
Laura Biagiotti > 2014 > Blu di Roma Uomo > ♂
Laura Biagiotti > 2016 > Roma Passione > ♀
Laura Biagiotti > 2016 > Roma Passione Uomo > ♂
Laura Biagiotti > 2017 > Roma Edt Rosa > ♀
Laura Biagiotti > 2017 > Roma Uomo Edt Cedro > ♂
Laura Biagiotti > 2018 > Romamor > ♀
Laura Biagiotti > 2018 > Romamor Uomo > ♂
Laura Biagiotti > 2019 > Forever > ♀
Laura Biagiotti > 2019 > Laura Tender > ♀
Laura Tonatto (Tonatto Profumi) > > >
Le Cult 1944 > 2014 > Anilina > ♂
Le Cult 1944 > 2014 > Arsenale > ♂

Le Cult 1944 > 2014 > Bastione > ♂
Le Cult 1944 > 2014 > Borneo > ♂
Le Cult 1944 > 2014 > Burano > ♂
Le Cult 1944 > 2014 > Cocco > ♂
Le Cult 1944 > 2014 > Cocco Vaniglia > ♂
Le Cult 1944 > 2014 > Doge > ♂
Le Cult 1944 > 2014 > Dolce > ♂
Le Cult 1944 > 2014 > Impero > ♂
Le Cult 1944 > 2014 > Monsù > ♂
Le Cult 1944 > 2014 > Moto Ondoso > ♂
Le Cult 1944 > 2014 > Oriente > ♂
Le Cult 1944 > 2014 > Porto Cesareo > ♂
Le Cult 1944 > 2014 > Spezzieria > ♂
L'Erbolario > 1996 > Il Profumo dei Piccoli > ♂
L'Erbolario > 1996 > Lavanda > ♀
L'Erbolario > 1996 > Magnolia > ♀
L'Erbolario > 1996 > Mandorla > ♀
L'Erbolario > 1996 > Mimosa > ♀
L'Erbolario > 1996 > Mirto > ♂
L'Erbolario > 1996 > Mughetto > ♀
L'Erbolario > 1996 > Muschio > ♂
L'Erbolario > 1996 > Muschio Bianco > ♂
L'Erbolario > 1999 > Acqua di Colonia Imperiale > ♂
L'Erbolario > 1999 > Acqua di Profumo al Muschio Bianco > ♂
L'Erbolario > 1999 > Ambra e Muschio > ♂
L'Erbolario > 1999 > Bergamotto > ♂
L'Erbolario > 1999 > Caprifoglio > ♀
L'Erbolario > 1999 > Cedro > ♂
L'Erbolario > 1999 > Fiorichiari > ♀
L'Erbolario > 1999 > Fioriscuri > ♀
L'Erbolario > 1999 > Garofano > ♀
L'Erbolario > 1999 > Nostos > ♂
L'Erbolario > 1999 > Rosa > ♀
L'Erbolario > 1999 > Sandalo > ♂
L'Erbolario > 1999 > Spezie > ♂
L'Erbolario > 1999 > Tè & Cedro > ♂
L'Erbolario > 1999 > Tuberosa > ♀
L'Erbolario > 1999 > Vaniglia > ♂
L'Erbolario > 1999 > Vaniglia e Zenzero > ♀
L'Erbolario > 1999 > Verde > ♂
L'Erbolario > 1999 > Vetiver de la Reunion > ♂
L'Erbolario > 2000 > Acqua di Colonia del Ponte > ♂
L'Erbolario > 2000 > Ambraliquida > ♂
L'Erbolario > 2000 > Assenzio > ♂
L'Erbolario > 2000 > Myrrhae > ♂
L'Erbolario > 2000 > Narciso Sublime > ♀
L'Erbolario > 2000 > Petali & Fiori > ♀
L'Erbolario > 2000 > Tè Bianco > ♂
L'Erbolario > 2000 > Tè Verde > ♂
L'Erbolario > 2000 > Rugiada d'Oriente > ♂
L'Erbolario > 2002 > China > ♂
L'Erbolario > 2002 > Corteccia > ♂
L'Erbolario > 2008 > Felci > ♂
L'Erbolario > 2009 > Citrus > ♂
L'Erbolario > 2009 > Legni Fruttati > ♂
L'Erbolario > 2009 > Patchouli > ♂
L'Erbolario > 2009 > Peonie > ♀
L'Erbolario > 2010 > Dolcelisir > ♀
L'Erbolario > 2010 > Fiore dell'Onda > ♀
L'Erbolario > 2010 > Frutto della Passione > ♀
L'Erbolario > 2010 > Periplo > ♀
L'Erbolario > 2010 > Acacia > ♀
L'Erbolario > 2010 > Tiaré > ♀
L'Erbolario > 2010 > Iris > ♀
L'Erbolario > 2010 > Méharées > ♂
L'Erbolario > 2011 > 3 Rosa > ♀
L'Erbolario > 2011 > Papavero Soave > ♀
L'Erbolario > 2011 > Primaverde > ♀
L'Erbolario > 2011 > Uomo > ♂
L'Erbolario > 2012 > Accordo Viola > ♀
L'Erbolario > 2012 > Acqua di More > ♀
L'Erbolario > 2012 > Hedera > ♂
L'Erbolario > 2012 > Iris Tenue > ♀
L'Erbolario > 2013 > All'olio di Argan > ♂
L'Erbolario > 2013 > Ibisco > ♀
L'Erbolario > 2013 > Ombra del Tiglio > ♀
L'Erbolario > 2013 > Ortensia > ♀
L'Erbolario > 2014 > Acordo Arancio > ♀
L'Erbolario > 2014 > Camelia > ♀
L'Erbolario > 2014 > Regine dei Prati > ♀
L'Erbolario > 2015 > Frescaessenza > ♂
L'Erbolario > 2015 > Gelsomino Indiano > ♀

L'Erbolario > 2015 > Goji > ♂
L'Erbolario > 2016 > Ginepro Nero > ♂
L'Erbolario > 2016 > Osmanthus > ♀
L'Erbolario > 2016 > Orangerie > ♀
L'Erbolario > 2017 > Indaco > ♂
L'Erbolario > 2017 > Lillà Lillà > ♀
L'Erbolario > 2017 > Tra i Ciliegi > ♀
L'Erbolario > 2018 > Dance of Flowers (Danza di Fiori) > ♀
L'Erbolario > 2018 > Fior di Salina > ♀
L'Erbolario > 2018 > Rabarbaro (Rhubarb) > ♂
L'Erbolario > 2018 > Neroli > ♀
L'Erbolario > 2019 > Accordo di Ebano > ♂
L'Erbolario > 2019 > Giada > ♀
L'Erbolario > 2019 > Sfumature di Dalia > ♀
Les Copains > 1998 > L'hommo > ♂
Les Copains > 1998 > Les Copains > ♀
Les Copains > 2000 > Le Bleu > ♂
Les Copains > 2001 > Trend Lei > ♀
Les Copains > 2001 > Trend Lui > ♂
Les Copains > 2004 > Papillon > ♀
Les Copains > 2005 > Pour Homme > ♂
Les Copains > 2007 > Femme > ♀
Les Voiles Dépliées > 2011 > Bayadere > ♀
Les Voiles Dépliées > 2011 > Des Salins > ♀
Les Voiles Dépliées > 2011 > Eau Saharienne > ♂
Les Voiles Dépliées > 2011 > Potiche > ♀
Les Voiles Dépliées > 2011 > Vanilla > ♀
Les Voiles Dépliées > 2011 > Tuberosa > ♂
Les Voiles Dépliées > 2013 > Agrakal > ♀
Les Voiles Dépliées > 2013 > Flower & Things > ♀
Les Voiles Dépliées > 2017 > Gato > ♂
Limonero Profumo d'Umbria > 2012 > Profumo d'Umbria > ♂
LIU.JO > 2014 > LIU.JO Eau de Parfum > ♀
LIU.JO > 2015 > Scent of LIU.JO > ♀
LIU.JO > 2016 > LIU.JO Gold > ♀
LIU.JO > 2017 > Lovely U > ♀
LIU.JO > 2018 > Lovely Me > ♀
LIU.JO > 2019 > LIU.JO Glam > ♀
LIU.JO > 2019 > LIU.JO Milano > ♀
Locherber > 2017 > Absolute Green Tea > ♂
Locherber > 2017 > Baltic Amber > ♂
Locherber > 2017 > Bourbon Vanilla > ♂
Locherber > 2017 > Dokki Cotton > ♂
Locherber > 2017 > Fig and Rose of Tabriz > ♂
Locherber > 2017 > Habana Tobacco > ♂
Locherber > 2017 > Hejaz Incense > ♂
Locherber > 2017 > Linen Buds > ♂
Locherber > 2017 > Malabar Pepper > ♂
Locherber > 2017 > Oudh > ♂
Locherber > 2017 > Rice Germs > ♂
Locherber > 2017 > Tropical Fruits > ♂
Locherber > 2017 > Venetiae > ♂
Locherber > 2018 > Inuit > ♂
Locherber > 2018 > Kyushu Rice > ♂
Locherber > 2018 > Medeleine Rose > ♂
Locherber > 2018 > Rhubarbe Royale > ♂
Locherber > 2019 > Mannequin > ♂
Lola Moods Parfums > 2013 > Red Carpet Attitude Angelina > ♀
Lola Moods Parfums > 2013 > Red Carpet Attitude Jennifer > ♀
Lola Moods Parfums > 2013 > Red Carpet Attitude Kate > ♀
Lola Moods Parfums > 2013 > Red Carpet Attitude Nicole > ♀
Lord Milano > 2019 > Adventure > ♂
Lord Milano > 2019 > Blue Water > ♂
Lord Milano > 2019 > Champs Elysées > ♂
Lord Milano > 2019 > His Highness > ♂
Lord Milano > 2019 > Imperial Oud > ♂
Lord Milano > 2019 > Je t'Aime > ♂
Lord Milano > 2019 > Light & Shadow > ♂
Lord Milano > 2019 > London > ♂
Lord Milano > 2019 > Love Story > ♂
Lord Milano > 2019 > Morrocan Oud > ♂
Lord Milano > 2019 > Occasion 6pm > ♂
Lord Milano > 2019 > Paradise > ♂
Lord Milano > 2019 > Phantom > ♂
Lord Milano > 2019 > Tuxedo > ♂
Lord Milano > 2019 > Velvet Rose > ♂
Lorenzo Villoresi > 1993 > Uomo > ♂
Lorenzo Villoresi > 1994 > Donna > ♀
Lorenzo Villoresi > 1994 > Spezie > ♂
Lorenzo Villoresi > 1994 > Vetiver > ♂
Lorenzo Villoresi > 1995 > Musk > ♂
Lorenzo Villoresi > 1995 > Sandalo > ♂

Lorenzo Villoresi > 1996 > Acqua di Colonia > ♀
Lorenzo Villoresi > 1996 > Patchouli > ♂
Lorenzo Villoresi > 1997 > Garofano > ♂
Lorenzo Villoresi > 1997 > Incensi > ♂
Lorenzo Villoresi > 1999 > Piper Nigrum > ♀
Lorenzo Villoresi > 2000 > Dilmun > ♂
Lorenzo Villoresi > 2000 > Teint de Neige > ♀
Lorenzo Villoresi > 2000 > Wild Lavender > ♂
Lorenzo Villoresi > 2001 > Yerbamate > ♂
Lorenzo Villoresi > 2006 > Alamut > ♀
Lorenzo Villoresi > 2010 > Iperborea > ♀
Lorenzo Villoresi > 2011 > Theseus > ♂
Lorenzo Villoresi > 2012 > Aura Maris > ♂
Lorenzo Villoresi > 2014 > Vintage Collection Ambra > ♂
Lorenzo Villoresi > 2014 > Vintage Collection Garofano > ♂
Lorenzo Villoresi > 2014 > Vintage Collection Incensi > ♂
Lorenzo Villoresi > 2014 > Vintage Collection Tropicana > ♀
Lorenzo Villoresi > 2014 > Vintage Collection Vetiver > ♂
Lorenzo Villoresi > 2014 > Vintage Collection Ylang Ylang > ♂
Lorenzo Villoresi > 2015 > Kamasurabhi > ♂
Lorenzo Villoresi > 2016 > 25 Insieme > ♂
Lorenzo Villoresi > 2018 > Atman Xaman > ♂
Loriblu > 2010 > Sensual Seduction Man > ♂
Loriblu > 2010 > Sensual Seduction Woman > ♀
Loriblu > 2016 > Mi Piaci Black > ♀
Loriblu > 2016 > Mi Piaci White > ♀
Lotto > 2005 > Lotto Man > ♂
Lotto > 2005 > Lotto Woman > ♀
Lotto > 2008 > Gravity Power for Men > ♂
Lotto > 2008 > Gravity Power for Women > ♀
Lotto > 2011 > Blue 2 > ♂
Lotto > 2011 > Lotto Air > ♂
Lotto > 2011 > Lotto Earth > ♂
Lotto > 2011 > Lotto Fire > ♂
Lotto > 2011 > Lotto Water > ♂
Lotto > 2011 > White 2 > ♀
Lú by Ludovica di Loreto > 2015 > Lú Lei > ♂
Lú by Ludovica di Loreto > 2015 > Lú Lui > ♂
Lú by Ludovica di Loreto > 2018 > Lú Cerere > ♀
Lú by Ludovica di Loreto > 2018 > Lú Iupiter > ♂
Lú by Ludovica di Loreto > 2018 > Lú Mercurio > ♂
Lú by Ludovica di Loreto > 2018 > Lú Minerva > ♀
Lú by Ludovica di Loreto > 2018 > Lú Numen > ♂
Luciano Soprani > 1987 > Luciano Soprani > ♀
Luciano Soprani > 1988 > Luciano Soprani Uomo > ♂
Luciano Soprani > 1992 > 2 > ♀
Luciano Soprani > 1995 > Active > ♂
Luciano Soprani > 1995 > Solo Soprani > ♂
Luciano Soprani > 1998 > Solo Blu > ♂
Luciano Soprani > 1998 > Solo Rosa > ♀
Luciano Soprani > 2002 > Strass > ♀
Luciano Soprani > 2004 > Jolie > ♀
Luciano Soprani > 2004 > Just Free > ♂
Luciano Soprani > 2004 > Luciano Soprani Donna > ♀
Luciano Soprani > 2005 > Sulky > ♂
Luciano Soprani > 2006 > Flirt Issimo > ♀
Luciano Soprani > 2006 > Solo Amore > ♀
Luciano Soprani > 2007 > D Luciano Soprani > ♀
Luciano Soprani > 2007 > Ls Man > ♂
Luciano Soprani > 2007 > Miss Soprani > ♀
Luciano Soprani > 2008 > Soprani Uomo > ♂
Luciano Soprani > 2009 > D Noir > ♂
Luciano Soprani > 2010 > Solo Soprani Rose > ♀
Luciano Soprani > 2011 > Luciano Soprani Her > ♀
Luciano Soprani > 2011 > Luciano Soprani Him > ♂
Luciano Soprani > 2012 > Solo Soprani Green > ♂
Luciano Soprani > 2012 > Sopranissima > ♀
Luciano Soprani > 2013 > D Rouge > ♀
Luciano Soprani > 2014 > Fico Pesca > ♂
Luciano Soprani > 2016 > Solo Soprani Dream > ♀
Luciano Soprani > 2016 > Solo Soprani Love > ♀
Luciano Soprani > 2016 > Solo Soprani Smile > ♀
Luciano Soprani > 2018 > Luciano Soprani D Moi > ♀
Luigi Borrelli Napoli > 2016 > Cashmere > ♂
Luigi Borrelli Napoli > 2016 > Cotton > ♂
Luigi Borrelli Napoli > 2016 > Vicunia Wool > ♂
Luigi Borrelli Napoli > 2019 > Silk > ♂
Luisa Spagnoli > 2013 > Luisa > ♀
Magdala Essenza di Benessere > 2011 > Armonia > ♂
Magdala Essenza di Benessere > 2011 > Concentrazione > ♂
Magdala Essenza di Benessere > 2011 > Energia > ♂
Magdala Essenza di Benessere > 2011 > Purezza > ♂

Maison des Rêves > 2011 > Gourmandise > ♀
Maison des Rêves > 2011 > Mousse au Café > ♀
Maison des Rêves > 2011 > Poudre > ♀
Mandarina Duck > 2004 > Mandarina Duck > ♀
Mandarina Duck > 2006 > Mandarina Duck Man > ♂
Mandarina Duck > 2007 > Mandarina Duck Cute Pink > ♀
Mandarina Duck > 2007 > Mandarina Duck Rouge Intense > ♀
Mandarina Duck > 2008 > Scarlet Rain > ♀
Mandarina Duck > 2009 > Pure Black > ♂
Mandarina Duck > 2011 > Mandarina Duck Blue > ♂
Mandarina Duck > 2011 > Mandarina Duck Cute Blue > ♀
Mandarina Duck > 2012 > All of Me for Her > ♀
Mandarina Duck > 2012 > All of Me for Him > ♂
Mandarina Duck > 2013 > Cool Black > ♂
Mandarina Duck > 2013 > Pink is in the Air > ♀
Mandarina Duck > 2014 > Black Extreme > ♂
Mandarina Duck > 2014 > M+ > ♂
Mandarina Duck > 2014 > Oh Bella > ♀
Mandarina Duck > 2016 > Black & Red > ♂
Mandarina Duck > 2016 > Black & White > ♀
Mandarina Duck > 2016 > So Bella! So Chic! > ♀
Mandarina Duck > 2017 > Let's Travel to New York for Man > ♂
Mandarina Duck > 2017 > Let's Travel to New York for Woman > ♀
Mandarina Duck > 2017 > Mandarina Duck for Man > ♂
Mandarina Duck > 2018 > Let's Travel to Paris for Men > ♂
Mandarina Duck > 2018 > Let's Travel to Paris for Women > ♀
Mandarina Duck > 2019 > Let's Travel to Miami for Men > ♂
Mandarina Duck > 2019 > Let's Travel to Miami for Women > ♀
Manila Grace > 2015 > Manila Grace > ♀
Manila Grace > 2016 > Manila Grace Eau Fraiche > ♀
Manila Grace > 2016 > Manila Grace Fleur Narcotique > ♀
Mansfield > 2000 > Georges Feghali Monte Carlo > ♂
Mansfield > 2000 > Georges Feghali Monte Carlo Atomes Crochus > ♂
Mansfield > 2000 > Georges Feghali Monte Carlo Coup de Foudre > ♂
Mansfield > 2002 > Piazzetta di Portofino > ♂
Mansfield > 2002 > Piazzetta di Portofino Acqua da Toaletta > ♂
Mansfield > 2002 > Piazzetta di Portofino Fragranza Classica > ♀
Mansfield > 2008 > Antonio De Curtis > ♂
Mansfield > 2011/2014 > Ame Noire > ♂
Mansfield > 2011/2014 > Bois Extreme > ♂
Mansfield > 2011/2014 > L'amant > ♀
Mansfield > 2011/2014 > Sortilège > ♂
Mansfield > 2011/2014 > Tam Tam > ♂
Mansfield > 2017 > Acqua Lunare > ♀
Mansfield > 2019 > Femelle > ♀
Mansfield > 2019 > Fusion à distance > ♀
Mansfield > 2019 > Oudamar > ♂
Mansfield > 2019 > Tattoo > ♂
Marella Ferrera > 1995 > Marella Ferrera > ♀
Marella Ferrera > 2003 > Ambre Ze > ♀
Maria Candida Gentile > 2009 > Cinabre > ♀
Maria Candida Gentile > 2009 > Exultat > ♂
Maria Candida Gentile > 2009 > Gershwin > ♂
Maria Candida Gentile > 2009 > Sideris > ♂
Maria Candida Gentile > 2010 > Barry Lyndon > ♂
Maria Candida Gentile > 2010 > Hanbury > ♂
Maria Candida Gentile > 2012 > Burlesque > ♀
Maria Candida Gentile > 2012 > Gentile > ♂
Maria Candida Gentile > 2012 > Lady Day > ♀
Maria Candida Gentile > 2012 > Luberon > ♂
Maria Candida Gentile > 2013 > Finisterre > ♂
Maria Candida Gentile > 2013 > Noir Tropical > ♂
Maria Candida Gentile > 2014 > Flight of the Bumblebee: Kitrea > ♂
Maria Candida Gentile > 2014 > Flight of the Bumblebee: Leucò > ♂
Maria Candida Gentile > 2014 > Flight of the Bumblebee: Syconium > ♂
Maria Candida Gentile > 2015 > Elephant & Roses > ♀
Maria Candida Gentile > 2016 > Lankaran Forest > ♂
Maria Candida Gentile > 2016 > Rrose Selavy > ♂
Marialux > 2012 > Deeply > ♀
Marialux > 2012 > Madly > ♀
Marialux > 2012 > Truly > ♀
Marialux > 2014 > Aramesh > ♂
Marialux > 2014 > Mogadess > ♂
Mariella Arduini > 2017 > Mariella > ♀
Mariella Burani > 1993 > Mariella Burani > ♀
Mariella Burani > 1996 > Mariella > ♀
Mariella Burani > 1997 > Eau Rosée > ♀
Mariella Burani > 1998 > Collection de Roses > ♀
Mariella Burani > 1999 > Amuleti > ♀
Mariella Burani > 2001 > Bouquet de Roses Refraichissante > ♀
Mariella Burani > 2001 > Bouquet de Roses Regenerante > ♀
Mariella Burani > 2001 > Bouquet de Roses Relaxante > ♀

Mariella Burani > 2001 > Bouquet de Roses Sensuelle > ♀
Mariella Burani > 2001 > Messages > ♀
Mariella Burani > 2002 > Bouquet d'Amour Malicieuse > ♀
Mariella Burani > 2002 > Bouquet d'Amour Mysterieuse > ♀
Mariella Burani > 2002 > Bouquet d'Amour Romantique > ♀
Mariella Burani > 2002 > Bouquet d'Amour Vitale > ♀
Mariella Burani > 2002 > Messages d'homme > ♂
Mariella Burani > 2003 > Mb > ♀
Mariella Martinato > 2015 > Black > ♀
Mariella Martinato > 2015 > White > ♀
Marina Spadafora > 2005 > Marina Spadafora > ♀
Marina Yachting > 2000 > Marina Yachting > ♂
Marina Yachting > 2005 > Marina > ♀
Mario Valentino > 1989 > Echo > ♀
Mario Valentino > 1990 > Ocean Rain > ♂
Mario Valentino > 1999 > Eau d'Essence > ♀
Marni > 2012 > Marni > ♀
Marni > 2013 > Marni Metallic > ♀
Marni > 2013 > Marni Rose > ♀
Marni > 2014 > Marni Luxury Edition Eau de Parfum > ♀
Marni > 2014 > Marni Luxury Edition Rose Eau de Parfum > ♀
Marni > 2015 > Marni Element > ♀
Marni > 2015 > Marni Spice > ♀
Mascalzone Latino > 2016 > Blu > ♂
Mascalzone Latino > 2016 > Maestrale > ♂
Mascalzone Latino > 2016 > Nero > ♂
Masone > 1986 > Xtsy Donna > ♀
Masone > 1995 > Greed > ♂
Masone > 1996 > Xtsy Uomo > ♂
Masone > 1998 > Live Love Laugh Donna > ♀
Masone > 1998 > Live Love Laugh Uomo > ♂
Masone > 1999 > Desire > ♀
Masone > 1999 > Imperiale Uomo > ♂
Masone > 1999 > La Storia > ♀
Masone > 1999 > Millennium > ♂
Masone > 1999 > Soave > ♀
Masone > 2001 > Dreams > ♀
Masone > 2003 > Adorable > ♀
Masone > 2003 > Sotto Zero Donna > ♀
Masone > 2003 > Sotto Zero Uomo > ♂
Masque Milano > 2012 > Dolceacqua > ♀
Masque Milano > 2012 > Petra > ♀
Masque Milano > 2013 > Act 1 – Montecristo > ♂
Masque Milano > 2013 > Act 1 – Terralba > ♀
Masque Milano > 2013 > Act 2 – Luci ed Ombre > ♂
Masque Milano > 2013 > Act 3 – Tango > ♀
Masque Milano > 2014 > Act 1 – Russian Tea > ♀
Masque Milano > 2015 > Act 3 – Romanza > ♀
Masque Milano > 2016 > Act 3 – L'attesa > ♀
Masque Milano > 2017 > Act 1 – Times Square > ♂
Masque Milano > 2017 > Act 2 – Mandala > ♀
Masque Milano > 2018 > Act 2 – (Homage to) Hemingway > ♂
Masque Milano > 2019 > Act 2 – Kintsugi > ♀
Masque Milano > 2019 > Act 3 – Love Kills > ♀
Massimiliano Il Profumiere > 2000 > Classic Collection: Passiflora Rouge > ♀
Massimiliano Il Profumiere > 2000 > Classic Collection: Melone Rosso > ♂
Massimiliano Il Profumiere > 2000 > Classic Collection: Primrose > ♀
Massimiliano Il Profumiere > 2000 > Classic Collection: Tuberosa Musk > ♀
Massimiliano Il Profumiere > 2000 > Patchouly Secco Indonesia > ♂
Massimiliano Il Profumiere > 2002 > Classic Collection: Conchiglie Verdi > ♂
Massimiliano Il Profumiere > 2003 > Classic Collection: Resina di Fico Verde > ♂
Massimiliano Il Profumiere > 2003 > Classic Collection: Vaniglia Bourbon > ♀
Massimiliano Il Profumiere > 2004 > Classic Collection: Rosa di Maggio e Aoud > ♂
Massimiliano Il Profumiere > 2004 > Classic Collection: Vaniglia Speziata Calda > ♀
Massimiliano Il Profumiere > 2005 > Pepe Bianco e Aoud > ♂
Massimiliano Il Profumiere > 2005 > Radica Aoud > ♂
Massimiliano Il Profumiere > 2005 > Resina Araba > ♂
Massimiliano Il Profumiere > 2005 > Tabacco Extreme > ♂
Massimiliano Il Profumiere > 2005 > Vanille Gourmand > ♀
Massimiliano Il Profumiere > 2006 > Classic Collection: Incenso e Frangipane > ♂
Massimiliano Il Profumiere > 2006 > Noix Champagne > ♂
Massimiliano Il Profumiere > 2007 > Ambra Nera > ♂
Massimiliano Il Profumiere > 2007 > Classic Collection: Cipria Bianca > ♂
Massimiliano Il Profumiere > 2007 > Classic Collection: Fiore del Thiaré > ♀
Massimiliano Il Profumiere > 2007 > Classic Collection: Frutta Rossa di Persia > ♂

Massimiliano Il Profumiere > 2007 > Classic Collection: Menta Verde del Marocco > ♂
Massimiliano Il Profumiere > 2007 > Classic Collection: Sweet Sugar > ♂
Massimiliano Il Profumiere > 2007 > Mandarine Mousse > ♂
Massimiliano Il Profumiere > 2007 > Miele Amaro > ♂
Massimiliano Il Profumiere > 2008 > Ambroxine > ♂
Massimiliano Il Profumiere > 2008 > Arabian Nektar > ♂
Massimiliano Il Profumiere > 2008 > Classic Collection: Dubai Sahara > ♀
Massimiliano Il Profumiere > 2008 > Classic Collection: Kabala Indù > ♂
Massimiliano Il Profumiere > 2008 > Classic Collection: Poudre e Iris > ♀
Massimiliano Il Profumiere > 2008 > Classic Collection: Sabbia Calda del Deserto > ♂
Massimiliano Il Profumiere > 2008 > Classic Collection: Tender Milk > ♀
Massimiliano Il Profumiere > 2008 > Classic Collection: Vaniglia Verde > ♂
Massimiliano Il Profumiere > 2008 > Radice Verde di Vetyver > ♂
Massimiliano Il Profumiere > 2008 > Whiskey Caldo > ♂
Massimiliano Il Profumiere > 2008 > Zephyros > ♂
Massimiliano Il Profumiere > 2009 > Cioccolato Amaro e Patchouli > ♂
Massimiliano Il Profumiere > 2009 > Classic Collection: Edera e Lattuga Verde > ♂
Massimiliano Il Profumiere > 2009 > Classic Collection: Latte di Fico > ♂
Massimiliano Il Profumiere > 2009 > Hot Rhum > ♂
Massimiliano Il Profumiere > 2009 > Lemon – Bah > ♂
Massimiliano Il Profumiere > 2009 > Orange Douce > ♂
Massimiliano Il Profumiere > 2009 > Oud Extreme > ♂
Massimiliano Il Profumiere > 2010 > Black Land > ♂
Massimiliano Il Profumiere > 2010 > Classic Collection: Boogie > ♂
Massimiliano Il Profumiere > 2010 > Classic Collection: Cannella Dolce > ♂
Massimiliano Il Profumiere > 2010 > Classic Collection: Cocco Vaniglia 18 > ♂
Massimiliano Il Profumiere > 2010 > Classic Collection: Vetyver Blu > ♂
Massimiliano Il Profumiere > 2010 > Gommoresina Araba > ♂
Massimiliano Il Profumiere > 2010 > Mexican Lyme > ♂
Massimiliano Il Profumiere > 2010 > Olibanum della Somalia > ♂
Massimiliano Il Profumiere > 2011 > Classic Collection: Bacca Verde di Cassis > ♂
Massimiliano Il Profumiere > 2011 > Classic Collection: Bois de Vanille > ♂
Massimiliano Il Profumiere > 2012 > Amyas Marakesh > ♂
Massimiliano Il Profumiere > 2012 > Bois de Cedrat > ♂
Massimiliano Il Profumiere > 2012 > Cacao Bianco d'Arabia > ♂
Massimiliano Il Profumiere > 2012 > Classic Collection: Ambra Orientale > ♂
Massimiliano Il Profumiere > 2012 > Classic Collection: Black Regressive > ♂
Massimiliano Il Profumiere > 2012 > Classic Collection: Camelia Flowers > ♀
Massimiliano Il Profumiere > 2012 > Classic Collection: Patchouli Indonesia 08 > ♂
Massimiliano Il Profumiere > 2012 > Classic Collection: Sublime > ♂
Massimiliano Il Profumiere > 2012 > Tobacco Flowers > ♂
Massimiliano Il Profumiere > 2013 > Classic Collection: Bois De Santal > ♂
Massimiliano Il Profumiere > 2013 > Classic Collection: Real Jack > ♂
Massimiliano Il Profumiere > 2013 > Jamila > ♀
Massimiliano Il Profumiere > 2013 > Sex Therapy > ♂
Massimiliano Il Profumiere > 2013 > Shaakar > ♂
Massimiliano Il Profumiere > 2013 > Sweet Jeazy > ♂
Massimiliano Il Profumiere > 2014 > Classic Collection: Melissa e Opoponax > ♂
Massimiliano Il Profumiere > 2014 > Classic Collection: San Salvador Thiaré > ♂
Massimiliano Il Profumiere > 2014 > Classic Collection: Vanille de Chantilly > ♀
Massimiliano Il Profumiere > 2014 > Cuir Oud > ♂
Massimiliano Il Profumiere > 2014 > Gambo di Rosa > ♂
Massimiliano Il Profumiere > 2014 > Jour de Rose > ♀
Massimiliano Il Profumiere > 2014 > Scent Green Bouquet > ♀
Massimiliano Il Profumiere > 2014 > Vanille Mimosa > ♀
Massimiliano Il Profumiere > 2015 > 10 O'Clock > ♂
Massimiliano Il Profumiere > 2015 > Ambra Spirituale > ♂
Massimiliano Il Profumiere > 2015 > Amyr > ♂
Massimiliano Il Profumiere > 2015 > Azhar > ♂
Massimiliano Il Profumiere > 2015 > Caribbean Beach > ♂
Massimiliano Il Profumiere > 2015 > Cox Royale > ♂
Massimiliano Il Profumiere > 2016 > Caramel Vanille > ♀
Massimiliano Il Profumiere > 2016 > Classic Collection: Cedar Helycrysium > ♂
Massimiliano Il Profumiere > 2016 > Classic Collection: Nettare della Malesia > ♂
Massimiliano Il Profumiere > 2016 > Classic Collection: Pompelmo Rosa Spremuto > ♂
Massimiliano Il Profumiere > 2016 > Classic Collection: Princess Blanche > ♀
Massimiliano Il Profumiere > 2016 > Classic Collection: Steli di Rugiada > ♂

Massimiliano Il Profumiere > 2016 > Payago > ♂
Massimiliano Il Profumiere > 2016 > Vaniglia 07 > ♀
Massimiliano Il Profumiere > 2017 > Classic Collection: Bergamotto Amber 09 > ♂
Massimiliano Il Profumiere > 2017 > Classic Collection: Violetta Bianca > ♀
Massimiliano Il Profumiere > 2017 > Dolci Sottoboschi > ♀
Massimiliano Il Profumiere > 2017 > Resinato Ylang > ♂
Massimiliano Il Profumiere > 2018 > Classic Collection: Ciclamino Rhum > ♂
Massimiliano Il Profumiere > 2018 > Classic Collection: Giunchiglia Selvatica > ♂
Massimiliano Il Profumiere > 2018 > Classic Collection: Platano Guinea > ♂
Massimiliano Il Profumiere > 2018 > Cumino Garofano > ♂
Massimiliano Il Profumiere > 2018 > Pimento Spice > ♂
Massimiliano Il Profumiere > 2018 > Sijux > ♂
Massimiliano Il Profumiere > 2108 > Classic Collection: Indaco Corallo > ♂
Masterpiece L'élite des Parfums > 2018 > First Breath > ♂
Masterpiece L'élite des Parfums > 2018 > My Way > ♀
Masterpiece L'élite des Parfums > 2018 > Nirvana > ♂
Masterpiece L'élite des Parfums > 2018 > Remember Me > ♂
Masterpiece L'élite des Parfums > 2018 > Shadow of Your Smile > ♂
Masterpiece L'élite des Parfums > 2018 > Stairway to Heaven > ♂
Mauro Lorenzi Profumi > 2017 > Aventinus > ♂
Mauro Lorenzi Profumi > 2017 > Caelius > ♂
Mauro Lorenzi Profumi > 2017 > Capitolium > ♂
Mauro Lorenzi Profumi > 2017 > Esquilinus > ♂
Mauro Lorenzi Profumi > 2017 > Palatinus > ♂
Mauro Lorenzi Profumi > 2017 > Quirinalis > ♂
Mauro Lorenzi Profumi > 2017 > Viminalis > ♂
Max Mara > 2004 > Max Mara > ♀
Max Mara > 2007 > Max Mara Gold Touch > ♀
Max Mara > 2007 > Max Mara Silk Touch > ♀
Max Mara > 2008 > Kashmina Touch > ♀
Max Mara > 2008 > Le Parfum > ♀
Max Mara > 2009 > Max Mara Le Parfum Zeste & Musc > ♀
Mazzolari > 2000 > Ambra > ♂
Mazzolari > 2000 > Fleurs d'Oranger > ♀
Mazzolari > 2000 > Marina > ♀
Mazzolari > 2000 > Musk > ♂
Mazzolari > 2000 > Patchouli > ♂
Mazzolari > 2000 > Vetiver > ♂
Mazzolari > 2000 > Zagara > ♀
Mazzolari > 2000 > Alessandro > ♂
Mazzolari > 2000 > Bergamotto Mediterraneo > ♂
Mazzolari > 2000 > Carolina > ♀
Mazzolari > 2000 > Le Rose > ♀
Mazzolari > 2006 > Lui > ♂
Mazzolari > 2006 > Mazzolari > ♂
Mazzolari > 2006 > Lei > ♀
Mazzolari > 2010 > Monforte > ♂
Mazzolari > 2014 > Augusto > ♂
Mazzolari > 2014 > Elena > ♀
Mazzolari > 2014 > Nero > ♂
Mazzolari > 2014 > Oud > ♂
Mazzolari > 2014 > Sofia > ♀
Mazzolari > 2014 > Vaniglia > ♂
Mazzolari > 2015 > Alchemico > ♂
Mazzolari > 2015 > Oriente > ♂
Melogranoantico Profumeria Botanica > 2019 > Come una Rosa > ♂
Melogranoantico Profumeria Botanica > 2019 > Eucalipto e Fiori Bianchi > ♂
Melogranoantico Profumeria Botanica > 2019 > Heliotropium > ♂
Memento – Italian Olfactive Landscapes > 2007 > 22 settembre 2007 ore 8 vaporetto per Il Lido di Venezia > ♀
Memento – Italian Olfactive Landscapes > 2008 > 6 marzo 2008 ore 11 piazza Duomo Ortigia Siracusa – Sicilia > ♀
Memento – Italian Olfactive Landscapes > 2010 > January 28th 3pm Hotel Cristallo – Cortina > ♀
Memento – Italian Olfactive Landscapes > 2010 > June 15th 10am on Porticciolo Beach Chia – Sardinia > ♀
Memento – Italian Olfactive Landscapes > 2010 > October 1st 6 pm Belvedere Villa Borghese – Roma > ♀
Mendittorosa > 2012 > Alfa > ♂
Mendittorosa > 2012 > Id > ♂
Mendittorosa > 2012 > Omega > ♂
Mendittorosa > 2013 > North > ♂
Mendittorosa > 2013 > South > ♂
Mendittorosa > 2014 > Talismans: Le Mat > ♂
Mendittorosa > 2015 > Talismans: Sogno Reale > ♂
Mendittorosa > 2016 > Talismans: Nettuno > ♂
Mendittorosa > 2017 > Archetipo > ♂
Mendittorosa > 2017 > Rituale > ♂

Mendittorosa > 2017 > Talismans: Osang > ♂
Mendittorosa > 2018 > Lacura > ♂
Mendittorosa > 2018 > Talismans: Sirio > ♂
Mendittorosa > 2019 > Ithaka > ♂
Mendittorosa > 2019 > Talento > ♂
Meo Fusciuni > 2010 > 1# Nota di Viaggio (Rites de Passage) > ♂
Meo Fusciuni > 2011 > 2# Nota di Viaggio (Shukran) > ♂
Meo Fusciuni > 2011 > 3# Nota di Viaggio (Ciavuru d'Amuri) > ♂
Meo Fusciuni > 2012 > Notturno > ♂
Meo Fusciuni > 2013 > Luce > ♂
Meo Fusciuni > 2015 > Narcotico > ♂
Meo Fusciuni > 2015 > Odor 93 > ♂
Meo Fusciuni > 2017 > L'oblio > ♂
Meo Fusciuni > 2018 > Little Song > ♂
Meo Fusciuni > 2019 > 3# Nota di Viaggio (Ciavuru d'Amuri) 2019 Edition > ♂
Meo Fusciuni > 2019 > Spirito > ♂
Micaelangelo > 2000 > Atlantide > ♀
Micaelangelo > 2000 > Bellagio > ♀
Micaelangelo > 2000 > Bellagio Uomo > ♂
Micaelangelo > 2001 > Aurora Acqua > ♀
Micaelangelo > 2001 > Aurora Aria > ♀
Micaelangelo > 2001 > Aurora Fuoco > ♀
Micaelangelo > 2001 > Aurora Terra > ♀
Micaelangelo > 2001 > Bellagio Glamour > ♀
Micaelangelo > 2001 > Sibilla > ♀
Micaelangelo > 2001 > Sibilla Oro > ♀
Milano Cento > 2016 > Milano Cento > ♂
Mila Schön > 1981 > Haute Couture > ♀
Mila Schön > 1981 > Mila Schön (Original) > ♀
Mila Schön > 1986 > Mila Schön Uomo (Original) > ♂
Mila Schön > 1990 > Y10 Avenue > ♀
Mila Schön > 1997 > Schön > ♀
Mila Schön > 2002 > Mila Schön Donna > ♀
Mila Schön > 2003 > Mila Schön Homme > ♂
Mila Schön > 2007 > LMila Schön Lui > ♂
Mila Schön > 2007 > Mila Schön Lei > ♀
Mila Schön > 2009 > 60 > ♀
Mila Schön > 2009 > 70 > ♀
Mila Schön > 2009 > 80 > ♀
Mila Schön > 2009 > 90 > ♀
Mila Schön > 2009 > Oo due Zeri > ♀
Mimmina > 1990 > M Mimmina > ♀
Mimmina > 1991 > M for Men > ♂
Mimmina > 1995 > Mimmina Blue > ♀
Mimmina > 1995 > Mimmina Exotic > ♀
Mimmina > 1995 > Mimmina Red > ♀
Mimmina > 1995 > More Musk > ♀
Mimmina > 1995 > Vanilla > ♀
Mimmina > 1995 > White Musk > ♀
Mimmina > 2013 > Flower Bouquet de Roses > ♀
Mimmina > 2013 > Flower Bouquet Extreme > ♀
Mimmina > 2013 > Flower Bouquet Melange > ♀
Mimmina > 2013 > Flower Bouquet Romantique > ♀
Mine Perfume Lab > 2012 > Cuoio > ♂
Mine Perfume Lab > 2012 > Isla > ♂
Mine Perfume Lab > 2012 > Muschio Bianko-20 > ♂
Mine Perfume Lab > 2012 > Rosa-22 > ♀
Mine Perfume Lab > 2013 > Ambra-4 > ♂
Mine Perfume Lab > 2013 > La Mora-18 > ♂
Mine Perfume Lab > 2013 > Patchouli-7 > ♂
Mine Perfume Lab > 2013 > Vetiver-30 > ♂
Mine Perfume Lab > 2014 > Fire-46 > ♂
Mine Perfume Lab > 2014 > Sun > ♂
Mine Perfume Lab > 2014 > Vaniglia-28 > ♂
Mine Perfume Lab > 2014 > Violetta-31 > ♂
Mine Perfume Lab > 2015 > Brise d'Agadir > ♂
Mine Perfume Lab > 2015 > Incenso-15 > ♂
Mine Perfume Lab > 2015 > Tuberose-26 > ♂
Mine Perfume Lab > 2015 > Vaniglia & Tabacco-29 > ♂
Mine Perfume Lab > 2016 > Acqua di Iris & Talco-23 > ♂
Mine Perfume Lab > 2016 > Chileme > ♂
Mine Perfume Lab > 2016 > Corteccia di Cedro-16 > ♂
Mine Perfume Lab > 2016 > Fico-11 > ♂
Mine Perfume Lab > 2016 > Iris & Talco-23 > ♂
Mine Perfume Lab > 2016 > Lo'verte > ♂
Mine Perfume Lab > 2016 > Santal-76 > ♂
Mine Perfume Lab > 2016 > Talco & Panna-2 > ♀
Mine Perfume Lab > 2016 > Vaniglia & Mou > ♂
Mine Perfume Lab > 2017 > Absque > ♂
Mine Perfume Lab > 2017 > Arancia Oud-6 > ♂
Mine Perfume Lab > 2017 > Fresia Orientale > ♂

Mine Perfume Lab > 2017 > Grace-56 > ♀
Mine Perfume Lab > 2017 > Hope-42 > ⚥
Mine Perfume Lab > 2017 > Hush > ⚥
Mine Perfume Lab > 2017 > Jasmine-75 > ♀
Mine Perfume Lab > 2017 > Legni & Agrumi-14 > ♂
Mine Perfume Lab > 2017 > Legni & Spezie-71 > ⚥
Mine Perfume Lab > 2017 > Melograno-13 > ⚥
Mine Perfume Lab > 2017 > Ollà-44 > ⚥
Mine Perfume Lab > 2017 > Oud > ⚥
Mine Perfume Lab > 2017 > Sale & Muschio-10 > ⚥
Mine Perfume Lab > 2018 > Acqua di Talco & Panna-2 > ⚥
Mine Perfume Lab > 2018 > Ambre Café > ⚥
Mine Perfume Lab > 2018 > Malabar Pepper's > ⚥
Mine Perfume Lab > 2018 > Nargilé > ⚥
M.INT > 2016 > 3-D Scent > ⚥
M.INT > 2016 > Affecting Mind > ⚥
M.INT > 2016 > Azure Haze > ⚥
M.INT > 2016 > Blue Waterfall > ⚥
M.INT > 2016 > Cashmere Beige > ⚥
M.INT > 2016 > Hit the Mark > ⚥
M.INT > 2016 > Irisation > ⚥
M.INT > 2016 > Joking Aside > ⚥
M.INT > 2016 > Meek Passion > ⚥
M.INT > 2016 > Mystic Treasure > ⚥
M.INT > 2016 > Neon Night > ⚥
M.INT > 2016 > No Coward > ⚥
M.INT > 2016 > Pitch and Toss > ⚥
M.INT > 2016 > Rainy City > ⚥
M.INT > 2016 > Refocus > ⚥
M.INT > 2016 > Ten Strike > ⚥
M.INT > 2016 > The Smart Set > ⚥
M.INT > 2016 > Time to Target > ⚥
M.INT > 2016 > Vibrant Scent > ⚥
M.INT > 2016 > Winged Heart > ⚥
M.INT > 2019 > Fashion Intervention > ⚥
M.INT > 2019 > Flight Mode > ⚥
Mirato > 2010 > Malizia Bon Bons Melody > ♀
Mirato > 2010 > Malizia Bon Bons Primobacio > ♀
Mirato > 2012 > Malizia Like: Free Spirit > ♀
Mirato > 2012 > Malizia Like: Hot Glam > ♀
Mirato > 2012 > Malizia Like: Neo Chic > ♀
Mirato > 2012 > Malizia Like: Secret Love > ♀
Mirato > 2012 > Malizia Like: So Sweet > ♀
Mirato > 2012 > Uomo Amber > ♂
Mirato > 2012 > Uomo Aqua > ♂
Mirato > 2012 > Uomo Black > ♂
Mirato > 2012 > Uomo Cobalt > ♂
Mirato > 2012 > Uomo Gold > ♂
Mirato > 2012 > Uomo Iron > ♂
Mirato > 2012 > Uomo Silver > ♂
Mirato > 2012 > Uomo Skyline > ♂
Mirato > 2012 > Uomo Vetyver > ♂
Mirato > 2012 > Uomo Wood > ♂
Mirato > 2013 > Malizia Bon Bons Butterfly > ♀
Mirato > 2013 > Malizia Bon Bons Cherry Up > ♀
Mirato > 2013 > Malizia Bon Bons Cotton Flower > ♀
Mirato > 2013 > Malizia Bon Bons Fashion Girl > ♀
Mirato > 2013 > Malizia Bon Bons Happiness > ♀
Mirato > 2013 > Malizia Bon Bons Milk Shake > ♀
Mirato > 2013 > Malizia Bon Bons Oxygen Bubble > ♀
Mirato > 2013 > Malizia Bon Bons Pesca Pop > ♀
Mirato > 2013 > Malizia Bon Bons Sweet Vanilla > ♀
Mirko Buffini Firenze > 2014 > Gods > ⚥
Mirko Buffini Firenze > 2014 > Haecceitas > ⚥
Mirko Buffini Firenze > 2014 > Haiku > ⚥
Mirko Buffini Firenze > 2014 > Ki > ⚥
Mirko Buffini Firenze > 2014 > Kirk > ♂
Mirko Buffini Firenze > 2014 > Klitò > ⚥
Mirko Buffini Firenze > 2014 > Moà > ⚥
Mirko Buffini Firenze > 2014 > Moxi > ⚥
Mirko Buffini Firenze > 2014 > Mu > ⚥
Mirko Buffini Firenze > 2014 > No. 31 > ⚥
Mirko Buffini Firenze > 2014 > Og > ⚥
Mirko Buffini Firenze > 2014 > Saba > ⚥
Mirko Buffini Firenze > 2016 > La Chute d'Eau > ⚥
Mirko Buffini Firenze > 2017 > Finnegan Hce > ⚥
Mirko Buffini Firenze > 2017 > From Hce > ⚥
Mirko Buffini Firenze > 2017 > Gigot Hce > ⚥
Mirko Buffini Firenze > 2017 > Herma Hce > ⚥
Mirko Buffini Firenze > 2017 > Mr Fry Hce > ⚥
Mirko Buffini Firenze > 2017 > Nnn Hce > ⚥
Mirko Buffini Firenze > 2017 > Wake Hce > ⚥

Mirko Buffini Firenze > 2017 > Woid Hce > ⚥
Mirko Buffini Firenze > 2017 > Youth Hce > ⚥
Mirko Buffini Firenze > 2017 > Zeit Hce > ⚥
Mirum > 2015 > Jimi > ⚥
Mirum > 2015 > Make Love no War > ♀
Mirum > 2015 > Not for Sale > ⚥
Mirum > 2015 > Veteran > ⚥
Mirum > 2015 > Warm Thrill > ⚥
Mirum > 2016 > Bye Bye > ⚥
Mirum > 2016 > Maredolce > ♀
Mirum > 2018 > Dominus > ⚥
Mirum > 2018 > Rubacuori > ♀
Mirum > 2018 > Spirito Libero > ⚥
Miss Sixty > 2005 > Miss Sixty > ♀
Miss Sixty > 2006 > Miss Sixty Elixir > ♀
Miss Sixty > 2007 > Miss Sixty Flower Power > ♀
Miss Sixty > 2007 > Miss Sixty Rock Muse > ♀
Miss Sixty > 2008 > Miss > ♀
Miss Sixty > 2008 > Miss Sixty Summer Collection 2008 > ♀
Missoni > 1981 > Missoni > ♀
Missoni > 1987 > Aria Missoni > ♀
Missoni > 1990 > Missoni Sport > ♂
Missoni > 1990 > Missoni Uomo > ♂
Missoni > 1990 > Molto Missoni > ♀
Missoni > 1993 > Noi Missoni > ♀
Missoni > 1994 > Olympios > ♂
Missoni > 2006 > Missoni > ♀
Missoni > 2007 > Missoni Qcqua > ♀
Missoni > 2008 > Missoni Colori – Arancio > ♀
Missoni > 2008 > Missoni Colori – Giallo > ♀
Missoni > 2008 > Missoni Colori – Gianduia > ♀
Missoni > 2008 > Missoni Colori – Rosa > ♀
Missoni > 2015 > Missoni > ♀
Missoni > 2016 > Missoni Edt > ♀
Missoni > 2017 > Missoni Parfum pour Homme > ♂
Miu Miu > 2015 > Miu Miu > ♀
Miu Miu > 2016 > Miu Miu L'Eau Bleue > ♀
Miu Miu > 2018 > Miu Miu Fleur d'Argent > ♀
Miu Miu > 2018 > Miu Miu L'Eau Rosée > ♀
Miu Miu > 2019 > Twist > ♀
Miu Miu > 2019 > Twist Edt > ♀
Modigliani > 1994 > Supreme > ♀
Modigliani > 1995 > Modigliani > ♀
Modigliani > 1996 > Paradiso > ♀
Momo Design > 2013 > Black > ♂
Momo Design > 2013 > White > ♂
Momo Design > 2015 > Gold > ♂
Momo Design > 2015 > Silver > ♂
Momo Design > 2015 > Violet > ♀
Monella Vagabonda > 2015 > Cuore Italiano > ♂
Monella Vagabonda > 2015 > Monella Vagabonda > ♀
Monella Vagabonda > 2015 > Monello Vagabondo > ♂
Monella Vagabonda > 2017 > Alone > ⚥
Monella Vagabonda > 2017 > Snob > ♀
Monella Vagabonda > 2017 > Vip Intense > ⚥
Monolab > 2015 > B-Zone > ⚥
Monolab > 2015 > Black Star > ⚥
Monolab > 2015 > Blood > ⚥
Monolab > 2015 > Gloom > ⚥
Monolab > 2015 > S-Line > ⚥
Monolab > 2015 > Slash > ⚥
Monolab > 2015 > White-Star > ⚥
Monolab > 2019 > Courage > ⚥
Monolab > 2019 > Hannibal > ⚥
Monolab > 2019 > Juicy > ⚥
Monolab > 2019 > Vandal > ⚥
Monolab > 2019 > W-Zone > ⚥
Monom > 2014 > Irmao > ⚥
Monom > 2014 > Nardo > ⚥
Monom > 2014 > Oscuro > ⚥
Monom > 2014 > Respiro > ⚥
Monom > 2014 > Rosalia > ⚥
Monom > 2014 > Sacro > ⚥
Monom > 2014 > Tari > ⚥
Monom > 2017 > Brama > ⚥
Monom > 2018 > Florea > ⚥
Monotheme Fine Fragrances Venezia > 2000 > Ciclamino > ♀
Monotheme Fine Fragrances Venezia > 2003 > Scottish Lavender > ♂
Monotheme Fine Fragrances Venezia > 2003 > Tabacco Latino > ⚥
Monotheme Fine Fragrances Venezia > 2003 > Vetiver Bourbon > ♂
Monotheme Fine Fragrances Venezia > 2005 > Orange Flowers > ♀
Monotheme Fine Fragrances Venezia > 2005 > Rose Petals > ♀

Monotheme Fine Fragrances Venezia > 2005 > Sweet Violet > ♀
Monotheme Fine Fragrances Venezia > 2005 > White Gardenia > ♀
Monotheme Fine Fragrances Venezia > 2006 > Tea Leaves: Green Tea & Bamboo > ♂
Monotheme Fine Fragrances Venezia > 2006 > Tea Leaves: Red Tea & Spices > ♂
Monotheme Fine Fragrances Venezia > 2006 > Tè Bianco & Riso > ♂
Monotheme Fine Fragrances Venezia > 2006 > Vanilla Blossom > ♀
Monotheme Fine Fragrances Venezia > 2006 > White Musk Pour Femme > ♀
Monotheme Fine Fragrances Venezia > 2006 > White Tea > ♀
Monotheme Fine Fragrances Venezia > 2008 > Frangipane delle Maldive > ♀
Monotheme Fine Fragrances Venezia > 2008 > Iris of Tuscany > ♀
Monotheme Fine Fragrances Venezia > 2010 > Talc Douceur > ♀
Monotheme Fine Fragrances Venezia > 2010 > Tè Nero & Vaniglia > ♀
Monotheme Fine Fragrances Venezia > 2010 > Tè Rosso & Spezie > ♀
Monotheme Fine Fragrances Venezia > 2010 > Tè Verde & Bamboo > ♂
Monotheme Fine Fragrances Venezia > 2011 > Black Jasmine > ♀
Monotheme Fine Fragrances Venezia > 2011 > Extrait d'Iris > ♀
Monotheme Fine Fragrances Venezia > 2011 > Black Coffee > ♂
Monotheme Fine Fragrances Venezia > 2011 > Black Musk > ♂
Monotheme Fine Fragrances Venezia > 2012 > Bio Line: Orange Blossom > ♂
Monotheme Fine Fragrances Venezia > 2012 > Bio Line: Vanilla Elixir > ♂
Monotheme Fine Fragrances Venezia > 2012 > Bio Line: White Musk > ♂
Monotheme Fine Fragrances Venezia > 2012 > Bio Line: White Tea Flowers > ♂
Monotheme Fine Fragrances Venezia > 2012 > Gelsomino dell'India > ♀
Monotheme Fine Fragrances Venezia > 2012 > Giglio delle Hawaii > ♀
Monotheme Fine Fragrances Venezia > 2012 > Ibiza Nightflowers > ♀
Monotheme Fine Fragrances Venezia > 2012 > Monoi della Polinesia > ♀
Monotheme Fine Fragrances Venezia > 2012 > Rio de Janeiro Passion Fruit > ♀
Monotheme Fine Fragrances Venezia > 2012 > Tiaré de Tahiti > ♀
Monotheme Fine Fragrances Venezia > 2012 > Vaniglia del Madagascar > ♀
Monotheme Fine Fragrances Venezia > 2012 > Ylang Ylang della Polinesia > ♀
Monotheme Fine Fragrances Venezia > 2012 > Orchidee d'Oriente > ♀
Monotheme Fine Fragrances Venezia > 2012 > Pure Cacao > ♂
Monotheme Fine Fragrances Venezia > 2012 > Pure Neroli > ♂
Monotheme Fine Fragrances Venezia > 2012 > Spicy > ♂
Monotheme Fine Fragrances Venezia > 2012 > Star Anise > ♂
Monotheme Fine Fragrances Venezia > 2012 > Tropical Bamboo > ♂
Monotheme Fine Fragrances Venezia > 2013 > Amber Wood > ♂
Monotheme Fine Fragrances Venezia > 2013 > Black Oud > ♂
Monotheme Fine Fragrances Venezia > 2013 > Daisy Daisy > ♀
Monotheme Fine Fragrances Venezia > 2013 > Leather > ♂
Monotheme Fine Fragrances Venezia > 2013 > Rose Oud > ♀
Monotheme Fine Fragrances Venezia > 2013 > Agrumi di Sicilia > ♂
Monotheme Fine Fragrances Venezia > 2013 > Apotheose de Rose > ♀
Monotheme Fine Fragrances Venezia > 2013 > Aqva Marina > ♂
Monotheme Fine Fragrances Venezia > 2013 > Cashmere Wood > ♂
Monotheme Fine Fragrances Venezia > 2013 > Grace Amber > ♀
Monotheme Fine Fragrances Venezia > 2013 > Green Tea > ♀
Monotheme Fine Fragrances Venezia > 2013 > Narciso Bianco > ♀
Monotheme Fine Fragrances Venezia > 2016 > Bergamotto > ♂
Monotheme Fine Fragrances Venezia > 2016 > Boccioli di Limone > ♀
Monotheme Fine Fragrances Venezia > 2016 > Magnolia > ♀
Monotheme Fine Fragrances Venezia > 2016 > Mandarino > ♂
Monotheme Fine Fragrances Venezia > 2016 > Pompelmo > ♀
Monotheme Fine Fragrances Venezia > 2016 > Verbena > ♂
Monotheme Fine Fragrances Venezia > 2016 > Verde d'Arancia > ♀
Monotheme Fine Fragrances Venezia > 2016 > Zagara > ♀
Monotheme Fine Fragrances Venezia > 2016 > Patchouli Leaves > ♂
Monotheme Fine Fragrances Venezia > 2017 > Mimosa > ♀
Monotheme Fine Fragrances Venezia > 2017 > Tuberose > ♀
Monotheme Fine Fragrances Venezia > 2018 > Macchia Mediterranea > ♂
Monotheme Fine Fragrances Venezia > 2018 > Mediterranean Coast > ♂
Monotheme Fine Fragrances Venezia > 2018 > Red Fig > ♂
Monotheme Fine Fragrances Venezia > 2019 > Bloom pour Femme > ♀
Monotheme Fine Fragrances Venezia > 2019 > Cherry Blossom > ♀
Monotheme Fine Fragrances Venezia > 2019 > Korea Exclusive Edition: Blackberry > ♀
Monotheme Fine Fragrances Venezia > 2019 > Korea Exclusive Edition: Citrusy Blossom > ♂
Monotheme Fine Fragrances Venezia > 2019 > Almond >
Monotheme Fine Fragrances Venezia > 2019 > Nymphea > ♀
Montegrappa > 2012 > Nerouno > ♂
Montegrappa > 2012 > Nerouno for Women > ♀
Moresque Parfum > 2000 > Ballerina > ♀
Moresque Parfum > 2015 > Al Andalus > ♂

Moresque Parfum > 2015 > Aristoqrati > ♂
Moresque Parfum > 2015 > Diadema > ♂
Moresque Parfum > 2015 > Emarati > ♂
Moresque Parfum > 2015 > Emiro > ♂
Moresque Parfum > 2015 > Moreta > ♂
Moresque Parfum > 2015 > Rand > ♂
Moresque Parfum > 2015 > Tamima > ♂
Moresque Parfum > 2016 > Aurum > ♂
Moresque Parfum > 2016 > Contessa > ♂
Moresque Parfum > 2016 > Fiamma > ♀
Moresque Parfum > 2016 > Fiore di Portofino > ♂
Moresque Parfum > 2016 > Oroluna > ♀
Moresque Parfum > 2016 > Regina > ♂
Moresque Parfum > 2017 > Rosa Ekaterina > ♀
Moresque Parfum > 2017 > Sandal Granada > ♂
Moresque Parfum > 2017 > Sole > ♂
Moresque Parfum > 2018 > Alma Pure > ♀
Moresque Parfum > 2018 > Harrods Exclusive: Midnight London > ♂
Moresque Parfum > 2018 > Jasminisha > ♂
Moresque Parfum > 2018 > Oro > ♂
Moresque Parfum > 2018 > Re Nero > ♂
Moresque Parfum > 2018 > Sahara Blue > ♂
Moresque Parfum > 2018 > Seta > ♂
Moresque Parfum > 2018 > Soul Batik > ♂
Moresque Parfum > 2018 > Ubar 1992 > ♂
Moresque Parfum > 2019 > Royal > ♂
Moresque Parfum > 2019 > White Duke > ♂
Morph > 2016 > Vision > ♂
Morph > 2017 > Axum > ♂
Morph > 2017 > Indomable > ♂
Morph > 2018 > Zeta > ♂
Morph > 2018 > Antigua > ♀
Morph > 2018 > Arles > ♀
Morph > 2018 > Cruda > ♀
Morph > 2018 > Kolonaki > ♀
Morph > 2018 > Malaga > ♀
Morph > 2018 > Montmartre > ♂
Morph > 2018 > Nudo > ♂
Morph > 2018 > Pure Soul > ♀
Morph > 2019 > A21 > ♂
Morph > 2019 > Animal >
Morph > 2019 > N. 8 > ♂
Morph > 2019 > Rose J. > ♀
Morris > 1975 > Morris > ♂
Morris > 1976 > Morris Sport > ♂
Morris > 1979 > Gocce di Napoleon > ♂
Morris > 1985 > Luna > ♀
Morris > 1991 > Gocce Gocce di Napoleon > ♂
Morris > 1995 > Occhi Verdi Batik > ♀
Morris > 2006 > Maria Amalia > ♀
Morris > 2010 > Morriselle Eau Fraiche > ♀
Morris > 2010 > Morriselle Eau Tendre > ♀
Morris > 2010 > Morriselle pour Elle > ♀
Morris > 2013 > Morriselle pour Elle Musc > ♀
Morris > 2014 > Black Intense > ♂
Morris > 2015 > Gocce di Amore > ♀
Morris > 2015 > Gocce di Passione > ♀
Morris > 2015 > Miss Gocce Romantic > ♀
Morris > 2015 > Miss Gocce Sensual > ♀
Morris > 2016 > Morriselle pour Elle le Parfum > ♀
Morris > 2017 > Morriselle pour Elle Moi > ♀
Morris > 2018 > The Wild Man > ♂
Moschino > 1987 > Moschino > ♀
Moschino > 1990 > Moschino pour Homme > ♂
Moschino > 1995 > Cheap & Chic > ♀
Moschino > 1996 > Oh! De Moschino > ♀
Moschino > 1998 > Uomo? > ♂
Moschino > 2001 > L'Eau de Cheap and Chic > ♀
Moschino > 2004 > Cheap and Chic – I Love Love > ♀
Moschino > 2004 > Couture! > ♀
Moschino > 2005 > Friends Men > ♂
Moschino > 2007 > Moschino Funny! > ♀
Moschino > 2008 > Cheap and Chic – Hippy Fizz > ♀
Moschino > 2008 > Glamour > ♀
Moschino > 2009 > Cheap and Chic – Light Clouds > ♀
Moschino > 2010 > Glamour – Toujours Glamour > ♀
Moschino > 2011 > Moschino Forever > ♂
Moschino > 2012 > Glamour Pink Bouquet > ♀
Moschino > 2013 > Cheap and Chic – Chic Petals > ♀
Moschino > 2013 > Moschino Forever Sailing > ♂
Moschino > 2014 > Stars > ♀
Moschino > 2014 > Toy > ♂

Moschino > 2015 > Fresh Couture > ♀
Moschino > 2017 > Fresh Couture Gold > ♀
Moschino > 2017 > Fresh Couture Pink > ♀
Moschino > 2017 > So Real Cheap & Chic > ♀
Moschino > 2018 > Toy 2 > ♀
Moschino > 2019 > Toy Boy > ♂
My Inner Island Parfums > 2014 > Muschio Marino e Sale > ♂
My Inner Island Parfums > 2014 > My Second Island – Absinthe Bleu Glaces > ♂
My Inner Island Parfums > 2014 > My Second Island – Ambre Exotique sur La Plage > ♂
My Inner Island Parfums > 2014 > My Second Island – Rose Amere du Desert > ♂
My Inner Island Parfums > 2014 > My Third Island – Cocco e Limone > ♀
My Inner Island Parfums > 2014 > My Third Island – Vaniglia, Cacao, Caffè > ♀
My Inner Island Parfums > 2014 > Pepe Extra e Lime > ♂
My Inner Island Parfums > 2014 > The Numbers – Eight Dangers > ♂
My Inner Island Parfums > 2014 > The Numbers – Nine Reasons > ♂
My Inner Island Parfums > 2014 > The Numbers – Seven Stars > ♂
My Inner Island Parfums > 2014 > Vaniglia Sopraffina E Rhum > ♂
Naj Oleari > 1999 > Naj Oleari > ♀
Narcotica Perfume > 2019 > Bright Black > ♀
Naso di Raza > 2015 > Aqua Maris > ♂
Naso di Raza > 2015 > Ask Me no More > ♀
Naso di Raza > 2015 > Cyrano > ♂
Naso di Raza > 2015 > Fin du Passe > ♂
Naso di Raza > 2015 > La Chaise Vide > ♂
Naso di Raza > 2015 > Than... White > ♀
Naso di Raza > 2017 > Cher Tetu > ♀
Naso di Raza > 2017 > Giuseppe > ♂
Naso di Raza > 2017 > Mozzafiato > ♀
Naso di Raza > 2017 > Ravi > ♂
Naso di Raza > 2019 > Esmeralda > ♂
Naso di Raza > 2019 > Use Black > ♂
Nasomatto > 2007 > Absinth > ♂
Nasomatto > 2007 > Duro > ♂
Nasomatto > 2007 > Silver Musk > ♂
Nasomatto > 2008 > China White > ♀
Nasomatto > 2008 > Hindu Grass > ♀
Nasomatto > 2009 > Black Afgano > ♂
Nasomatto > 2009 > Narcotic Venus > ♀
Nasomatto > 2010 > Nuda > ♀
Nasomatto > 2011 > Pardon > ♂
Nasomatto > 2014 > Blamage > ♂
Nasomatto > 2016 > Baraonda > ♀
Nasomatto > 2018 > Nudiflorum > ♀
Natur Milano > 2014 > Adorami > ♀
Natur Milano > 2014 > Armonia > ♂
Natur Milano > 2014 > Gioia > ♀
Natur Milano > 2014 > Horus Cinza Concreto > ♂
Nature's > 2017 > Assoluta di Rosa > ♀
Nature's > 2017 > Boccioli > ♀
Nature's > 2017 > Cedro Donna > ♀
Nature's > 2017 > Cedro Uomo > ♂
Nature's > 2017 > Elisia > ♀
Nature's > 2017 > Fiori di Osmanto > ♀
Nature's > 2017 > Fiori di Zenzero > ♂
Nature's > 2017 > Gelsomino Adorabile > ♀
Nature's > 2017 > Giardino d'Agrumi > ♂
Nature's > 2017 > Hematite > ♂
Nature's > 2017 > Legni > ♂
Nature's > 2017 > Lillà > ♀
Nature's > 2017 > Malaquite > ♀
Nature's > 2017 > Muschio d'Acqua > ♀
Nature's > 2017 > Passione d'Africa > ♀
Nature's > 2017 > Pepe Fondente > ♂
Nature's > 2017 > Pomelia > ♀
Nature's > 2017 > Vaniglia Bianca > ♀
Nature's > 2017 > Vetiverde > ♂
Nature's > 2017 > Zucchero d'Ambra > ♀
Nautilus > 1998 > Aqua Nautilus > ♂
Nautilus > 2000 > Donna Nautilus > ♀
Nautilus > 2000 > Pois > ♀
Nautilus > 2001 > Black Marlin > ♂
Nautilus > 2005 > Blazer > ♂
Nazareno Gabrielli > 1996 > Nazareno Gabrielli > ♀
Nazareno Gabrielli > 1996 > Nazareno Gabrielli > ♂
Nazareno Gabrielli > 2000 > Nazareno > ♀
Nazareno Gabrielli > 2004 > Nazarenogabrielli > ♀
Nazareno Gabrielli > 2004 > Nazarenogabrielli > ♂
Nazareno Gabrielli > 2004 > Tu > ♀

Nazareno Gabrielli > 2004 > Tu > ♂
Nazareno Gabrielli > 2015 > Details for Her > ♀
Nazareno Gabrielli > 2015 > Details for Him > ♂
Niyo&Co. > 2017 > Fiori del Mediterraneo: Magnolia Blumei > ♀
Niyo&Co. > 2017 > Fiori del Mediterraneo: Rosa Acquarello > ♀
Niyo&Co. > 2017 > Giardini d'Italia: Fico > ♀
Niyo&Co. > 2017 > Giardini d'Italia: Mirto > ♀
Niyo&Co. > 2017 > Grandi Classici: Ambra > ♀
Niyo&Co. > 2017 > Grandi Classici: Muschio Bianco > ♀
Niyo&Co. > 2017 > Grandi Classici: Patchouly > ♀
Niyo&Co. > 2017 > Grandi Classici: Tuberosa > ♀
Niyo&Co. > 2017 > Grandi Classici: Vaniglia > ♀
Niyo&Co. > 2017 > Grandi Classici: Vetiver > ♀
Niyo&Co. > 2017 > L'Essenziere Estratto 1 > ♀
Niyo&Co. > 2017 > L'Essenziere Estratto 2 > ♀
Niyo&Co. > 2017 > L'Essenziere Estratto 3 > ♀
Niyo&Co. > 2017 > L'Essenziere Estratto 4 > ♀
Niyo&Co. > 2017 > L'Essenziere Estratto 5 > ♀
Niyo&Co. > 2017 > L'Essenziere Estratto 6 > ♀
Niyo&Co. > 2017 > L'Essenziere Estratto 7 > ♀
Niyo&Co. > 2017 > L'Essenziere Estratto 8 > ♀
Niyo&Co. > 2017 > L'Essenziere Estratto 9 > ♀
Niyo&Co. > 2017 > L'Essenziere Estratto 10 > ♀
Niyo&Co. > 2017 > L'Essenziere Estratto 11 > ♀
Niyo&Co. > 2017 > L'Essenziere Estratto 12 > ♀
Niyo&Co. > 2017 > L'Essenziere Estratto 13 > ♀
Niyo&Co. > 2017 > L'Essenziere Estratto 14 > ♀
Niyo&Co. > 2017 > L'Essenziere Estratto 15 > ♀
Niyo&Co. > 2017 > L'Essenziere Intenso 01 Velvet Oud > ♀
Niyo&Co. > 2017 > L'Essenziere Intenso 02 Cashmere Sea > ♀
Niyo&Co. > 2017 > L'Essenziere Intenso 03 Damask Wood > ♀
Nobile 1942 > 2000 > I Rigati: Ambra Nobile > ♂
Nobile 1942 > 2005 > Pontevecchio > ♂
Nobile 1942 > 2005 > Vespri Esperidati Women > ♀
Nobile 1942 > 2006 > Anonimo Veneziano > ♂
Nobile 1942 > 2008 > I Rigati: Acqua Nobile > ♀
Nobile 1942 > 2008 > I Rigati: Lavanda Nobile > ♀
Nobile 1942 > 2008 > Vespri Esperidati > ♂
Nobile 1942 > 2009 > Alla Corte del Re: Cedro Atlas I Superhero > ♂
Nobile 1942 > 2009 > Alla Corte del Re: Cedro Atlas II Cola > ♂
Nobile 1942 > 2009 > Alla Corte del Re: Cedro Atlas III Robinson > ♂
Nobile 1942 > 2009 > Alla Corte del Re: Rosa Incantevole I Julie Coeur > ♀
Nobile 1942 > 2009 > Alla Corte del Re: Rosa Incantevole II Vanille > ♀
Nobile 1942 > 2009 > Alla Corte del Re: Rosa Incantevole III Rose Iris > ♀
Nobile 1942 > 2009 > Casta Diva > ♀
Nobile 1942 > 2009 > Castadiva Estratto > ♀
Nobile 1942 > 2009 > I Rigati: Patchouli Nobile > ♂
Nobile 1942 > 2009 > Pontevecchio > ♂
Nobile 1942 > 2009 > Vaniglia Estratto > ♂
Nobile 1942 > 2010 > Anonimo Veneziano Estratto > ♂
Nobile 1942 > 2010 > Estroverso > ♀
Nobile 1942 > 2010 > Profumo Imperiale > ♀
Nobile 1942 > 2011 > Alla Corte del Re: Le Petit Chocolatier I Confiture > ♀
Nobile 1942 > 2011 > Alla Corte del Re: Le Petit Chocolatier II Praline > ♀
Nobile 1942 > 2011 > Alla Corte del Re: Le Petit Chocolatier III Noir Intense > ♀
Nobile 1942 > 2011 > Ambra Estratto > ♂
Nobile 1942 > 2011 > Chypre 1942 > ♀
Nobile 1942 > 2011 > Chypre Estratto > ♀
Nobile 1942 > 2011 > I Rigati: Muschio Nobile > ♀
Nobile 1942 > 2011 > Patchouli Estratto > ♂
Nobile 1942 > 2011 > Pontevecchio Estratto > ♂
Nobile 1942 > 2011 > Pontevecchio Estratto > ♀
Nobile 1942 > 2012 > Alla Corte del Re: Piccoli Nobili > ♀
Nobile 1942 > 2012 > La Danza delle Libellule > ♀
Nobile 1942 > 2013 > Café Chantant > ♀
Nobile 1942 > 2013 > Infinito > ♂
Nobile 1942 > 2013 > Vespri Aromatico > ♂
Nobile 1942 > 2013 > Vespri Orientale > ♂
Nobile 1942 > 2013 > Vespri Orientali Estratto > ♂
Nobile 1942 > 2014 > Alla Corte del Re: Bon Bon I Zucchero Candito > ♂
Nobile 1942 > 2014 > Alla Corte del Re: Bon Bon II Alla Fragola > ♀
Nobile 1942 > 2014 > Alla Corte del Re: Bon Bon III Altea > ♀
Nobile 1942 > 2014 > Rudis > ♂
Nobile 1942 > 2015 > Café Chantant Exceptional Edition > ♂
Nobile 1942 > 2015 > Casta Diva Exceptional Edition > ♀
Nobile 1942 > 2015 > I Rigati: Fougère Nobile > ♂
Nobile 1942 > 2015 > La Danza delle Libellule Exceptional Edition > ♀
Nobile 1942 > 2015 > Malia > ♀
Nobile 1942 > 2015 > Pontevecchio Exceptional Edition > ♂
Nobile 1942 > 2015 > Pontevecchio Exceptional Edition > ♀
Nobile 1942 > 2015 > Vespri Esperidati Estratto > ♀
Nobile 1942 > 2016 > I Rigati: Sandalo Nobile > ♂

Nobile 1942 > 2016 > Perdizione > ⚥
Nobile 1942 > 2017 > 1001 > ♂
Nobile 1942 > 2017 > Levante > ⚥
Nobile 1942 > 2018 > Il Capriccio del Maestro > ⚥
Nobile 1942 > 2018 > Il Sentiero degli Dei > ⚥
Nobile 1942 > 2018 > Malvs > ♀
Nobile 1942 > 2018 > Shamal > ⚥
Note di Profumum > 2016 > Amante > ⚥
Note di Profumum > 2016 > Lvce > ⚥
Note di Profumum > 2016 > Lvce dell'Est > ⚥
Note di Profumum > 2016 > Meraviglia-Re > ⚥
Note di Profumum > 2016 > Osa-Re > ⚥
Note di Profumum > 2016 > Vet-G16 > ⚥
Note di Profumum > 2018 > Vetta > ⚥
Notebook Fragrances > 2019 > Bergamot & Sandalwood > ⚥
Notebook Fragrances > 2019 > Cassis & Pink Pepper > ⚥
Notebook Fragrances > 2019 > Citrus & Green Tea > ⚥
Notebook Fragrances > 2019 > Patchouli & Cedarwood > ⚥
Notebook Fragrances > 2019 > Peony & White Musk > ⚥
Notebook Fragrances > 2019 > Rose Musk & Vanilla > ⚥
Notebook Fragrances > 2019 > White Wood & Vetiver > ⚥
Od – Onediffusion > 2009 > One Diffusion 53-63 > ⚥
Od – Onediffusion > 2009 > One Diffusion A-080 > ⚥
Od – Onediffusion > 2009 > One Diffusion C-090 > ♀
Od – Onediffusion > 2009 > One Diffusion F-051 > ♀
Od – Onediffusion > 2009 > One Diffusion F-055 > ♀
Od – Onediffusion > 2009 > One Diffusion F-070 > ♀
Od – Onediffusion > 2009 > One Diffusion F-075 > ♀
Od – Onediffusion > 2009 > One Diffusion W-101 > ♂
Od – Onediffusion > 2009 > One Diffusion W-102 > ♂
Od – Onediffusion > 2009 > One Diffusion W-108 > ♂
Od – Onediffusion > 2009 > One Diffusion W-110 > ♂
Odori – Profumo di Firenze > 2008 > Cuoio 2008 > ⚥
Odori – Profumo di Firenze > 2008 > Gli Odori 2008 > ⚥
Odori – Profumo di Firenze > 2008 > Iris 2008 > ⚥
Odori – Profumo di Firenze > 2008 > Spigo 2008 > ⚥
Odori – Profumo di Firenze > 2008 > Tabacco 2008 > ⚥
Odori – Profumo di Firenze > 2008 > Zafferano 2008 > ⚥
O'driu > 2011 > Alchimia di Profumo – Lalfegrigio > ⚥
O'driu > 2011 > Alchimia di Profumo – Lalfeorosa > ♀
O'driu > 2011 > Alchimia di Profumo – Laltrove 1001 > ♂
O'driu > 2011 > Alchimia di Profumo – Laltrove 1002 > ⚥
O'driu > 2011 > Alchimia di Profumo – Linfedele 1003 > ♂
O'driu > 2011 > Alchimia di Profumo – Linfedele 1004 > ⚥
O'driu > 2011 > Alchimia di Profumo – Londa 1005 > ♂
O'driu > 2011 > Alchimia di Profumo – Londa 1006 > ♀
O'driu > 2011 > Genesi – Ladamo > ♂
O'driu > 2011 > Genesi – Leva > ♀
O'driu > 2012 > Vetiver Experience – Supercilium > ⚥
O'driu > 2013 > Eva Kant > ♀
O'driu > 2013 > Peety > ⚥
O'driu > 2014 > L'infedele Haiku > ⚥
O'driu > 2014 > Pathetique > ⚥
O'driu > 2015 > Angel Collection – Italian Angel > ⚥
O'driu > 2015 > Captivus > ⚥
O'driu > 2015 > L'inferno-2 > ⚥
O'driu > 2015 > Satyricon > ⚥
O'driu > 2015 > Vendetta – Det > ⚥
O'driu > 2015 > Vendetta – Ta > ⚥
O'driu > 2015 > Vendetta – Ven > ⚥
O'driu > 2016 > Angel Collection – Gothic Angel > ⚥
O'driu > 2016 > Kiss my Ass Angelorraziopregoni > ⚥
O'driu > 2016 > Kiss my Ass Basenotes > ⚥
O'driu > 2016 > Kiss my Ass Scent and Chemistry > ⚥
O'driu > 2017 > Angel Collection – Sea Angel > ⚥
Officina delle Essenze > 2006 > Puro Lino > ⚥
Officina delle Essenze > 2008 > Puro Neroli > ⚥
Officina delle Essenze > 2008 > Puro Talco > ⚥
Officina delle Essenze > 2010 > Musc Pure > ⚥
Officina delle Essenze > 2012 > Caldo Gourmand > ⚥
Officina delle Essenze > 2012 > Caldo Legnoso > ⚥
Officina delle Essenze > 2012 > Caldo Orientale > ⚥
Officina delle Essenze > 2012 > Puro Fico > ⚥
Officina delle Essenze > 2014 > Caldo Encens > ⚥
Officina delle Essenze > 2014 > Caldo Fruttato > ⚥
Officina delle Essenze > 2014 > Osmarine (Osmanto Marino) > ⚥
Officina delle Essenze > 2018 > Oud Gourmand > ⚥
Officine del Profumo > 2005 > Argento > ♀
Officine del Profumo > 2008 > Passiflora > ♀
Officine del Profumo > 2009 > Aquamarina > ⚥
Officine del Profumo > 2009 > Artemisia > ♂
Officine del Profumo > 2009 > Fresia di Portofino > ♀
Officine del Profumo > 2009 > Gelsomino Viola > ♀
Officine del Profumo > 2009 > Ginepro di Calabria > ♂
Officine del Profumo > 2009 > Incenso di Toscana > ♂
Officine del Profumo > 2009 > Lavanda di Roma > ♂
Officine del Profumo > 2009 > Mandorla di Sicilia > ♀
Officine del Profumo > 2009 > Rosa Primula > ♀
Officine del Profumo > 2009 > A Sud del Mondo > ⚥
Officine del Profumo > 2009 > Agrumi Mediterranei > ⚥
Officine del Profumo > 2009 > Ambra d'Oriente > ⚥
Officine del Profumo > 2009 > Hiera > ⚥
Officine del Profumo > 2009 > Juanito > ♂
Officine del Profumo > 2009 > Mandarino e Spezie > ⚥
Officine del Profumo > 2009 > Mojito > ⚥
Officine del Profumo > 2009 > Mughetto delle Cinque Terre > ⚥
Officine del Profumo > 2009 > Musk > ⚥
Officine del Profumo > 2009 > Notti del Golfo > ⚥
Officine del Profumo > 2009 > Orchidea della Costa Rica > ♀
Officine del Profumo > 2009 > Patchouli d'Italia > ⚥
Officine del Profumo > 2009 > Wood > ⚥
Officine del Profumo > 2009 > Zaahra > ⚥
Officine del Profumo > 2013 > Giacinto Imperiale > ♀
Officine del Profumo > 2013 > Lei > ♀
Officine del Profumo > 2013 > Magnolia Imperiale > ♀
Officine del Profumo > 2013 > Ribes Nero Imperiale > ♀
Officine del Profumo > 2013 > Tuberosa Imperiale > ♀
Officine del Profumo > 2017 > Imperio > ⚥
Officine del Profumo > 2017 > Incanto > ⚥
Officine del Profumo > 2017 > Meraviglioso Istante > ⚥
Olfattology > 2015 > Clux Edition – Ot 11 > ⚥
Olfattology > 2015 > Clux Edition – Ot 23 > ⚥
Olfattology > 2015 > Itenez > ⚥
Olfattology > 2015 > Kasai > ⚥
Olfattology > 2015 > Parana > ⚥
Olfattology > 2015 > Sagami > ⚥
Olfattology > 2015 > Tamaki > ⚥
Olfattology > 2015 > Yacuma > ⚥
Olivares & Ribero > 2015 > Acacia & Unicità > ⚥
Olivares & Ribero > 2015 > Bois de Rose & Grazia > ⚥
Olivares & Ribero > 2015 > Ebano & Forza > ⚥
Olivares & Ribero > 2015 > Palissandro & Nobiltà > ⚥
Olivares & Ribero > 2017 > Ciliegio & Passione > ⚥
Olivier Strelli > 2005 > Olivier Strelli > ♂
Olivier Strelli > 2007 > The World is Wonderful > ♀
Omnia Profumi > 2004 > Ambra > ♀
Omnia Profumi > 2004 > Granato > ♀
Omnia Profumi > 2005 > Acquamarina > ♀
Omnia Profumi > 2005 > Onice > ♀
Omnia Profumi > 2006 > Opale > ♀
Omnia Profumi > 2007 > Madera > ♀
Omnia Profumi > 2011 > Oro > ♀
Omnia Profumi > 2012 > Argento > ♂
Omnia Profumi > 2012 > Rame 29 > ♂
Omnia Profumi > 2013 > Cristallo di Rocca > ♀
Omnia Profumi > 2013 > Peridoto > ♀
Omnia Profumi > 2013 > Platino > ♀
Omnia Profumi > 2013 > Titanio > ♀
Omnia Profumi > 2014 > Bronzo > ♀
Omnia Profumi > 2015 > White Madera > ♀
Omnia Profumi > 2016 > Cristallo di Rocca New Edition > ⚥
Omnia Profumi > 2016 > White Ambra > ⚥
Omnia Profumi > 2017 > Ferro > ♂
Omnia Profumi > 2018 > Diamante > ♀
Omnia Profumi > 2019 > Animanobile > ⚥
Omnia Profumi > 2019 > Evodia > ⚥
Omnia Profumi > 2019 > Fabrizio Tagliacarne – Icio > ⚥
One of Those (Ex Nube) > 2012 > Carbon (6C) > ⚥
One of Those (Ex Nube) > 2012 > Helium (2He) > ⚥
One of Those (Ex Nube) > 2012 > Hydrogen (1H) > ⚥
One of Those (Ex Nube) > 2012 > Lithium (3Li) > ⚥
One of Those (Ex Nube) > 2012 > Oxygen (8O) > ⚥
One of Those (Ex Nube) > 2013 > Mercury (HOHg) > ⚥
One of Those (Ex Nube) > 2013 > Sulphur (16S) > ⚥
One of Those (Ex Nube) > 2016 > Curium (Cm96) > ⚥
Onyrico > 2015 > Empireo > ⚥
Onyrico > 2015 > Enygma > ⚥
Onyrico > 2015 > Michelangelo > ⚥
Onyrico > 2015 > Rossa Boheme > ⚥
Onyrico > 2015 > Tau > ♂
Onyrico > 2015 > Unguentum > ⚥
Onyrico > 2015 > Zephiro > ⚥
Onyrico > 2016 > Itineris > ⚥
Onyrico > 2018 > Artimitia > ⚥

Onyrico > 2019 > Ingenium > ♀
O.P.S.O. > 2013 > Araia > ♀
O.P.S.O. > 2013 > Baiana > ♀
O.P.S.O. > 2013 > Carminia > ♀
O.P.S.O. > 2013 > Dalila > ♀
O.P.S.O. > 2013 > Edgar > ♂
Opsobjects > 2015 > Ops! Love > ♀
Optico L'arte del Profumo > 2016 > Optico.cr > ♂
Optico L'arte del Profumo > 2016 > Optico.it > ♀
Optico L'arte del Profumo > 2016 > Optico.lk > ♂
Optico L'arte del Profumo > 2016 > Optico.re > ♂
Optico L'arte del Profumo > 2019 > BSX > ♂
Orobianco > 2011 > 417 > ♂
Orobianco > 2011 > 418 > ♀
Orobianco > 2013 > Eccessive > ♀
Orobianco > 2013 > Estetiko > ♂
Orobianco > 2013 > Kattiva > ♀
Orobianco > 2013 > Kattivo > ♂
Orobianco > 2013 > Lalibela > ♀
Orobianco > 2013 > Sadyca > ♀
Ortigia Sicilia > 2006 > Ambra Nera > ♀
Ortigia Sicilia > 2006 > Bergamotto > ♀
Ortigia Sicilia > 2006 > Fico d'India > ♀
Ortigia Sicilia > 2006 > Geranio > ♀
Ortigia Sicilia > 2006 > Melograno > ♀
Ortigia Sicilia > 2006 > Neroli > ♂
Ortigia Sicilia > 2006 > Sandalo > ♀
Ortigia Sicilia > 2006 > Zagara > ♀
Ortigia Sicilia > 2007 > Corallo > ♀
Ortigia Sicilia > 2008 > Florio > ♀
Ortigia Sicilia > 2008 > Lime > ♂
Ortigia Sicilia > 2009 > Lavanda > ♂
Ortigia Sicilia > 2009 > Mandorla > ♀
Ortigia Sicilia > 2014 > Gelsomino > ♀
Orto Parisi > 2014 > Bergamask > ♂
Orto Parisi > 2014 > Boccanera > ♂
Orto Parisi > 2014 > Brutus > ♂
Orto Parisi > 2014 > Stercus > ♀
Orto Parisi > 2014 > Viride > ♀
Orto Parisi > 2016 > Seminalis > ♂
Orto Parisi > 2017 > Terroni > ♂
Orto Parisi > 2019 > Megamare > ♂
Paglieri > 2015 > Paglieri Essenza Autentica > ♀
Paglieri > 2016 > Agrigentum > ♂
Paglieri > 2016 > Amalphia > ♀
Paglieri > 2016 > Florentia > ♀
Paglieri > 2016 > Genua > ♀
Paglieri > 2016 > Romae > ♂
Paglieri > 2016 > Venetiae > ♀
Paglieri > 2017 > Bononia > ♀
Paglieri > 2017 > Mediolanum > ♂
Pal Zileri > 2002 > Pal Zileri > ♂
Pal Zileri > 2005 > Concept N. 18 > ♂
Pal Zileri > 2005 > Sartoriale > ♂
Pal Zileri > 2006 > Lab > ♂
Pal Zileri > 2008 > Lab I-White > ♂
Pal Zileri > 2010 > Collezione Privata: Blu di Provenza > ♂
Pal Zileri > 2010 > Collezione Privata: Cashmere e Ambra > ♂
Pal Zileri > 2010 > Collezione Privata: Colonia Purissima > ♂
Pal Zileri > 2010 > Collezione Privata: Viaggio d'Africa > ♂
Pal Zileri > 2011 > Uomo > ♂
Pal Zileri > 2011 > Uomo Essenza di Capri > ♂
Pal Zileri > 2012 > Collezione Privata: Cuoio > ♂
Pal Zileri > 2012 > Collezione Privata: Fougère e Legni > ♂
Pal Zileri > 2012 > Venice Cup > ♂
Pal Zileri > 2013 > Cerimonia Pour Femme > ♀
Pal Zileri > 2013 > Collezione Privata: Essenza di Aoud > ♂
Pancaldi > 1988 > Pancaldi & B > ♀
Pancaldi > 1988 > Pancaldi & B > ♂
Pancaldi > 1989 > Pancaldi > ♂
Pantheon Roma > 2013 > Donna Margherita > ♀
Pantheon Roma > 2013 > Il Giardino > ♂
Pantheon Roma > 2013 > Notte d'Amore > ♂
Pantheon Roma > 2013 > Raffaello > ♂
Pantheon Roma > 2015 > Trastevere > ♂
Pantheon Roma > 2016 > Dolce Passione > ♀
Pantheon Roma > 2017 > Così Blu > ♀
Pantheon Roma > 2018 > Annone > ♀
Pantheon Roma > 2019 > Harrod's Exclusive: Sempre Mio > ♀
Paolo Gigli Firenze > 2008 > Grecale > ♀
Paolo Gigli Firenze > 2008 > Libeccio > ♀
Paolo Gigli Firenze > 2008 > Maestrale > ♀

Paolo Gigli Firenze > 2008 > Scirocco > ♀
Paolo Gigli Firenze > 2008 > Niagara > ♀
Paolo Gigli Firenze > 2009 > Acqua > ♀
Paolo Gigli Firenze > 2009 > Aria > ♀
Paolo Gigli Firenze > 2009 > Excentrique pour Femme > ♀
Paolo Gigli Firenze > 2009 > Excentrique pour Homme > ♂
Paolo Gigli Firenze > 2009 > Fuoco > ♀
Paolo Gigli Firenze > 2009 > Terra > ♀
Paolo Gigli Firenze > 2010 > Alhambra > ♂
Paolo Gigli Firenze > 2010 > Bahamas > ♀
Paolo Gigli Firenze > 2010 > Barbados > ♀
Paolo Gigli Firenze > 2010 > Jamaica > ♀
Paolo Gigli Firenze > 2010 > Martinique > ♀
Paolo Gigli Firenze > 2010 > Rubino > ♀
Paolo Gigli Firenze > 2010 > Sardegna > ♀
Paolo Gigli Firenze > 2010 > Sicilia > ♀
Paolo Gigli Firenze > 2010 > Smeraldo > ♀
Paolo Gigli Firenze > 2010 > Topazio > ♀
Paolo Gigli Firenze > 2010 > Toscana > ♀
Paolo Gigli Firenze > 2010 > Zaffiro > ♀
Paolo Gigli Firenze > 2012 > Final Touch for Man > ♂
Paolo Gigli Firenze > 2012 > Final Touch for Woman > ♀
Paolo Gigli Firenze > 2012 > Sunrise > ♀
Paolo Gigli Firenze > 2012 > Sunset > ♀
Paolo Gigli Firenze > 2013 > Oro Rosso > ♂
Paolo Gigli Firenze > 2016 > Desiderio > ♂
Paolo Gigli Firenze > 2016 > Desiderio Extract > ♂
Paolo Gigli Firenze > 2016 > Emozione > ♀
Paolo Gigli Firenze > 2016 > Emozione Extract > ♀
Paolo Gigli Firenze > 2016 > Orgoglio > ♂
Paolo Gigli Firenze > 2016 > Orgoglio Extract > ♂
Paolo Gigli Firenze > 2016 > Passione > ♀
Paolo Gigli Firenze > 2016 > Passione Extract > ♀
Paolo Gigli Firenze > 2016 > Morning > ♀
Paolo Gigli Firenze > 2016 > Night > ♀
Paolo Gigli Firenze > 2016 > Più Tardi > ♀
Paolo Gigli Firenze > 2016 > Prima > ♂
Paolo Pecora Milano > 2015 > Bigli > ♂
Paolo Pecora Milano > 2015 > Magenta > ♂
Paolo Pecora Milano > 2015 > Nirone > ♂
Paolo Pecora Milano > 2015 > Senato > ♂
Paolo Pecora Milano > 2019 > Fiori Chiari > ♂
Paolo Pecora Milano > 2019 > Solferino > ♀
Parah > 1996 > Parah > ♀
Parah > 1999 > Essenza di Mediterraneò > ♀
Parah > 1999 > Essenza Di Mediterraneò > ♂
Parah > 2003 > Pur H > ♂
Parah > 2007 > Parah Man > ♂
Parah > 2007 > Parah Woman > ♀
Parah > 2007 > Really Parah > ♀
Parah > 2010 > Black Touch > ♀
Parah > 2010 > Noir > ♀
Parco 1923 > 2016 > Parco 1923 > ♀
Parco 1923 > 2018 > Scarpetta di Venere > ♀
Parfums Bombay 1950 > 2014 > Ambra 304 Tangeri > ♀
Parfums Bombay 1950 > 2014 > Capri > ♂
Parfums Bombay 1950 > 2014 > Panarea > ♀
Parfums Bombay 1950 > 2014 > Ponza > ♀
Patrizia Pepe > 2011 > Patrizia > ♀
Patrizia Pepe > 2011 > Pepe > ♀
Patrizia Pepe > 2015 > In Vogue > ♀
Patrizia Pepe > 2015 > Sophia > ♀
Patrizia Pepe > 2015 > White & Sexy > ♀
Peccato Originale > 2013 > Emulsione Libera > ♀
Peccato Originale > 2013 > Eros > ♂
Peccato Originale > 2013 > Essenza Miracolosa > ♂
Peccato Originale > 2013 > Estratto di Follia > ♂
Peccato Originale > 2013 > Iniezione di Morfina > ♀
Peccato Originale > 2014 > Antidoto Reattivo > ♂
Peccato Originale > 2014 > Cantaride > ♀
Peccato Originale > 2014 > Tintura Spiritosa > ♂
Peccato Originale > 2017 > Gas Antisociale > ♂
Peccato Originale > 2018 > Polvere di Etere > ♂
Perlier > 2000 > Caribbean Original Vanilla > ♀
Perlier > 2000 > Nature's One Fresia > ♀
Perlier > 2002 > Caribbean Vanilla & Coffee > ♀
Perlier > 2002 > Caribbean Vanilla & Green Apple > ♀
Perlier > 2002 > Caribbean Vanilla & Orange > ♀
Perlier > 2002 > Caribbean Vanilla Lime > ♀
Perlier > 2002 > Caribbean Vanilla Mango > ♀
Perlier > 2002 > Vanilla Strawberry > ♀
Perlier > 2010 > Bouquet de Coquelicots > ♀

Perlier > 2010 > Bouquet de Gardenia > ♀
Perlier > 2010 > Bouquet de Violettes > ♀
Perlier > 2010 > Bucaneve delle Alpi > ♀
Perlier > 2012 > L'Iris > ♀
Perlier > 2012 > La Calla > ♀
Perlier > 2012 > La Rosa > ♀
Perlier > 2012 > Peonia Rosa di Luoyang > ♀
Perlier > 2013 > Ginepro della Corsica > ♂
Perlier > 2013 > Vetiver di Java > ♂
Perlier > 2014 > Angelic Snowdrop > ♀
Perlier > 2014 > Ricette Mediterranee Bois de Grece > ♀
Perlier > 2014 > Ricette Mediterranee Brise de Capri > ♀
Perlier > 2014 > Ricette Mediterranée Petales de Rhodes > ♀
Perlier > 2015 > White Honey > ♀
Pineider > 2011 > Cuoio Nobile > ♂
Pineider > 2012 > Assoluta di Neroli e Gelsomino > ♀
Pineider > 2012 > Bianco di Bulgaria > ♂
Pineider > 2012 > Classica di Magnolia > ♀
Pineider > 2012 > Colonia Ambrata > ♂
Pineider > 2012 > Estratto di Colonia > ♂
Pineider > 2014 > Orchidea Reale > ♀
Pineider > 2014 > Oud Assoluto > ♂
Pineider > 2016 > Luxury Collection: Giglio di Firenze > ♀
Pineider > 2018 > Luxury Collection: Nero Incenso > ♂
Pininfarina > 2015 > Lumina > ♀
Pininfarina > 2015 > Segno > ♀
Pininfarina > 2015 > Segno > ♀
Pininfarina > 2017 > Acqua Lunare > ♂
Pino Silvestre > 1992 > Ice Water > ♂
Pino Silvestre > 1998 > Green Generation > ♂
Pino Silvestre > 1998 > Green Generation Her > ♀
Pino Silvestre > 1998 > Green Generation Him > ♂
Pino Silvestre > 1998 > Pino Silvestre Extreme > ♂
Pino Silvestre > 2005 > Pino Fifty > ♂
Pino Silvestre > 2008 > Pino Silvestre Sport Cologne > ♂
Pino Silvestre > 2010 > Pine Gems Essence > ♂
Pino Silvestre > 2010 > Mediterraneo > ♂
Pino Silvestre > 2010 > Muschi di Bosco > ♂
Pino Silvestre > 2014 > Oud Absolute > ♂
Pino Silvestre > 2014 > Rainforest > ♂
Pino Silvestre > 2014 > Underwood > ♂
Pino Silvestre > 2018 > Black Musk > ♂
Pino Silvestre > 2018 > Deep Charisma > ♂
Pino Silvestre > 2018 > Modern Dandy > ♂
Pino Silvestre > 2018 > Perfect Gentleman > ♂
Pino Silvestre > 2000 > Pino Blue > ♂
Pino Silvestre > 2000 > Soffio di Talco > ♂
Pnina Tornai > 2013 > Pnina Tornai > ♀
Police > 1998 > Police Original > ♂
Police > 2001 > Interactive pour Femme > ♀
Police > 2001 > Interactive pour Homme > ♂
Police > 2002 > Dark Men > ♂
Police > 2003 > Naked pour Femme > ♀
Police > 2003 > Naked pour Homme > ♂
Police > 2004 > Contemporary > ♂
Police > 2004 > Cosmopolitan > ♂
Police > 2004 > Eyes Feminine > ♀
Police > 2004 > Uomo Police > ♂
Police > 2005 > Eyes for You > ♀
Police > 2006 > B-Cool > ♂
Police > 2006 > Silver Wings > ♂
Police > 2006 > Wings Femme > ♀
Police > 2007 > Police Caribbean > ♀
Police > 2008 > Freedom > ♂
Police > 2008 > Pure Man > ♂
Police > 2008 > Pure Woman > ♀
Police > 2008 > Wings pour Homme > ♂
Police > 2009 > Pure Dna Femme > ♀
Police > 2009 > Pure Dna Homme > ♂
Police > 2009 > Pure London Femme > ♀
Police > 2009 > Pure London Homme > ♂
Police > 2010 > Frozen > ♂
Police > 2010 > Gold Wings > ♂
Police > 2010 > Instinct > ♂
Police > 2010 > Passion > ♂
Police > 2010 > Passion > ♂
Police > 2010 > Royal Black > ♂
Police > 2010 > Glamorous pour Femme > ♀
Police > 2010 > Glamorous pour Homme > ♂
Police > 2011 > Dark Women > ♀
Police > 2011 > Pure New York Man > ♂
Police > 2011 > Pure New York Woman > ♀

Police > 2011 > Titanium Wings > ♂
Police > 2011 > To Be > ♂
Police > 2012 > The Illusionist > ♂
Police > 2012 > To Be Woman > ♀
Police > 2013 > Sunscent > ♀
Police > 2013 > To Be The King > ♂
Police > 2013 > To Be The Queen > ♀
Police > 2014 > Icon > ♂
Police > 2014 > The Sinner > ♂
Police > 2014 > The Sinner for Women > ♀
Police > 2015 > Daydream > ♀
Police > 2015 > Exotic > ♀
Police > 2015 > Icon Intense > ♂
Police > 2015 > Imperial Patchouli > ♂
Police > 2015 > To Be Camouflage > ♂
Police > 2015 > Wings Blue > ♂
Police > 2016 > Icon Gold > ♂
Police > 2016 > Patchouli > ♀
Police > 2016 > The Sinner Forbidden > ♀
Police > 2016 > The Sinner Forbidden > ♂
Police > 2016 > To Be Rebel > ♂
Police > 2016 > To Be Rose Blossom > ♀
Police > 2017 > Police Legend for Man > ♂
Police > 2017 > Police Legend for Woman > ♀
Police > 2017 > To Be Camouflage Pink > ♀
Police > 2017 > To Be Miss Beat > ♀
Police > 2017 > To Be Mr. Beat > ♂
Police > 2017 > To Be Tattooart > ♀
Police > 2017 > To Be Tattooart > ♂
Police > 2019 > Icon Platinum > ♂
Police > 2019 > Shock-in-Scent for Men > ♂
Police > 2019 > Shock-in-Scent for Women > ♀
Police > 2019 > To Be Exotic Jungle for Man > ♂
Police > 2019 > To Be Exotic Jungle for Woman > ♀
Pomellato > 1989 > Pomellato Donna > ♀
Pomellato > 1990 > Pomellato Uomo > ♂
Pomellato > 1995 > Pomellato II > ♀
Pomellato > 2013 > Nudo Amber > ♀
Pomellato > 2013 > Nudo Blue > ♀
Pomellato > 2013 > Nudo Rose > ♀
Pomellato > 2014 > 67 Artemisia > ♀
Pomellato > 2014 > Nudo Amber Intense > ♀
Pomellato > 2014 > Nudo Blue Intense > ♀
Pomellato > 2014 > Nudo Rose Intense > ♀
Porsche Design > 2008 > The Essence > ♂
Porsche Design > 2009 > The Essence Intense > ♂
Porsche Design > 2010 > The Essence Summer Ice > ♂
Porsche Design > 2012 > Porsche Design Sport > ♂
Porsche Design > 2012 > Porsche Titan > ♂
Porsche Design > 2013 > Porsche Design Sport L'eau > ♂
Porsche Design > 2015 > Palladium > ♂
Porsche Design > 2018 > Porsche Design 180 > ♂
Porsche Design > 2019 > Porsche Woman > ♀
Porsche Design > 2019 > Porsche Woman Black > ♀
Prada > 1990 > Prada > ♀
Prada > 2003 > Prada Exclusives: N. 1 Iris > ♀
Prada > 2003 > Prada Exclusives: N. 2 Oeillet > ♀
Prada > 2003 > Prada Exclusives: N. 3 Cuir Amber > ♀
Prada > 2003 > Prada Exclusives: N. 4 Fleurs d'Oranger > ♀
Prada > 2004 > Prada (Amber) > ♀
Prada > 2005 > Prada Intense > ♀
Prada > 2006 > Prada Amber pour Homme > ♂
Prada > 2007 > Prada Exclusives: N. 5 Narciso > ♀
Prada > 2007 > Prada Exclusives: N. 6 Tubereuse > ♀
Prada > 2007 > Prada Exclusives: N. 7 Violette > ♀
Prada > 2007/2015 > Infusion d'Iris > ♀
Prada > 2008 > Infusion d'homme > ♂
Prada > 2008 > Prada Exclusives: N. 8 Opoponax > ♀
Prada > 2008 > Prada Exclusives: N. 9 Benjoin > ♀
Prada > 2008 > Prada Exclusives: N. 10 Myrrhe > ♀
Prada > 2009 > L'Eau Ambrée > ♀
Prada > 2009/2015 > Infusion de Fleur d'Oranger > ♀
Prada > 2010 > Infusion d'Iris Edt > ♀
Prada > 2010 > Infusion de Tubereuse > ♀
Prada > 2010/2015 > Infusion de Vetiver > ♂
Prada > 2011 > Prada Amber pour Homme Intense > ♂
Prada > 2011 > Prada Candy > ♀
Prada > 2011 > Prada Exclusives: N. 11 Cuir Styrax > ♀
Prada > 2011/2017 > Infusion de Rose > ♀
Prada > 2012 > Infusion d'Iris edp Absolue > ♀
Prada > 2012 > Luna Rossa > ♂
Prada > 2012 > Prada Exclusives: N. 14 Rossetto > ♀

Pupa > 1998 > Violet Glycine > ♀
Pupa > 2000 > Eau Active Minerale > ♂
Pupa > 2000 > Eau Active Thermale > ♂
Pupa > 2003 > Jailia > ♀
Pupa > 2007 > Yes Gold > ♀
Pupa > 2008 > Plumes > ♀
Pupa > 2008 > Puposhka Gold > ♀
Pupa > 2008 > Very Flower Fiore Tahiti > ♀
Pupa > 2008 > Very Flower Iris > ♀
Pupa > 2008 > Very Flower Orchidea > ♀
Pupa > 2008 > Very Flower Rosa > ♀
Pupa > 2009 > Yes Silver > ♀
Pupa > 2010 > In Case of Love > ♀
Pupa > 2011 > Air de Fio N. 1 > ♀
Pupa > 2011 > Air de Fio N. 2 > ♀
Pupa > 2011 > Air de Fio N. 3 > ♀
Pupa > 2011 > Air de Fio N. 4 > ♀
Pupa > 2011 > Air de Fio N. 5 > ♀
Pupa > 2011 > Air de Fio N. 6 > ♀
Pupa > 2011 > Air de Fio Passion Pois > ♀
Pupa > 2012 > Puposhka > ♀
Pupa > 2013 > I'm Fio Acid Green > ♀
Pupa > 2013 > I'm Fio Cloudy Violet > ♀
Pupa > 2013 > I'm Fio Deep Coral > ♀
Pupa > 2013 > I'm Fio Emerald Dream > ♀
Pupa > 2013 > I'm Fio Glam Fuchsia > ♀
Pupa > 2013 > I'm Fio Watermarin > ♀
Pupa > 2014 > Miss Princess – Tè Verde > ♀
Pupa > 2014 > Miss Princess – Confetti di Zucchero > ♀
Pupa > 2014 > Miss Princess – Gelsomino > ♀
Pupa > 2014 > Miss Princess – Petali di Rosa > ♀
Pupa > 2014 > Miss Princess – Tè Bianco > ♀
Pupa > 2014 > Miss Princess – Vaniglia > ♀
Pupa > 2015 > I'm > ♀
Pupa > 2019 > Red Queen Amber Treasure > ♀
Pupa > 2019 > Red Queen Citrusy Blossom > ♀
Pupa > 2019 > Red Queen Extravagant Chypre > ♀
Pupa > 2019 > Red Queen Fresh Aldehydes > ♀
Pupa > 2019 > Red Queen Rich Flowery > ♀
Pupa > 2019 > Red Queen Sophisticated Fruity > ♀
Pure Gold Perfumes > 2016 > African Gold > ♀
Pure Gold Perfumes > 2016 > American Gold > ♂
Pure Gold Perfumes > 2016 > Australian Gold > ♀
Pure Gold Perfumes > 2016 > Mexican Gold > ♀
Pure Gold Perfumes > 2016 > Russian Gold > ♂
Pure Gold Perfumes > 2016 > Suisse Gold > ♂
Rajani > 2018 > Ashanti > ♀
Rajani > 2018 > Goa > ♂
Rajani > 2018 > Narjis > ♀
Rajani > 2018 > Oltrenero > ♂
Rajani > 2019 > Morocco > ♂
Rajani > 2019 > O-Fu-Jing > ♂
Regina Schrecker > 1987 > Regina Schrecker > ♀
Renato Balestra > 1978 > Balestra > ♀
Renato Balestra > 1991/2006 > Renato Balestra Classic pour Femme > ♀
Renato Balestra > 1991/2006 > Renato Balestra Classic pour Homme > ♂
Renato Balestra > 1997 > Argento pour Homme > ♂
Renato Balestra > 1997 > Oro > ♀
Renato Balestra > 2001 > Via Sistina 67 Femme > ♀
Renato Balestra > 2001 > Via Sistina 67 Homme > ♂
Renato Balestra > 2007 > Diamante > ♀
Renato Balestra > 2009 > Diamante Nero > ♀
Renato Balestra > 2011 > Diamante Nero Homme > ♂
Renato Balestra > 2012 > Colonia Sport > ♂
Renato Balestra > 2012 > Essenza Divina > ♀
Renato Balestra > 2012 > Fiori di Essenza Divina > ♀
Renato Balestra > 2013 > Colonia Chic > ♀
Renato Balestra > 2013 > Colonia Cuoio > ♂
Renato Balestra > 2015 > Caesar > ♂
Replay Fragrances > 2008 > Replay for Her > ♀
Replay Fragrances > 2008 > Replay for Him > ♂
Replay Fragrances > 2009 > Replay Intense for Her > ♀
Replay Fragrances > 2009 > Replay Intense for Him > ♂
Replay Fragrances > 2009 > Replay your Fragrance! For Her > ♀
Replay Fragrances > 2009 > Replay your Fragrance! For Him > ♂
Replay Fragrances > 2010 > Replay your Fragrance! For Her > ♀
Replay Fragrances > 2010 > Replay your Fragrance! Refresh for Her > ♀
Replay Fragrances > 2011 > Jeans Spirit! For Her > ♀
Replay Fragrances > 2011 > Jeans Spirit! For Him > ♂
Replay Fragrances > 2012 > Replay Jeans Original for Her > ♀
Replay Fragrances > 2012 > Replay Jeans Oroginal for Him > ♂
Replay Fragrances > 2014 > Essential for Her > ♀

Replay Fragrances > 2014 > Essential for Him > ♂
Replay Fragrances > 2014 > Relover > ♂
Replay Fragrances > 2015 > Stone for Her > ♀
Replay Fragrances > 2015 > Stone for Him > ♂
Replay Fragrances > 2015 > True Replay for Her > ♀
Replay Fragrances > 2015 > True Replay for Him > ♂
Replay Fragrances > 2016 > Stone Supernova for Her > ♀
Replay Fragrances > 2016 > Stone Supernova for Him > ♂
Replay Fragrances > 2017 > #Tank for Her > ♀
Replay Fragrances > 2017 > #Tank for Him > ♂
Replay Fragrances > 2017 > Replay Signature for Men > ♂
Replay Fragrances > 2017 > Replay Signature for Women > ♀
Replay Fragrances > 2018 > #Tank for Her > ♀
Replay Fragrances > 2018 > #Tank for Him > ♂
Replay Fragrances > 2018 > Replay Signature Red Dragon > ♂
Replay Fragrances > 2018 > Replay Signature Secret > ♀
Replay Fragrances > 2019 > #Tank Custom for Her > ♀
Replay Fragrances > 2019 > #Tank Custom for Him > ♂
Replay Fragrances > 2019 > Replay Signature Re-Verse for Her > ♀
Replay Fragrances > 2019 > Replay Signature Re-Verse for Him > ♂
Re Profumo Venezia > 2014 > Adone > ♂
Re Profumo Venezia > 2014 > Alexandros > ♂
Re Profumo Venezia > 2014 > Ekstasis > ♂
Re Profumo Venezia > 2014 > Sogno Damore > ♂
Re Profumo Venezia > 2014 > Superuomo > ♂
Re Profumo Venezia > 2015 > Meraviglia > ♂
Re Profumo Venezia > 2016 > Aqva Meravigliosa > ♂
Re Profumo Venezia > 2016 > Aqva Narcotica > ♂
Re Profumo Venezia > 2016 > Aqva Passionale > ♂
Rhizome > 2019 > Rhizome 01 > ♂
Rhizome > 2019 > Rhizome 02 > ♂
Rhizome > 2019 > Rhizome 03 > ♂
Rhizome > 2019 > Rhizome 04 > ♂
Rhizome > 2019 > Rhizome 05 > ♂
Rick Owens > 2017 > Lamyland > ♂
Riva > 2007 > L'altra Follia di Aquarama Light > ♀
Riva > 2007 > Rivarama > ♀
Riva > 2008 > Follia di Aquarama > ♂
Riva > 2008 > L'altra Follia > ♀
Roberta di Camerino > 1993 > L'uomo R > ♂
Roberta di Camerino > 1995 > Donna R > ♀
Roberta di Camerino > 1995 > Protagonista pour Femme > ♀
Roberta di Camerino > 1995 > Protagonista pour Homme > ♂
Roberta di Camerino > 1998 > Roberta > ♀
Roberta di Camerino > 1998 > Roberta di Camerino pour Homme > ♂
Roberta di Camerino > 2002 > Roberta di Camerino pour Femme > ♀
Roberta Girl > 2017 > Candy Girl > ♀
Roberta Girl > 2017 > Chili Pepper Girl > ♀
Roberta Girl > 2017 > Funny Girl > ♀
Roberta Girl > 2017 > Happy Girl > ♀
Roberta Girl > 2017 > Naughty Girl > ♀
Roberta Girl > 2017 > Solar Girl > ♀
Roberto Capucci > 1974 > Yendi > ♀
Roberto Capucci > 1979 > Punjab > ♂
Roberto Capucci > 1980 > Corps Fou > ♂
Roberto Capucci > 1980 > L'atelier de Capucci pour Elle > ♀
Roberto Capucci > 1980 > L'atelier de Capucci pour Lui > ♂
Roberto Capucci > 1983 > Filly > ♀
Roberto Capucci > 1985 > R de Capucci > ♂
Roberto Capucci > 1987 > Capucci de Capucci > ♀
Roberto Capucci > 1996 > Ballade à Venise > ♀
Roberto Capucci > 1999 > Opera III > ♂
Roberto Capucci > 2000 > Opera IV > ♂
Roberto Capucci > 2000 > Capucci N. 3 pour Femme > ♀
Roberto Capucci > 2006 > Nuance > ♀
Roberto Capucci > 2006 > Nuance > ♂
Roberto Capucci > 2015 > Roberto Capucci Her > ♀
Roberto Capucci > 2015 > Roberto Capucci Him > ♂
Roberto Capucci > 2016 > L'Homme Suave > ♂
Roberto Cavalli > 2002 > Roberto Cavalli > ♀
Roberto Cavalli > 2003 > Roberto Cavalli Man > ♂
Roberto Cavalli > 2004 > Just Cavalli Her > ♀
Roberto Cavalli > 2004 > Just Cavalli Him > ♂
Roberto Cavalli > 2004 > Roberto Cavalli Oro > ♀
Roberto Cavalli > 2005 > Serpentine > ♀
Roberto Cavalli > 2006 > Just Cavalli Blue > ♂
Roberto Cavalli > 2006 > Just Cavalli Pink > ♀
Roberto Cavalli > 2006 > Roberto Cavalli Black > ♂
Roberto Cavalli > 2008 > Serpentine Silver > ♀
Roberto Cavalli > 2010 > Anniversary > ♀
Roberto Cavalli > 2010 > Just Cavalli I Love Her > ♀
Roberto Cavalli > 2010 > Just Cavalli I Love Him > ♂

Roberto Cavalli > 2012 > Roberto Cavalli Edp > ♀
Roberto Cavalli > 2013 > Just Cavalli – Just > ♂
Roberto Cavalli > 2013 > Just Cavalli- Just > ♂
Roberto Cavalli > 2013 > Roberto Cavalli Acqua > ♀
Roberto Cavalli > 2013 > Roberto Cavalli Nero Assoluto > ♀
Roberto Cavalli > 2013 > Roberto Cavalli Oud Edition > ♀
Roberto Cavalli > 2013 > Roberto Cavalli Tiger Oud > ♂
Roberto Cavalli > 2014 > Just Cavalli – Gold for Her > ♀
Roberto Cavalli > 2014 > Just Cavalli – Gold for Him > ♂
Roberto Cavalli > 2014 > Oud Al Qasr > ♀
Roberto Cavalli > 2014 > Roberto Cavalli Exotica > ♀
Roberto Cavalli > 2014 > Roberto Cavalli Gold Edition > ♀
Roberto Cavalli > 2014 > Roberto Cavalli Nero Assoluto Exclusive Edition > ♀
Roberto Cavalli > 2015 > Paradiso > ♀
Roberto Cavalli > 2015 > Paradiso Assoluto > ♀
Roberto Cavalli > 2015 > Roberto Cavalli Essenza > ♀
Roberto Cavalli > 2016 > Baroque Musk > ♀
Roberto Cavalli > 2016 > Divine Oud > ♂
Roberto Cavalli > 2016 > Golden Amber > ♀
Roberto Cavalli > 2016 > Paradiso Azzurro > ♀
Roberto Cavalli > 2016 > Roberto Cavalli Uomo > ♂
Roberto Cavalli > 2016 > Royal Iris > ♀
Roberto Cavalli > 2016 > Sumptuous Rose > ♀
Roberto Cavalli > 2016 > Supreme Sandal > ♂
Roberto Cavalli > 2017 > Florence > ♀
Roberto Cavalli > 2017 > Roberto Cavalli La Notte Uomo Silver Essence > ♂
Roberto Cavalli > 2018 > Gemma di Paradiso > ♀
Roberto Cavalli > 2018 > Imperial Hyacinth > ♀
Roberto Cavalli > 2018 > Precious Leather > ♂
Roberto Cavalli > 2018 > Roberto Cavalli La Notte > ♀
Roberto Cavalli > 2018 > Roberto Cavalli Uomo La Notte > ♂
Roberto Cavalli > 2019 > Florence Amber > ♀
Roberto Cavalli > 2019 > Florence Blossom > ♀
Roberto Cavalli > 2019 > Roberto Cavalli Deep Desire > ♀
Roberto Cavalli > 2019 > Roberto Cavalli Uomo Deep Desire > ♂
Roberto Cavalli > 2019 > Splendid Vanilla > ♀
Roberto Dario Esperienze Olfattive > 2011 > A Come > ♂
Roberto Dario Esperienze Olfattive > 2011 > Attimi > ♀
Roberto Dario Esperienze Olfattive > 2011 > Lavanda d'Oriente > ♂
Roberto Dario Esperienze Olfattive > 2011 > Lavanda Fizz > ♂
Roberto Dario Esperienze Olfattive > 2011 > Spicy Lavender > ♂
Roberto Dario Esperienze Olfattive > 2012 > Dolce Desiderio > ♀
Roberto Dario Esperienze Olfattive > 2014 > Living Lavender > ♂
Roberto Ugolini > 2019 > Blue Suede Shoes > ♂
Roberto Ugolini > 2019 > High Heel White > ♀
Roberto Ugolini > 2019 > Kitten Heel > ♀
Roberto Ugolini > 2019 > Loafer > ♂
Roberto Ugolini > 2019 > Oxford > ♂
Roberto Ugolini > 2019 > Rosso 17 > ♂
Roca Perfums > 2011 > Nuvol de Llimona > ♀
Roccobarocco > 1986 > Uno > ♀
Roccobarocco > 1987 > Roccobarocco (Rinominato Roccobarocco Uno) > ♀
Roccobarocco > 1989 > Eau de Toilette pour Homme > ♂
Roccobarocco > 1991 > Tre > ♀
Roccobarocco > 1993 > Joint pour Femme > ♀
Roccobarocco > 1993 > Joint pour Homme > ♂
Roccobarocco > 1993 > Vetiver > ♂
Roccobarocco > 1995 > Silver Jeans > ♀
Roccobarocco > 1995 > Silver Jeans Men > ♂
Roccobarocco > 1996 > Black Jeans Homme > ♂
Roccobarocco > 1997 > Gold Jeans > ♂
Roccobarocco > 1997 > Gold Jeans Cologne > ♂
Roccobarocco > 1998 > Black Jeans Femme > ♀
Roccobarocco > 1998 > Piazza di Spagna Uomo > ♂
Roccobarocco > 2000 > Extraordinary > ♀
Roccobarocco > 2000 > Extraordinary for Men > ♂
Roccobarocco > 2000 > Jeans pour Femme > ♀
Roccobarocco > 2000 > Jeans pour Homme > ♂
Roccobarocco > 2000 > Souvenir d'Italie > ♀
Roccobarocco > 2001 > Mouse > ♀
Roccobarocco > 2001 > Mouse Cologne > ♂
Roccobarocco > 2001 > Tre Tendre > ♀
Roccobarocco > 2009 > Fashion Man > ♂
Roccobarocco > 2009 > Fashion Woman > ♀
Roccobarocco > 2012 > Roccobarocco Black for Women > ♀
Roccobarocco > 2014 > Jardin de Capri Lilac > ♀
Roccobarocco > 2014 > Jardin de Capri Rose > ♀
Roccobarocco > 2014 > Jardin de Capri Violet > ♀
Roccobarocco > 2014 > Rocco White for Men > ♂
Roccobarocco > 2014 > Roccobarocco White for Women > ♀

Roccobarocco > 2015 > Rubino > ♀
Roccobarocco > 2015 > Scirocco > ♂
Roccobarocco > 2017 > Oriental Collection: Halima > ♂
Roccobarocco > 2017 > Oriental Collection: Haroa > ♂
Roccobarocco > 2017 > Oriental Collection: Jamila > ♀
Roccobarocco > 2017 > Oriental Collection: Malai > ♂
Roccobarocco > 2017 > Oriental Collection: Nadira > ♂
Roccobarocco > 2018 > Gold Queen > ♀
Roccobarocco > 2018 > My Sir > ♂
Rocco Ragni > 2017 > Cashmere Cedar > ♂
Rocco Ragni > 2017 > Cashmere Orchid > ♀
Rocco Ragni > 2017 > Cashmere Sandalwood > ♂
Rocco Ragni > 2017 > Cashmere Tuberose > ♀
Rockford > 1990 > Blurock > ♂
Rockford > 2015 > Wildwhite > ♂
Romeo Gigli > 1989 > Romeo > ♀
Romeo Gigli > 1990 > Romeo Eau Fraiche > ♀
Romeo Gigli > 1991 > Romeo Gigli for Man > ♂
Romeo Gigli > 1991 > Romeo Gigli per Uomo > ♂
Romeo Gigli > 1994 > G Gigli > ♀
Romeo Gigli > 1995 > Sud Est > ♂
Romeo Gigli > 1999 > Di Romeo Gigli > ♀
Romeo Gigli > 1999 > Di Romeo Gigli Uomo > ♂
Romeo Gigli > 2000 > Laki Edp > ♀
Romeo Gigli > 2000 > Laki Edt > ♂
Romeo Gigli > 2003 > Romeo Gigli > ♀
Romeo Gigli > 2004 > Romeo Gigli Man > ♂
Romeo Gigli > 2012 > Romeo Gigli Women > ♀
Romeo Gigli > 2014 > Celebration Man > ♂
Romeo Gigli > 2014 > Celebration Woman > ♀
Roveri & Aura > 1989 > Valentina di Guido Crepax > ♀
Roveri & Aura > 1989 > Valentina di Guido Crepax Uomo > ♂
Royal Cosmetic > 2015 > Ego > ♂
Royal Cosmetic > 2015 > Energy > ♂
Royal Cosmetic > 2015 > Exclusive West > ♂
Royal Cosmetic > 2015 > Extreme > ♂
Royal Cosmetic > 2015 > Hilton > ♂
Royal Cosmetic > 2015 > Platinum Air > ♂
Royal Cosmetic > 2015 > Platinum Bordo > ♂
Royal Cosmetic > 2015 > Platinum Crystal > ♂
Royal Cosmetic > 2015 > Platinum E.g. > ♂
Royal Cosmetic > 2015 > Platinum Gold > ♂
Royal Cosmetic > 2015 > Platinum Noir > ♂
Royal Cosmetic > 2015 > Polar > ♂
Royal Cosmetic > 2015 > Safari > ♂
Royal Cosmetic > 2015 > Superman > ♂
Royal Cosmetic > 2015 > Superman The Best > ♂
Royal Cosmetic > 2015 > Voyager > ♂
Royal Cosmetic > 2015 > Wall Street > ♂
Royal Cosmetic > 2015 > Yachting > ♂
Royal Crown > 2011 > Celebration > ♀
Royal Crown > 2011 > Musk Ubar > ♂
Royal Crown > 2011 > Noor > ♀
Royal Crown > 2011 > Poudre de Fleurs > ♀
Royal Crown > 2011 > Rain > ♂
Royal Crown > 2011 > Tabac Royal > ♂
Royal Crown > 2011 > Tenebra > ♀
Royal Crown > 2012 > Al Kimya > ♂
Royal Crown > 2012 > Les Petits Coquins > ♀
Royal Crown > 2012 > My Oud > ♂
Royal Crown > 2014 > Habanos > ♂
Royal Crown > 2014 > Ytzma > ♂
Royal Crown > 2015 > Black Bay: Adventure > ♂
Royal Crown > 2015 > Black Bay: Capture > ♂
Royal Crown > 2015 > Black Bay: Flying Dutch > ♂
Royal Crown > 2015 > Reflextion > ♂
Royal Crown > 2016 > Absolute > ♂
Royal Crown > 2016 > Ambrosia > ♂
Royal Crown > 2016 > Flair > ♀
Royal Crown > 2016 > Oud Collection: Oud Al Melka > ♀
Royal Crown > 2016 > Oud Collection: Oud Jasmine > ♀
Royal Crown > 2016 > Oud Collection: Oud Santal > ♂
Royal Crown > 2016 > Rose Masquat > ♀
Royal Crown > 2016 > Upper Class > ♂
Royal Crown > 2017 > Aurum Collection: Azhar > ♂
Royal Crown > 2017 > Aurum Collection: Azimuth > ♂
Royal Crown > 2017 > Aurum Collection: Chimera > ♂
Royal Crown > 2017 > Aurum Collection: Narkao > ♂
Royal Crown > 2017 > Aurum Collection: Oblivio > ♂
Royal Crown > 2017 > Aurum Collection: Oud Al Ain > ♂
Royal Crown > 2017 > Aurum Collection: So Gold > ♂
Royal Crown > 2018 > Black Bay: Mary Red > ♂

Royal Crown > 2018 > Imperial Collection: Imperator > ♀
Royal Crown > 2018 > Imperial Collection: K'abel > ♀
Royal Crown > 2018 > Imperial Collection: Khan > ♂
Royal Crown > 2018 > Imperial Collection: Sultan > ♂
Royal Crown > 2018 > Imperial Collection: Tzar > ♂
Royal Crown > 2019 > Imperial Collection: Isabella > ♀
Rubeus Milano > 2018 > Rouge > ♂
Rubeus Milano > 2019 > Blue > ♂
Rubeus Milano > 2019 > Vert > ♂
Rubini > 2015 > Fundamental > ♂
Rubini > 2018 > Tambour Sacre > ♂
Rubino Cosmetics > 2009 > Cosmo > ♂
Rubino Cosmetics > 2009 > Providence > ♀
Rubino Cosmetics > 2009 > Room 726 Black > ♀
Rubino Cosmetics > 2009 > Room 726 Red > ♀
Rubino Cosmetics > 2009 > Room 726 White > ♂
Rubino Cosmetics > 2009 > Shock > ♂
Rubino Cosmetics > 2010 > Predateur or Proie > ♂
Rudy Profumi > 2013 > Fior d'Arancio > ♂
Rudy Profumi > 2013 > Ibisco > ♀
Rudy Profumi > 2013 > Lavanda > ♀
Rudy Profumi > 2013 > Magnolia > ♀
Rudy Profumi > 2013 > Peonia > ♀
Rudy Profumi > 2013 > Rosa > ♀
Rudy Profumi > 2015 > Citrus Fruits > ♂
Rudy Profumi > 2015 > Cocoa Strawberry > ♀
Rudy Profumi > 2015 > Coconut Vanilla > ♀
Rudy Profumi > 2015 > Nectarine Peach > ♀
Rudy Profumi > 2015 > Red Apple > ♀
Rudy Profumi > 2015 > Wild Fig > ♀
Rudy Profumi > 2017 > Lavender & Vanilla > ♂
Rudy Profumi > 2017 > Lilly of The Valley & Fern > ♂
Rudy Profumi > 2017 > Orange & Verbena > ♀
Rudy Profumi > 2017 > Orchid & Lavender > ♂
Rudy Profumi > 2017 > Osmanthus Flowers & Honeysuckle > ♀
Rudy Profumi > 2017 > Rose & Figue > ♀
Rudy Profumi > 2017 > Rose & Rhubarb > ♀
Rudy Profumi > 2017 > Tangerine & Ginger > ♂
Rudy Profumi > 2017 > White Tea & Verbena > ♂
S4p > 2012 > Aurisse > ♂
S4p > 2012 > Laawan > ♂
S4p > 2012 > Sharky > ♂
S4p > 2012 > Skiron > ♂
Salvatore Ferragamo > 1960/2019 > Gilio > ♀
Salvatore Ferragamo > 1971 > F de Ferragamo > ♀
Salvatore Ferragamo > 1976 > Monsieur F > ♂
Salvatore Ferragamo > 1976 > Monsieur F de Ferragamo > ♂
Salvatore Ferragamo > 1998 > Salvatore Ferragamo pour Femme > ♀
Salvatore Ferragamo > 1999 > Salvatore Ferragamo pour Homme > ♂
Salvatore Ferragamo > 2002 > Parfum Subtil > ♀
Salvatore Ferragamo > 2003 > Incanto > ♀
Salvatore Ferragamo > 2003 > Incanto pour Homme > ♂
Salvatore Ferragamo > 2003 > Subtil pour Homme > ♂
Salvatore Ferragamo > 2005 > Incanto Dream > ♀
Salvatore Ferragamo > 2006 > F by Ferragamo > ♀
Salvatore Ferragamo > 2006 > Incanto Charms > ♀
Salvatore Ferragamo > 2006 > Incanto Essential pour Homme > ♂
Salvatore Ferragamo > 2007 > F by Ferragamo pour Homme > ♂
Salvatore Ferragamo > 2007 > F for Fascinating > ♀
Salvatore Ferragamo > 2007 > Incanto Heaven > ♀
Salvatore Ferragamo > 2007 > Incanto Shine > ♀
Salvatore Ferragamo > 2008 > Tuscan Soul > ♂
Salvatore Ferragamo > 2009 > F by Ferragamo Black > ♂
Salvatore Ferragamo > 2009 > F for Fascinating Night > ♀
Salvatore Ferragamo > 2009 > Incanto Bliss > ♀
Salvatore Ferragamo > 2010 > Attimo > ♀
Salvatore Ferragamo > 2010 > Incanto Bloom > ♀
Salvatore Ferragamo > 2011 > Attimo L'Eau Florale > ♀
Salvatore Ferragamo > 2011 > Attimo pour Homme > ♂
Salvatore Ferragamo > 2011 > F by Ferragamo Free Time > ♂
Salvatore Ferragamo > 2011 > F for Fascinating Crystal Edition > ♀
Salvatore Ferragamo > 2011 > Signorina > ♀
Salvatore Ferragamo > 2012 > Incanto Lovely Flower > ♀
Salvatore Ferragamo > 2012 > Signorina Edt > ♀
Salvatore Ferragamo > 2013 > Acqua Essenziale > ♂
Salvatore Ferragamo > 2013 > Signorina Limited Edition > ♀
Salvatore Ferragamo > 2013 > Tuscan Soul Bianco di Carrara > ♂
Salvatore Ferragamo > 2013 > Tuscan Soul Convivio > ♂
Salvatore Ferragamo > 2013 > Tuscan Soul Vendemmia > ♂
Salvatore Ferragamo > 2013 > Tuscan Soul Viola Essenziale > ♀
Salvatore Ferragamo > 2014 > Acqua Essenziale Blu > ♂
Salvatore Ferragamo > 2014 > Attimo Black Musk pour Homme > ♂

Salvatore Ferragamo > 2014 > Harrods Salon de Parfum: Signorina Edp > ♀
Salvatore Ferragamo > 2014 > Harrods Salon de Parfum: Signorina Eleganza Limited Edition > ♀
Salvatore Ferragamo > 2014 > Incanto Amity > ♀
Salvatore Ferragamo > 2014 > Incanto Bloom > ♀
Salvatore Ferragamo > 2014 > Signorina Eleganza > ♀
Salvatore Ferragamo > 2014 > Signorina Leather Edition > ♀
Salvatore Ferragamo > 2014 > Tuscan Scent Acacia > ♂
Salvatore Ferragamo > 2014 > Tuscan Scent Incense Suede > ♂
Salvatore Ferragamo > 2014 > Tuscan Scent White Mimosa > ♂
Salvatore Ferragamo > 2014 > Tuscan Soul Punta Ala > ♂
Salvatore Ferragamo > 2014 > Tuscan Soul Terra Rossa > ♂
Salvatore Ferragamo > 2015 > Acqua Essenziale Colonia > ♂
Salvatore Ferragamo > 2015 > Emozione > ♀
Salvatore Ferragamo > 2016 > Emozione Dolce Fiore > ♀
Salvatore Ferragamo > 2016 > Incanto Heaven Gold Petals Edition > ♀
Salvatore Ferragamo > 2016 > Signorina In Rosso > ♀
Salvatore Ferragamo > 2016 > Signorina Misteriosa > ♀
Salvatore Ferragamo > 2016 > Tuscan Scent Leather Rose > ♂
Salvatore Ferragamo > 2016 > Tuscan Soul La Corte > ♀
Salvatore Ferragamo > 2016 > Uomo > ♂
Salvatore Ferragamo > 2017 > Emozione Dolce Fiore Edp > ♀
Salvatore Ferragamo > 2017 > Emozione Rosa Orientale > ♀
Salvatore Ferragamo > 2017 > Signorina in Fiore > ♀
Salvatore Ferragamo > 2017 > Tuscan Soul La Commedia > ♂
Salvatore Ferragamo > 2017 > Uomo Casual Life > ♂
Salvatore Ferragamo > 2018 > Amo Ferragamo > ♀
Salvatore Ferragamo > 2018 > Amo Ferragamo Limited Edition > ♀
Salvatore Ferragamo > 2018 > Signorina in Fiore Fashion Edition > ♀
Salvatore Ferragamo > 2018 > Signorina Limited Edition 2018 > ♀
Salvatore Ferragamo > 2018 > Tuscan Creations Bianco di Carrara > ♂
Salvatore Ferragamo > 2018 > Tuscan Creations Calimala > ♂
Salvatore Ferragamo > 2018 > Tuscan Creations Convivio > ♂
Salvatore Ferragamo > 2018 > Tuscan Creations La Commedia > ♂
Salvatore Ferragamo > 2018 > Tuscan Creations La Corte > ♂
Salvatore Ferragamo > 2018 > Tuscan Creations Punta Ala > ♂
Salvatore Ferragamo > 2018 > Tuscan Creations Rinascimento > ♂
Salvatore Ferragamo > 2018 > Tuscan Creations Rinascimento > ♂
Salvatore Ferragamo > 2018 > Tuscan Creations Terra Rossa > ♂
Salvatore Ferragamo > 2018 > Tuscan Creations Testa di Moro > ♂
Salvatore Ferragamo > 2018 > Tuscan Creations Vendemmia > ♂
Salvatore Ferragamo > 2018 > Tuscan Creations Viola Essenziale > ♂
Salvatore Ferragamo > 2018 > Uomo Limited Edition > ♂
Salvatore Ferragamo > 2018 > Uomo Signature > ♂
Salvatore Ferragamo > 2019 > Amo Ferragamo Flowerful > ♀
Salvatore Ferragamo > 2019 > Amo Ferragamo Holiday Edition 2019 > ♀
Salvatore Ferragamo > 2019 > Signorina Edp Holiday Edition 2019 > ♀
Salvatore Ferragamo > 2019 > Signorina Ribelle > ♀
Salvatore Ferragamo > 2019 > Tuscan Creations Bianco di Carrara Limited Edition 2019 > ♂
Salvatore Ferragamo > 2019 > Tuscan Creations Gentil Suono > ♂
Salvatore Ferragamo > 2019 > Uomo Urban Feel > ♂
Salvatore Ferragamo > 2020 > Ferragamo > ♂
Sandalia > 2017 > Boeli > ♂
Sandalia > 2017 > Coros > ♂
Sandalia > 2017 > Karaly > ♀
Sandalia > 2017 > Lò > ♂
Sandalia > 2017 > Miana > ♂
Sandalia > 2017 > Othoca > ♂
Sandalia > 2019 > Nixias > ♂
Santa Maria Novella > 1996 > Zagara > ♀
Santa Maria Novella > 1997 > Acqua di Sicilia > ♂
Santa Maria Novella > 1997 > Caprifoglio > ♀
Santa Maria Novella > 1998 > Acqua di Cuba > ♂
Santa Maria Novella > 1999 > Calicantus > ♀
Santa Maria Novella > 1999 > Rosa > ♀
Santa Maria Novella > 2001 > Ginestra > ♀
Santa Maria Novella > 2002 > Eva > ♀
Santa Maria Novella > 2002 > Nostalgia > ♂
Santa Maria Novella > 2005 > Città di Kyoto > ♂
Santa Maria Novella > 2006 > Angeli di Firenze > ♂
Santa Maria Novella > 2006 > Gardenia > ♀
Santa Maria Novella > 2007 > Toscano > ♂
Santa Maria Novella > 2008 > Tabacco Toscano > ♂
Santa Maria Novella > 2010 > Ottone > ♂
Santa Maria Novella > 2010 > Porcellana > ♂
Santa Maria Novella > 2012 > Alba di Seoul > ♂
Santa Maria Novella > 2014 > Cala Rossa > ♂
Santa Maria Novella > 2015 > Acqua di Colonia Cinquanta > ♂
Santa Maria Novella > 2017 > Acqua di Colonia Lana > ♂
Sartoria Chiussi 1868 > 2020 > Aqva Robinia > ♂
Scentbar > 2012 > 300 > ♂

Scentbar > 2014 > 400 > ⚥
Scentbar > 2015 > 600 > ⚥
Scentbar > 2016 > 700 > ⚥
Scentbar > 2016 > 100 > ⚥
Scentbar > 2016 > 101 > ⚥
Scentbar > 2016 > 102 > ⚥
Scentbar > 2016 > 103 > ⚥
Scentbar > 2016 > 104 > ⚥
Scentbar > 2016 > 105 > ⚥
Scentbar > 2016 > 106 > ⚥
Scentbar > 2016 > 107 > ⚥
Scentbar > 2016 > 108 > ⚥
Scentbar > 2016 > 109 > ⚥
Scentbar > 2016 > 110 > ⚥
Scentbar > 2016 > 111 > ⚥
Scentbar > 2016 > 200 > ⚥
Scentbar > 2016 > 500 > ⚥
Scentbar > 2017 > 800 > ⚥
Scentbar > 2017 > 900 > ⚥
Scentbar > 2018 > 329 > ⚥
Segreti di Lucca > 2004 > Bohème > ⚥
Segreti di Lucca > 2004 > Elisa > ♀
Segreti di Lucca > 2010 > Carib – Spiriti del Tabacco > ⚥
Segreti di Lucca > 2010 > Luludi – Fiori Nomadi > ♀
Segreti di Lucca > 2011 > Koh-Do > ⚥
Sergio Nero > 2003 > Woman > ♀
Sergio Nero > 2006 > Girl > ♀
Sergio Nero > 2006 > Sergio Nero pour Homme > ♂
Sergio Nero > 2012 > Russian Police Clean Hands > ♂
Sergio Nero > 2012 > Russian Police Cold Head > ♂
Sergio Nero > 2012 > Russian Police Hot Heart > ♂
Sergio Nero > 2014 > Admiral > ♂
Sergio Nero > 2015 > Admiral Andreyevskiy Flag > ♂
Sergio Nero > 2015 > Admiral Pobedonosets > ♂
Sergio Nero > 2015 > Lost Paradise Mystery > ♀
Sergio Nero > 2015 > Lost Paradise Seduction > ♀
Sergio Nero > 2015 > Lost Paradise Serene > ♀
Sergio Nero > 2015 > Russian Present Blue > ♀
Sergio Nero > 2015 > Russian Present Magic > ♀
Sergio Nero > 2015 > Russian Present Red > ♀
Sergio Nero > 2015 > Admiral Patriot > ♂
Sergio Nero > 2015 > Admiral Posledniy Geroy > ♂
Sergio Nero > 2015 > Admiral Russkiy Kharakter > ♂
Sergio Nero > 2015 > Boy Green Apple > ♂
Sergio Nero > 2015 > Boy Orange Coffee > ♂
Sergio Nero > 2015 > Cappuccino > ♀
Sergio Nero > 2015 > Chocolate > ♀
Sergio Nero > 2015 > Coffee > ♀
Sergio Nero > 2015 > Russian Flowers Blossom > ♀
Sergio Nero > 2015 > Russian Flowers Bright > ♀
Sergio Nero > 2016 > My Pearl Divine > ♀
Sergio Nero > 2016 > My Pearl Romantic > ♀
Sergio Nero > 2016 > My Pearl Sensual > ♀
Sergio Nero > 2017 > Fleurs de La Demoiselle d'honneur > ♀
Sergio Nero > 2017 > Fleurs de Mariage > ♀
Sergio Nero > 2017 > Fleurs pour La Belle-Mère > ♀
Sergio Nero > 2017 > Red Moon pour Femme > ♀
Sergio Nero > 2017 > Sputnik > ♂
Sergio Nero > 2018 > Rose Silver Violette > ♀
Sergio Nero > 2019 > Russian Flowers Exciting > ♀
Sergio Scaglietti > 2017 > Racing Green > ♂
Sergio Scaglietti > 2017 > Racing Orange > ♂
Sergio Scaglietti > 2017 > Racing Steel > ♂
Sergio Scaglietti > 2017 > Racing Yellow > ♂
Sergio Soldano > 1985 > Sergio Soldano Black > ♂
Sergio Soldano > 1986 > Sergio Soldano White > ♂
Sergio Soldano > 1988 > Atelier > ♀
Sergio Soldano > 1988 > Atelier Noir > ♀
Sergio Soldano > 1991 > Proibito > ♀
Sergio Soldano > 1991 > Proibito for Men > ♂
Sergio Soldano > 1991 > Sergio Soldano > ♂
Sergio Soldano > 1992 > Via Venti > ♀
Sergio Soldano > 1995 > Via Venti Fresh Lady > ♀
Sergio Soldano > 1995 > Via Venti Luxe Lady > ♀
Sergio Soldano > 2011 > Sergio Soldano de Luxe Men N. 30 > ♂
Sergio Tacchini > 1987 > Sergio Tacchini > ♂
Sergio Tacchini > 1988 > Sergio Tacchini Donna > ♀
Sergio Tacchini > 1993 > Sergio Tacchini Sport Extreme > ♂
Sergio Tacchini > 1996 > Sergio Tacchini Uomo > ♂
Sergio Tacchini > 2000 > O-Zone Woman > ♀
Sergio Tacchini > 2003 > Stile > ♂
Sergio Tacchini > 2004 > Stile Donna > ♀

Sergio Tacchini > 2005 > Active Water > ♂
Sergio Tacchini > 2006 > Feel Good Man > ♂
Sergio Tacchini > 2006 > Feel Good Woman > ♀
Sergio Tacchini > 2007 > Sport Ego > ♂
Sergio Tacchini > 2008 > Be – St > ♀
Sergio Tacchini > 2009 > Experience Discovery > ♂
Sergio Tacchini > 2009 > Experience Sailing > ♂
Sergio Tacchini > 2009 > Precious Pink > ♀
Sergio Tacchini > 2011 > Donna Blooming Flowers > ♀
Sergio Tacchini > 2011 > O-Zone Blue Spirit > ♂
Sergio Tacchini > 2011 > O-Zone Green Wave > ♂
Sergio Tacchini > 2011 > O-Zone Pink Spirit > ♀
Sergio Tacchini > 2011 > O-Zone Pink Wave > ♀
Sergio Tacchini > 2012 > Club > ♂
Sergio Tacchini > 2012 > Precious Purple > ♀
Sergio Tacchini > 2012 > Sergio Tacchini Donna South Beach Essence > ♀
Sergio Tacchini > 2012 > With You > ♀
Sergio Tacchini > 2013 > Always With You > ♀
Sergio Tacchini > 2014 > Fantasy Forever > ♀
Sergio Tacchini > 2014 > Precious White > ♀
Sergio Tacchini > 2014 > Whit Style > ♀
Sergio Tacchini > 2015 > Club Intense > ♂
Sergio Tacchini > 2015 > Fantasy Forever Eau Romantique > ♀
Sergio Tacchini > 2015 > Precious Jade > ♀
Sergio Tacchini > 2016 > Club Edition Monte-Carlo > ♂
Sergio Tacchini > 2017 > Smash > ♂
Sergio Tacchini > 2018 > La Volee > ♀
Sergio Tacchini > 2019 > Club For Her > ♀
Serra & Fonseca > 2014 > Il Narciso > ♀
Serra & Fonseca > 2014 > Il Patchouli > ♂
Serra & Fonseca > 2014 > Il Vetyver > ♂
Serra & Fonseca > 2014 > La Rosa > ♀
Serra & Fonseca > 2014 > La Violetta > ♀
Serra & Fonseca > 2014 > La Zagara > ♀
Serra & Fonseca > 2016 > Eau de Moi > ♀
Sigilli > 2000 > Asprosa > ♀
Sigilli > 2000 > Athunis > ♂
Sigilli > 2000 > Claudiae > ♀
Sigilli > 2000 > Ea > ♀
Sigilli > 2000 > Ferfaen > ♀
Sigilli > 2000 > Hesperia > ♀
Sigilli > 2000 > Thu > ♂
Sigilli > 2000 > Tuscia > ♀
Sigilli > 2000 > Tyrsenoi > ♀
Sigilli > 2000 > Volumna > ♀
Sigilli > 2011 > Electra > ♀
Sigilli > 2011 > Pyrgos > ♂
Sigilli > 2012 > Bayan Mulak > ♂
Sigilli > 2012 > Hymba > ♀
Sigilli > 2013 > Khanbaliq > ♂
Sileno Cheloni Maestro Profumiere Firenze > 2019 > Sangue Blu > ♂
Simone Andreoli > 2011 > Business Man > ♂
Simone Andreoli > 2011 > Camouflage > ♀
Simone Andreoli > 2011 > Deep Island > ♂
Simone Andreoli > 2011 > Sentosa > ♀
Simone Andreoli > 2015 > Silenzio > ♂
Simone Andreoli > 2016 > Eterno > ♂
Simone Andreoli > 2016 > Moorea > ♂
Simone Andreoli > 2017 > Don't Ask me Permission > ♂
Simone Andreoli > 2017 > L'Or du Sillage > ♂
Simone Andreoli > 2018 > Malibu – Party in the Bay > ♂
Simone Andreoli > 2018 > Pacific Park > ♂
Simone Andreoli > 2018 > Smoke of God > ♂
Simone Andreoli > 2019 > Italian Heritage: Fico Nero di Sardegna > ♂
Simone Andreoli > 2019 > Italian Heritage: Mandorla di Noto > ♀
Simone Andreoli > 2019 > Italian Heritage: Zest di Sorrento > ♂
Simone Cosac Profumi > 2008 > Perle di Bianca > ♀
Simone Cosac Profumi > 2010 > Trama > ♀
Simone Cosac Profumi > 2012 > Trama Nera > ♀
Simone Cosac Profumi > 2014 > Bianca > ♀
Simone Cosac Profumi > 2014 > Osè > ♀
Simone Cosac Profumi > 2014 > Peccato > ♀
Simone Cosac Profumi > 2014 > Sublime > ♀
Simone Cosac Profumi > 2016 > Amore Proibito > ♀
Sinfonia di Note > 2000 > Blanc des Cotons > ♀
Sinfonia di Note > 2000 > Bouquet de Bois > ♂
Sinfonia di Note > 2000 > Coeur de Noisette > ♂
Sinfonia di Note > 2000 > Ecorce d'Orange > ♂
Sinfonia di Note > 2000 > Fleur de Santal > ♀
Sinfonia di Note > 2000 > Jardin d'Orient > ♂
Sinfonia di Note > 2000 > Petale Rose > ♀
Sinfonia di Note > 2000 > Poudre d'Épices > ♂

Sinfonia di Note > 2000 > Saveur d'Artichaut > ♀
Sinfonia di Note > 2000 > Toujours Verts > ♀
Sinfonia di Note > 2000 > Amande Sucrée > ♀
Sinfonia di Note > 2012 > Dolce Vaniglia > ♀
Sinfonia di Note > 2015 > Bianco Cotone > ♀
Sinfonia di Note > 2015 > Caldi Legni > ♀
Sinfonia di Note > 2015 > Dea Bianca > ♀
Sinfonia di Note > 2015 > Fiore Narcotico > ♀
Sinfonia di Note > 2015 > La Rotta del Mare > ♀
Sinfonia di Note > 2015 > La Via delle Spezie > ♀
Sinfonia di Note > 2015 > Nuvola Talcata > ♀
Sinfonia di Note > 2015 > Zucchero di Mandorla > ♀
Sinfonia di Note > 2015 > Bateau > ♀
Sinfonia di Note > 2016 > Patchouli > ♀
Sinfonia di Note > 2016 > Pepe & Menta > ♀
Sinfonia di Note > 2017 > Ambra del Cashmere > ♀
Sinfonia di Note > 2017 > Soffio d'Iris > ♀
Sinfonia di Note > 2017 > The Nero > ♀
Sinfonia di Note > 2017 > Vetyver > ♀
Smemoranda > 2016 > Rosa > ♀
Smemoranda > 2016 > Verde > ♂
Sofia Balestra > 2009 > Blue > ♀
Sofia Balestra > 2009 > Green > ♀
Sofia Balestra > 2009 > Pink > ♀
Sofia Balestra > 2011 > Sofia en Bleu > ♀
Sofia Balestra > 2011 > Sofia en Rose > ♀
Sorelle Fontana > 1990 > If for Women > ♀
Sorelle Fontana > 1991 > Micol > ♀
Sorelle Fontana > 2000 > If > ♂
Sorelle Fontana > 2000 > If Jeans > ♂
Sorelle Fontana > 2000 > If Jeans for Women > ♀
Sospiro Perfumes > 2011 > Chapter I Accento > ♀
Sospiro Perfumes > 2011 > Chapter I Allegro > ♀
Sospiro Perfumes > 2011 > Chapter I Capriccio > ♀
Sospiro Perfumes > 2011 > Chapter I Duetto > ♀
Sospiro Perfumes > 2011 > Chapter I Laylati (Afgano Puro) > ♀
Sospiro Perfumes > 2011 > Chapter I Vivace > ♀
Sospiro Perfumes > 2012 > Chapter I Wardasina (Rosso Afgano) > ♀
Sospiro Perfumes > 2013 > Chapter II Adagio > ♀
Sospiro Perfumes > 2013 > Chapter II Andante > ♀
Sospiro Perfumes > 2013 > Chapter II Erba Pura > ♀
Sospiro Perfumes > 2013 > Chapter II Grazioso > ♀
Sospiro Perfumes > 2013 > Chapter II Melodia > ♀
Sospiro Perfumes > 2013 > Chapter II Misterioso > ♀
Sospiro Perfumes > 2014 > Classica > ♀
Sospiro Perfumes > 2014 > Opera > ♀
Sospiro Perfumes > 2014 > Rosso Afgano > ♀
Sospiro Perfumes > 2015 > Sospiro Anniversary > ♀
Sospiro Perfumes > 2015 > Verde Accento > ♀
Sospiro Perfumes > 2016 > Ouverture > ♀
Sospiro Perfumes > 2016 > Purple Accento > ♀
Sospiro Perfumes > 2016 > Rosso Accento > ♀
Sospiro Perfumes > 2016 > Selfridges Exclusive Erba Gold > ♂
Sospiro Perfumes > 2017 > Diapason > ♀
Sospiro Perfumes > 2017 > Ensemble > ♀
Sospiro Perfumes > 2018 > Muse > ♀
Soul Couture > 2017 > Fil Rouge > ♀
Soul Couture > 2017 > Gender Ginger > ♀
Soul Couture > 2017 > Love Twist > ♀
Soul Couture > 2017 > Morphosis > ♀
Soul Couture > 2017 > Votum > ♀
Soul Couture > 2017 > Weekend Postmoderno > ♀
Sprezzatura > 2018 > 707 Dolce Amoretto > ♀
Sprezzatura > 2018 > 721 Ritorno di Fiamma > ♀
Sprezzatura > 2018 > 746 Amore Segreto > ♀
Sprezzatura > 2019 > 730 Amore Sviscerato > ♀
Sprezzatura > 2019 > 732 Cascante D'amore > ♀
Sprezzatura > 2019 > 751 Amori Erranti > ♀
Sprezzatura > 2019 > 768 Ars Amandi > ♀
Ssc Napoli > 2010 > Marek Ssn Napoli > ♂
Stefano Ricci > 2016 > Aureum > ♂
Stefano Ricci > 2016 > Classic > ♂
Stefano Ricci > 2016 > Platinum > ♂
Stefano Ricci > 2016 > Royal Eagle Black > ♂
Stefano Ricci > 2016 > Royal Eagle Gold > ♂
Stefano Ricci > 2016 > Royal Eagle Silver > ♂
Stefano Ricci > 2016 > Royal Eagle Sport > ♂
Stefano Ricci > 2017 > Sr Eight >
Stefano Ricci > 2017 > Sr Eight Limited Edition > ♂
Step Aboard > 2008 > Bosco Sospeso > ♀
Step Aboard > 2018 > 3D sul Duomo > ♀
Step Aboard > 2018 > Cuoio di Thaon > ♀

Step Aboard > 2018 > Menta sui Navigli > ♀
Step Aboard > 2018 > Milano Centrale > ♀
Strega del Castello > 1975 > Mistero > ♀
Strega del Castello > 1975 > Talco > ♀
Strega del Castello > 1976 > Muschio > ♂
Strega del Castello > 1977 > Mora e Muschio > ♂
Strega del Castello > 1978 > Habit Noir > ♂
Strega del Castello > 1979 > Colonia di Genova > ♀
Strega del Castello > 1979 > Rosa > ♀
Strega del Castello > 1979 > Violetta > ♀
Strega del Castello > 1980 > Neroli > ♀
Strega del Castello > 1980 > Tuberosa > ♀
Strega del Castello > 1981 > Vetiver > ♂
Strega del Castello > 1983 > Acqua di Genova > ♀
Strega del Castello > 1983 > Sandalo > ♂
Strega del Castello > 1990 > Arancia Cannella > ♀
Strega del Castello > 1996 > Macadam > ♂
Strega del Castello > 2003 > Ambra > ♀
Strega del Castello > 2003 > Vaniglia Bianca > ♀
Strega del Castello > 2005 > Fico > ♀
Strega del Castello > 2006 > Acqua di Panna > ♀
Strega del Castello > 2007 > Black Patchouli > ♀
Strega del Castello > 2007 > Colonia al Sale > ♀
Strega del Castello > 2008 > Acqua di Cotone > ♀
Strega del Castello > 2009 > Acqua di Confetto > ♀
Strega del Castello > 2009 > Confetto > ♀
Strega del Castello > 2010 > Acqua di Tè Verde > ♀
Strega del Castello > 2010 > Acqua di Tiglio > ♀
Strega del Castello > 2010 > Vaniglia e Tabacco > ♀
Strega del Castello > 2013 > Amore e Psiche > ♀
Strega del Castello > 2014 > Agrumi di Sicilia > ♀
Strega del Castello > 2015 > Granato Nero > ♀
Strega del Castello > 2016 > Fico > ♀
Strega del Castello > 2016 > Legno di Cedro > ♀
Strega del Castello > 2017 > Muschi e Pepe > ♀
Strega del Castello > 2018 > Elena Rossini > ♀
Strega del Castello > 2018 > Gemma di Sale > ♀
Strega del Castello > 2018 > Incenso > ♀
Strega del Castello > 2018 > Patchouli Nero > ♀
Strega del Castello > 2019 > Es Parfum > ♀
Strega del Castello > 2020 > Vaniglia Verde > ♀
Sulmona Essenza > 2018 > Sulmona Essenza > ♀
Sulmona Essenza > 2018 > Sulmona Essenza Homme > ♂
Sweet Years > 2006 > Funny Days > ♀
Sweet Years > 2006 > Funny Days Man > ♂
Sweet Years > 2006 > Sweet Years Man > ♂
Sweet Years > 2006 > Sweet Years Women > ♀
Sweet Years > 2007 > Sweet Years Privé > ♀
Sweet Years > 2012 > Choose Your Style – I'm Funny > ♀
Sweet Years > 2012 > Choose Your Style – I'm Funny > ♀
Sweet Years > 2012 > Choose Your Style – I'm Rock > ♀
Sweet Years > 2012 > Choose Your Style – I'm Rock > ♀
Sweet Years > 2012 > Choose Your Style – I'm Sexy > ♀
Sweet Years > 2012 > Choose Your Style – I'm Strong > ♂
Sweet Years > 2012 > Choose Your Style – I'm Trendy > ♂
Sweet Years > 2014 > Just Me > ♀
Tauleto > 2007 > Tauleto Wine Fragrance > ♀
Teaology > 2017 > Black Rose Tea > ♀
Teaology > 2019 > Matcha Lemon > ♀
Teatro Fragranze Uniche > 2016 > Black Divine > ♀
Teatro Fragranze Uniche > 2016 > Mimì > ♀
Teatro Fragranze Uniche > 2016 > Rodolfo > ♂
Teatro Fragranze Uniche > 2016 > Tabacco > ♀
Tesori d'Oriente > 2010 > Marrakech Ibisco e Pepe Rosa > ♀
Tesori d'Oriente > 2010 > Marrakech Neroli e Cardamomo > ♀
Tesori d'Oriente > 2010 > Marrakech Patchouli e Ginger > ♀
Tesori d'Oriente > 2010 > White Musk > ♀
Tesori d'Oriente > 2010 > Zenzero > ♀
Tesori d'Oriente > 2011 > Marrakech Ambra e Zafferano > ♀
Tesori d'Oriente > 2011 > Africa > ♀
Tesori d'Oriente > 2011 > Frangipani delle Indie > ♀
Tesori d'Oriente > 2011 > Legno di Guajaco > ♂
Tesori d'Oriente > 2011 > Orchidea della Cina > ♀
Tesori d'Oriente > 2011 > Sandalo del Kashmir & Vetiver > ♂
Tesori d'Oriente > 2011 > Tè Verde > ♀
Tesori d'Oriente > 2011 > Vaniglia e Zenzero del Madagascar > ♀
Tesori d'Oriente > 2013 > Royal Oud Dello Yemen > ♂
Tesori d'Oriente > 2013 > Tiaré delle Indie > ♀
Tesori d'Oriente > 2013 > Viola del Nepal > ♀
Tesori d'Oriente > 2015 > Japanese Rituals > ♀
Tesori d'Oriente > 2015 > Baobab > ♂
Tesori d'Oriente > 2015 > Fior di Loto > ♀

Tesori d'Oriente > 2015 > Hammam > U
Tesori d'Oriente > 2016 > Byzantium > ♀
Tesori d'Oriente > 2017 > Ayurveda > ♀
Tesori d'Oriente > 2017 > Aegyptus > ♀
Tesori d'Oriente > 2017 > Ambra Indiana > ♀
Tesori d'Oriente > 2017 > Fiore del Dragone > ♀
Tesori d'Oriente > 2017 > Jasmin di Giava > ♀
Tesori d'Oriente > 2017 > Papavero del Tibet > ♀
Tesori d'Oriente > 2019 > Matcha Green Tea > ♀
Tesori d'Oriente > 2019 > Thai Spa > ♀
Tezenis > 2013 > Fluo > ♀
Tezenis > 2013 > Fuxia > ♀
The Merchant of Venice > 2013 > Murano Collection: Asian Inspiration > ♂
The Merchant of Venice > 2013 > Murano Collection: Byzantium Saffron > ♂
The Merchant of Venice > 2013 > Murano Collection: Flower Fusion > ♀
The Merchant of Venice > 2013 > Murano Collection: Mandarin Carnival > ♀
The Merchant of Venice > 2013 > Murano Collection: Noble Potion > ♂
The Merchant of Venice > 2013 > Murano Collection: Suave Petals > ♀
The Merchant of Venice > 2015 > Dalmatian Sage > ♂
The Merchant of Venice > 2015 > Esperidi Water > ♂
The Merchant of Venice > 2015 > Murano Art Collection: Ardent Oud > ♂
The Merchant of Venice > 2015 > Murano Art Collection: Leather in Nude > ♂
The Merchant of Venice > 2015 > Murano Art Collection: Myrrh Oud > ♂
The Merchant of Venice > 2015 > Murano Art Collection: Oudelight > ♂
The Merchant of Venice > 2015 > Murano Art Collection: Oudrageous > ♂
The Merchant of Venice > 2015 > Murano Art Collection: Secret Rose > ♀
The Merchant of Venice > 2015 > Murano Exclusive: Arabesque > ♂
The Merchant of Venice > 2015 > Murano Exclusive: Craquele > ♂
The Merchant of Venice > 2015 > Murano Exclusive: Fenicia > ♂
The Merchant of Venice > 2015 > Murano Exclusive: Liberty > ♂
The Merchant of Venice > 2015 > Murano Exclusive: Rococò > ♂
The Merchant of Venice > 2015 > Murano Exclusive: Vinegia > ♂
The Merchant of Venice > 2015 > Ottoman Amber > ♂
The Merchant of Venice > 2015 > Sultan Leather > ♂
The Merchant of Venice > 2016 > La Fenice pour Femme > ♀
The Merchant of Venice > 2016 > La Fenice pour Homme > ♂
The Merchant of Venice > 2016 > Murano Art Collection: Divine Rose > ♂
The Merchant of Venice > 2016 > Murano Art Collection: Orchid Oud > ♂
The Merchant of Venice > 2016 > Murano Art Collection: Pearl Bouquet > ♂
The Merchant of Venice > 2016 > Murano Collection: Rosa Moceniga > ♀
The Merchant of Venice > 2016 > Venetian Blue > ♂
The Merchant of Venice > 2016 > Amber Crystal > ♂
The Merchant of Venice > 2016 > Arabian Myrrh > ♂
The Merchant of Venice > 2016 > Bergamot > ♂
The Merchant of Venice > 2016 > Black Musk > ♂
The Merchant of Venice > 2016 > Black Oud > ♂
The Merchant of Venice > 2016 > Black Pepper > ♂
The Merchant of Venice > 2016 > Blue Island > ♂
The Merchant of Venice > 2016 > Cedarwood > ♂
The Merchant of Venice > 2016 > Daisy Bloom > ♀
The Merchant of Venice > 2016 > Delirious Orange > ♂
The Merchant of Venice > 2016 > Egyptian Linen > ♂
The Merchant of Venice > 2016 > Frangipani Blossom > ♀
The Merchant of Venice > 2016 > Incense Mist > ♂
The Merchant of Venice > 2016 > Indian Jasmine > ♀
The Merchant of Venice > 2016 > Lemon Splash > ♂
The Merchant of Venice > 2016 > Light Cotton > ♂
The Merchant of Venice > 2016 > Lily > ♀
The Merchant of Venice > 2016 > Majestic Rose > ♂
The Merchant of Venice > 2016 > Mandarin > ♂
The Merchant of Venice > 2016 > Natural Cyclamen > ♀
The Merchant of Venice > 2016 > Orange Flowers > ♂
The Merchant of Venice > 2016 > Oriental Delice > ♀
The Merchant of Venice > 2016 > Osmanthus > ♀
The Merchant of Venice > 2016 > Passion Fruit > ♂
The Merchant of Venice > 2016 > Patchouli Vintage > ♂
The Merchant of Venice > 2016 > Pink Grapefruit > ♂
The Merchant of Venice > 2016 > Precious Woods > ♂
The Merchant of Venice > 2016 > Pure Leather > ♂
The Merchant of Venice > 2016 > Rose Oud > ♂
The Merchant of Venice > 2016 > Sandalwood > ♂
The Merchant of Venice > 2016 > Sicilian Citruses > ♂
The Merchant of Venice > 2016 > Spicy > ♂
The Merchant of Venice > 2016 > Timeless Lavender > ♂
The Merchant of Venice > 2016 > Vanilla Orchid > ♂
The Merchant of Venice > 2016 > Vetiver Bourbon > ♂
The Merchant of Venice > 2016 > Violet Petals > ♂
The Merchant of Venice > 2016 > White Gardenia > ♀
The Merchant of Venice > 2016 > White Musk > ♂
The Merchant of Venice > 2016 > White Tea > ♂
The Merchant of Venice > 2016 > Wild Musk > ♂
The Merchant of Venice > 2017 > Murano Art Collection: Oud Illusion > ♂

The Merchant of Venice > 2017 > Murano Art Collection: Oudelicious > ♂
The Merchant of Venice > 2017 > Murano Art Collection: Rose Cloud > ♂
The Merchant of Venice > 2017 > Venezia Essenza pour Femme > ♀
The Merchant of Venice > 2017 > Venezia Essenza pour Homme > ♂
The Merchant of Venice > 2018 > Blue Tea > ♂
The Merchant of Venice > 2018 > Murano Collection: Andalusian Soul > ♂
The Merchant of Venice > 2018 > Murano Collection: Mystic Incense > ♂
The Merchant of Venice > 2018 > Venetian Blue Intense > ♂
The Merchant of Venice > 2019 > Murano Collection: Red Potion > ♂
The Merchant of Venice > 2019 > Murano Exclusive: Imperial Emerald > ♂
The Party > 2000 > The Garden Party Frangipane > ♀
The Party > 2000 > The Garden Party Iris > ♀
The Party > 2000 > The Garden Party Tuberose > ♀
The Party > 2000 > The Garden Party Wistaria > ♀
The Party > 2000 > The Garden Party Wistaria > ♀
The Party > 2008 > The Party in Manhattan > ♀
The Party > 2008 > The Ten Party 1986 > ♀
The Party > 2010 > The Party in Paris > ♀
The Social Parfum > 2004 > The Social Parfum > ♀
Tino Cosma > 1993 > Tino Cosma > ♂
Tiziana Terenzi > 2012 > Ecstasy > ♂
Tiziana Terenzi > 2012 > Gold Rose Oudh > ♂
Tiziana Terenzi > 2012 > White Fire > ♂
Tiziana Terenzi > 2012 > XIX March > ♂
Tiziana Terenzi > 2013 > Lillipur > ♂
Tiziana Terenzi > 2013 > Maremma > ♂
Tiziana Terenzi > 2014 > Arethusa > ♂
Tiziana Terenzi > 2014 > Bianco Puro > ♂
Tiziana Terenzi > 2014 > Casanova > ♂
Tiziana Terenzi > 2014 > Chimaera > ♂
Tiziana Terenzi > 2014 > Laudano Nero > ♂
Tiziana Terenzi > 2015 > Al Contrario > ♂
Tiziana Terenzi > 2015 > Andromeda > ♂
Tiziana Terenzi > 2015 > Cassiopea > ♂
Tiziana Terenzi > 2015 > Draco > ♂
Tiziana Terenzi > 2015 > Kirkè > ♂
Tiziana Terenzi > 2015 > Orion > ♂
Tiziana Terenzi > 2015 > Ursa > ♂
Tiziana Terenzi > 2016 > Adhil > ♂
Tiziana Terenzi > 2016 > Bigia > ♂
Tiziana Terenzi > 2016 > Dubhe > ♂
Tiziana Terenzi > 2016 > Gumin > ♂
Tiziana Terenzi > 2016 > Harrods Exclusive: Oud Alshain > ♂
Tiziana Terenzi > 2016 > Harrods Exclusive: Oud Nihal > ♂
Tiziana Terenzi > 2016 > Harrods Exclusive: Oud Tarazed > ♂
Tiziana Terenzi > 2016 > Harrods Exclusive: Oud Wasat > ♂
Tiziana Terenzi > 2016 > Saiph Attar > ♂
Tiziana Terenzi > 2016 > Tabit Attar > ♂
Tiziana Terenzi > 2016 > Tabit Extrait de Parfum > ♂
Tiziana Terenzi > 2016 > Tyl > ♂
Tiziana Terenzi > 2017 > Barney's Ny Exclusive: Lunanera > ♂
Tiziana Terenzi > 2017 > Cas > ♂
Tiziana Terenzi > 2017 > Cas Attar > ♂
Tiziana Terenzi > 2017 > Delox > ♂
Tiziana Terenzi > 2017 > Eclix > ♂
Tiziana Terenzi > 2017 > Foconero > ♂
Tiziana Terenzi > 2017 > Harrods Exclusive: Kuma > ♂
Tiziana Terenzi > 2017 > Harrods Exclusive: Oud Mira > ♂
Tiziana Terenzi > 2017 > Harvey Nichols Exclusive: Lucenera > ♂
Tiziana Terenzi > 2017 > Kaff > ♂
Tiziana Terenzi > 2017 > Kaff Attar > ♂
Tiziana Terenzi > 2017 > Porpora > ♂
Tiziana Terenzi > 2017 > Saiph > ♂
Tiziana Terenzi > 2017 > Vele > ♂
Tiziana Terenzi > 2017 > Velorum > ♂
Tiziana Terenzi > 2018 > Afrodite > ♂
Tiziana Terenzi > 2018 > Alioth > ♂
Tiziana Terenzi > 2018 > Caput Mundi > ♂
Tiziana Terenzi > 2018 > Dionisio > ♂
Tiziana Terenzi > 2018 > Harrods Exclusive: La Superba Rossa > ♂
Tiziana Terenzi > 2018 > Lince > ♂
Tiziana Terenzi > 2018 > Mirach > ♂
Tiziana Terenzi > 2018 > Sirrah > ♂
Tiziana Terenzi > 2019 > Arrakis > ♂
Tiziana Terenzi > 2019 > Borea > ♂
Tiziana Terenzi > 2019 > Draconis > ♂
Tiziana Terenzi > 2019 > Hale Bopp > ♂
Tiziana Terenzi > 2019 > Halley > ♂
Tiziana Terenzi > 2019 > Harrods Exclusive: Mizar > ♂
Tiziana Terenzi > 2019 > Lyncis > ♂
Tiziana Terenzi > 2019 > Nero Oudh > ♂
Tiziana Terenzi > 2019 > Orionis > ♂

Tiziana Terenzi > 2019 > Selfridges Exclusive: Encke > ♂
Tiziana Terenzi > 2019 > Siene > ♀
Tiziana Terenzi > 2019 > Spirito Fiorentino > ⚥
Tiziana Terenzi > 2019 > Tempel > ♂
Tiziana Terenzi > 2019 > Wirtaner > ⚥
Tokidoki > 2016 > Latte > ♀
Tokidoki > 2016 > Milk > ♀
Tom Rebl > 2012 > Bordello > ♂
Tonatto Profumi > 2000 > 24.08.00 > ⚥
Tonatto Profumi > 2000 > 2624 > ♀
Tonatto Profumi > 2000 > Albi > ♂
Tonatto Profumi > 2000 > Ambrosia > ♀
Tonatto Profumi > 2000 > Amir > ♀
Tonatto Profumi > 2000 > Anena > ♀
Tonatto Profumi > 2000 > Anni Venti > ♀
Tonatto Profumi > 2000 > Antò Portami a Palmarola > ⚥
Tonatto Profumi > 2000 > Arco > ♀
Tonatto Profumi > 2000 > D'Eau de Parfum > ♀
Tonatto Profumi > 2000 > Flor d'Arancio > ♂
Tonatto Profumi > 2000 > Il Risveglio/The Awakening > ⚥
Tonatto Profumi > 2000 > Magnifico > ♀
Tonatto Profumi > 2000 > Nerola > ♀
Tonatto Profumi > 2000 > Oropuro > ♀
Tonatto Profumi > 2000 > Osa > ♀
Tonatto Profumi > 2000 > Palmarola > ♂
Tonatto Profumi > 2000 > Plaisir > ♀
Tonatto Profumi > 2000 > Safram > ♀
Tonatto Profumi > 2000 > Sandalo per Teti > ♂
Tonatto Profumi > 2002 > Aura Acqua > ⚥
Tonatto Profumi > 2002 > Dama > ♀
Tonatto Profumi > 2002 > M'amo > ♀
Tonatto Profumi > 2002 > M'oma > ♀
Tonatto Profumi > 2002 > Tuda > ♂
Tonatto Profumi > 2003 > Iss > ♂
Tonatto Profumi > 2003 > Re > ♂
Tonatto Profumi > 2010 > Eleonora Duse > ♀
Tonatto Profumi > 2010 > Solista > ♀
Tonatto Profumi > 2010 > Il Cammino/The Path > ⚥
Tonatto Profumi > 2010 > Notte a Taif > ♀
Tonatto Profumi > 2010 > Soglie > ♂
Tonatto Profumi > 2011 > Profumo di Fumne > ♀
Tonatto Profumi > 2012 > Bianco > ♀
Tonatto Profumi > 2012 > Oro > ♂
Tonatto Profumi > 2012 > Oud d'Arabia: Bianco > ♂
Tonatto Profumi > 2012 > Oud d'Arabia: Oro > ♂
Tonatto Profumi > 2012 > Oud d'Arabia: Rosso > ♂
Tonatto Profumi > 2012 > Oud d'Arabia: Ruscia > ♂
Tonatto Profumi > 2012 > Oud d'Arabia: Viola > ♂
Tonatto Profumi > 2012 > Rosso > ♀
Tonatto Profumi > 2012 > Ruscia > ♂
Tonatto Profumi > 2012 > Viola > ♂
Tonatto Profumi > 2013 > Violette a Sidney > ⚥
Tonatto Profumi > 2015 > Apeiron > ♂
Tonatto Profumi > 2015 > Il Profumo del Cielo/The Scent of Sky > ⚥
Tonatto Profumi > 2016 > Viburnum > ♂
Tonatto Profumi > 2017 > Profumo di Vita > ♂
Tonatto Profumi > 2017 > Profumo di Vita > ♂
Tonatto Profumi > 2018 > Freyja > ♂
Tonatto Profumi > 2020 > Palosanto > ⚥
Tonelli > 2011 > Tonelli Femme > ♀
Tonelli > 2011 > Tonelli Homme > ♂
Tonino Lamborghini > 1979 > Lamborghini Convertibile > ♂
Tonino Lamborghini > 1999 > Lamborghini pour Homme > ♂
Tonino Lamborghini > 2000 > Lamborghini pour Femme > ♀
Tonino Lamborghini > 2001 > Titanium > ♂
Tonino Lamborghini > 2004 > Overall > ♀
Tonino Lamborghini > 2004 > Overall pour Homme > ♂
Tonino Lamborghini > 2008 > Feroce > ♂
Tonino Lamborghini > 2008 > Forza > ♂
Tonino Lamborghini > 2008 > Mitico > ♂
Tonino Lamborghini > 2009 > Esplosivo > ♂
Tonino Lamborghini > 2010 > Intenso > ♂
Tonino Lamborghini > 2011 > Azione > ♂
Tonino Lamborghini > 2011 > Prestigio > ♂
Tonino Lamborghini > 2012 > Sportivo > ♂
Tonino Lamborghini > 2013 > Classico > ♂
Tonino Lamborghini > 2018 > Invincibile > ♂
Torre del Garda > 2015 > Ora > ♀
Torre del Garda > 2015 > Peler > ♂
Torre del Garda > 2016 > Bali > ♂
Torre del Garda > 2016 > Vinessa > ♀
Torre del Garda > 2017 > Isola del Garda > ♀

Torre of Tuscany > 2011 > Colonia Toscana > ♂
Torre of Tuscany > 2011 > Corpi Caldi > ♀
Torre of Tuscany > 2011 > Mughetto Verde > ♀
Torre of Tuscany > 2011 > Muschio Marino > ♂
Torre of Tuscany > 2011 > Vetiver Moderno > ♂
Torre of Tuscany > 2012 > Berkana > ♂
Torre of Tuscany > 2012 > Colonia Esperidea > ♀
Torre of Tuscany > 2012 > Dolce Narciso > ♀
Torre of Tuscany > 2012 > Savane Oud > ♂
Triquetra > 2014 > Anymus > ⚥
Triquetra > 2015 > Anymus La Sera > ♂
Triquetra > 2015 > Mystico > ♀
True Diamond Perfume > 2019 > Perfect Match > ♀
Trussardi > 1983 > Trussardi Uomo > ♂
Trussardi > 1984 > Trussardi > ♀
Trussardi > 1990 > Action Donna > ♀
Trussardi > 1990 > Action Uomo > ♂
Trussardi > 1993 > Action Sport > ♂
Trussardi > 1994 > Donna > ♀
Trussardi > 1995 > L'uomo > ♂
Trussardi > 1997 > Light Her > ♀
Trussardi > 1997 > Light Him > ♂
Trussardi > 1999 > Fresh > ♀
Trussardi > 1999 > Python > ♀
Trussardi > 2000 > Fresh > ♂
Trussardi > 2001 > Python Uomo > ♂
Trussardi > 2002 > Trussardi Skin > ♀
Trussardi > 2003 > Trussardi Jeans > ♀
Trussardi > 2004 > Trussardi Jeans Men > ♂
Trussardi > 2005 > Bianco > ♀
Trussardi > 2006 > Inside for Men > ♂
Trussardi > 2006 > Inside for Women > ♀
Trussardi > 2008 > Essenza del Tempo > ♂
Trussardi > 2008 > Inside Delight > ♀
Trussardi > 2009 > Inside Iced > ♂
Trussardi > 2011 > Donna Trussardi > ♀
Trussardi > 2011 > Trussardi Uomo > ♂
Trussardi > 2012 > Delicate Rose > ♀
Trussardi > 2012 > My Land > ♂
Trussardi > 2013 > My Name > ♀
Trussardi > 2014 > Black Extreme > ♂
Trussardi > 2014 > Trussardi a Way for Her > ♀
Trussardi > 2014 > Trussardi a Way for Him > ♂
Trussardi > 2015 > My Scent > ♀
Trussardi > 2016 > Amber Oud > ♂
Trussardi > 2016 > Trussardi Donna Edt > ♀
Trussardi > 2016 > Trussardi Uomo the Red > ♂
Trussardi > 2017 > Riflesso > ♂
Trussardi > 2017 > The Black Rose > ♀
Trussardi > 2017 > Trussardi Donna Goccia a Goccia > ♀
Trussardi > 2017 > Trussardi my Name Goccia a Goccia > ♀
Trussardi > 2018 > Riflesso Streets of Milano > ♂
Trussardi > 2018 > Scent of Gold > ♀
Trussardi > 2018 > Sound of Donna > ♀
Trussardi > 2019 > Riflesso Blue Vibe > ♂
Trussardi > 2019 > Trussardi Donna Edp Intense > ♀
Trussardi > 2019 > Trussardi Uomo Edp > ♂
Tuttotondo > 2016 > Castagna > ♂
Tuttotondo > 2016 > Chinotto > ♂
Tuttotondo > 2016 > Erbe Alpine > ♂
Tuttotondo > 2016 > Fico d'India > ♂
Tuttotondo > 2016 > Mirto > ♂
Tuttotondo > 2017 > Golf > ♂
Tuttotondo > 2017 > Scherma > ♂
Tuttotondo > 2018 > Vela > ♂
Twinset Milano > 2019 > Twinset > ♀
UèrMì > 2014 > Ab+-Cashmere > ♂
UèrMì > 2014 > No+-Suede > ♂
UèrMì > 2014 > Oh+-Denim > ♂
UèrMì > 2014 > Ur+-Silk > ♂
UèrMì > 2014 > Ve+-Velvet > ♂
UèrMì > 2014 > We+-Tweed > ♂
UèrMì > 2014 > Xx+-Latex > ♂
UèrMì > 2015 > Do+-Washi > ♂
UèrMì > 2016 > Collection Extraordinaire: Or White > ♀
UèrMì > 2016 > Collection Extraordinaire: Or+-Ange > ♂
UèrMì > 2016 > Collection Extraordinaire: Or+-Cashmere > ♂
UèrMì > 2017 > Collection Extraordinaire: Or+-Kanabo > ♂
UèrMì > 2018 > Collection Extraordinaire: Or+-Damask > ♀
UèrMì > 2018 > So+-Satin > ♂
UèrMì > 2018 > Ur+-Silk19 > ♂
UèrMì > 2019 > Nu Leather > ♂

Unique	2016	Kaleidoscope	♀
Unique	2016	Lumiere du Ciel	♂
Unique	2016	Royal Amber Oud	♂
Unique	2016	Woodmanity	♂
Valentina by Guido Crepax	2018	Valentina	♀
Valentino	1978	Valentino	♀
Valentino	1991	Vendetta Donna	♀
Valentino	1991	Vendetta Uomo	♂
Valentino	1998	Very Valentino	♀
Valentino	1998	Very Valentino Edt	♀
Valentino	1999	Very Valentino for Men	♂
Valentino	2002	Valentino Gold	♀
Valentino	2005	V	♀
Valentino	2005	V Absolu	♀
Valentino	2006	Rock'n Rose	♀
Valentino	2006	V Eté	♀
Valentino	2006	V pour Homme	♂
Valentino	2007	Rock'n Rose Couture	♀
Valentino	2008	Rock'n Rose Prêt-à-Porter	♀
Valentino	2009	Rock'n Dreams	♀
Valentino	2009	Valentino Edp	♂
Valentino	2011	Valentina	♀
Valentino	2012	Valentina Assoluto	♀
Valentino	2013	Valentina Acqua Floreale	♀
Valentino	2013	Valentina Oud Assoluto	♀
Valentino	2014	Valentina Rosa Assoluto	♀
Valentino	2014	Valentino Uomo	♂
Valentino	2015	Valentina Pink	♀
Valentino	2015	Valentino Donna	♀
Valentino	2015	Valentino Uomo	♂
Valentino	2016	Valentina Myrrh Assoluto	♀
Valentino	2016	Valentina Poudre	♀
Valentino	2016	Valentino Uomo Intense	♂
Valentino	2017	Valentina Blush	♀
Valentino	2017	Valentino Donna Acqua	♀
Valentino	2017	Valentino Donna Noir Absolu	♀
Valentino	2017	Valentino Uomo Acqua	♂
Valentino	2017	Valentino Uomo Noir Absolu	♂
Valentino	2018	Valentino Donna Verde	♀
Valentino	2018	Valentino Noir Absolu Musc Essence	♂
Valentino	2018	Valentino Noir Absolu Oud Essence	♂
Valentino	2019	Valentino Donna Born in Roma	♀
Valentino	2019	Valentino Uomo Born in Roma	♂
Vapro International	2015	Corvette Red	♂
Vapro International	2015	Rampage 100% Love	♀
Veejaga	1983	Hascisch Femme	♀
Veejaga	1983	Hascisch Homme	♂
Veejaga	1985	Black Hascish	♂
Veejaga	1988	Eau de Hascish	♀
Veejaga	1990	Christie	♀
Veejaga	1990	Harley Davidson	♂
Veejaga	1992	Hascish Musk	♀
Veejaga	1994	Hascish Royal	♀
Venezia 1920	2019	Divine	♀
Venezia 1920	2019	Grey Velvet	♂
Venezia 1920	2019	Lido	♀
Venezia 1920	2019	Oud Royale	♀
Versace	1981	Gianni Versace	♀
Versace	1986	Versace L'homme	♂
Versace	1989	V'e	♀
Versace	1991	Versus Uomo	♂
Versace	1992	Versus Donna	♀
Versace	1994	Blue Jeans	♂
Versace	1994	Red Jeans	♀
Versace	1995	Baby Blue Jeans	♂
Versace	1995	Baby Rose Jeans	♀
Versace	1995	Blonde	♀
Versace	1996	Dreamer	♂
Versace	1996	Green Jeans	♂
Versace	1996	Yellow Jeans	♀
Versace	1997	Black Jeans	♂
Versace	1997	White Jeans	♀
Versace	1998	V/S Femme	♀
Versace	2000	V/S Homme	♂
Versace	2000	Versace 2 Thousand	♀
Versace	2000	Versace Essence Emotional	♀
Versace	2000	Versace Essence Ethereal	♀
Versace	2000	Versace Essence Exciting	♀
Versace	2000	Versace Woman	♀
Versace	2001	Metal Jeans Women	♀
Versace	2001	Versus Time for Energy	♀
Versace	2001	Versus Time for Relax	♂

Versace	2002	Jeans Couture Man	♂
Versace	2002	Jeans Couture Woman	♀
Versace	2002	Versace Woman Summer	♀
Versace	2003	Jeans Couture Glam	♀
Versace	2003	Versace Man	♂
Versace	2003	Versus Time for Action	♂
Versace	2003	Versus Time for Pleasure	♀
Versace	2004	Crystal Noir	♀
Versace	2004	Jeans Woman	♀
Versace	2006	Bright Crystal	♀
Versace	2006	Versace Man Eau Fraiche	♂
Versace	2007	Versace pour Femme	♀
Versace	2008	Couture Violet	♀
Versace	2008	Versace pour Homme	♂
Versace	2009	Versense	♀
Versace	2010	The Dreamer	♂
Versace	2010	Versus	♀
Versace	2011	Metal Jeans Men	♂
Versace	2011	Vanitas	♀
Versace	2011	Yellow Diamond	♀
Versace	2012	Eros	♂
Versace	2012	Vanitas Edt	♀
Versace	2013	Bright Crystal Absolu	♀
Versace	2013	Versace pour Homme Oud Noir	♂
Versace	2014	Couture Jasmine	♀
Versace	2014	Couture Tuberose	♀
Versace	2014	Eros Pour Femme	♀
Versace	2014	Versace pour Femme Oud Oriental	♀
Versace	2014	Yellow Diamond Intense	♀
Versace	2016	Eros pour Femme Edt	♀
Versace	2016	Versace pour Homme Dylan Blue	♂
Versace	2017	Versace pour Femme Dylan Blue	♀
Versace	2018	Eros Flame	♂
Versace	2019	Atelier Versace Cedrat de Diamante	♂
Versace	2019	Atelier Versace Eclat de Rose	♀
Versace	2019	Atelier Versace Figue Blanche	♀
Versace	2019	Atelier Versace Jasmin au Soleil	♂
Versace	2019	Atelier Versace Santal Boisé	♂
Versace	2019	Atelier Versace Vanille Rouge	♀
Vespa	2014	Vespa for Her	♀
Vespa	2014	Vespa for Him	♂
Vespa	2015	Vespa Sensazione for Her	♀
Vespa	2015	Vespa Sensazione for Him	♂
Via dei Mille Sicilia	2017	Ianco Collection: Gelsomino	♀
Via dei Mille Sicilia	2017	Ianco Collection: Mandorlo	♀
Via dei Mille Sicilia	2017	Ianco Collection: Zagara	♀
Vicini	2015	Land of Fashion	♀
Vicini	2015	Private Collection	♀
Victor	1972	V by Victor	♂
Victor	1974	Signor Victor	♂
Victor	1980	Victor Club	♂
Victor	1984	Wall Street	♂
Victor	1995	Fresco Absolute	♂
Victor	1996	Off Shore	♂
Victor	1996	Green Tea	♂
Victor	1999	Spirit of Victor	♂
Victor	2000	Fresco	♂
Victor	2006	Torino 06	♂
Victor	2006	Torino 06	♂
Violin Fragrance	2013	Violin Eau de Parfum	♀
Wally	2005	Attar - Eau de Cologne Classica	♀
Wally	2005	Eau de Cologne Cuoio di Russia	♀
Wally	2005	Eau de Cologne Fougère	♀
Wally	2005	Eau de Cologne Lavanda	♀
Wally	2005	Eau de Cologne Pelle di Spagna	♀
Wally	2005	Eau de Cologne Rosa d'Italia	♀
Wally	2005	Incenso Nobile	♀
Wally	2005	Oud Absolu	♀
Wally	2005	Pape Satan	♀
Wally	2005	Tuscan Perfumery: Brezza Marina	♀
Wally	2005	Tuscan Perfumery: Fiorile	♀
Wally	2005	Tuscan Perfumery: Le Maremme	♀
Wally	2005	Tuscan Perfumery: Memorabilia	♀
Wally	2005	Tuscan Perfumery: Meriggi	♀
Wally	2005	Tuscan Perfumery: Prima Neve	♀
Wally	2005	Vero Toscano Bianco Eau de Parfum	⚥
Wally	2005	Vero Toscano Nero Eau de Parfum	
Womo	2014	Black Amber	♂
Womo	2014	Black Cologne	♂
Womo	2014	Black Oud	♂
Womo	2014	Black Powder	♂
Womo	2014	Black Spice	♂

Womo > 2014 > Black Tobacco > ♂
Womo > 2014 > Blue Linen > ♂
Womo > 2014 > Coiba > ♂
Womo > 2014 > Green Tweed > ⚥
Womo > 2014 > Red Velvet > ♂
Womo > 2016 > Koh Tao > ♂
Womo > 2016 > Samoa > ♂
Womo > 2016 > Sifnos > ♂
Womo > 2016 > Sport Collection: Blow In > ♂
Womo > 2016 > Sport Collection: Cool Down > ♂
Womo > 2016 > Sport Collection: Splash Out > ♂
Womo > 2016 > Sport Collection: Stand Up > ♂
Womo > 2016 > Sport Collection: Warm Up > ♂
Womo > 2016 > Sport Collection: Work Out > ♂
Womo > 2016 > Unexpected > ♂
Womo > 2016 > Xcel > ♂
Womo > 2016 > Xcentric > ♂
Womo > 2016 > Xcite > ♂
Womo > 2016 > Xplore > ♂
Womo > 2016 > Xpressive > ♂
Womo > 2017 > Incense+Cardamom > ⚥
Womo > 2017 > Leather+Benzoin > ⚥
Womo > 2017 > Vetiver+Chestnut > ⚥
Womo > 2018 > Juniper+Salt > ⚥
Words Firenze > 2016 > Addiction > ⚥
Words Firenze > 2016 > Bye Bye Baby > ⚥
Words Firenze > 2016 > Single > ⚥
Words Firenze > 2016 > The Best > ⚥
Wycon > 2016 > The Secret Potion of Glory > ♀
Wycon > 2016 > The Secret Potion of Happiness > ♀
Wycon > 2016 > The Secret Potion of Love > ♀
Wycon > 2016 > The Secret Potion of Seduction > ♀
Wycon > 2016 > The Secret Potion of Sensuality > ♀
Xerjoff > 2007 > Elle > ♀
Xerjoff > 2007 > Homme > ♂
Xerjoff > 2007 > Emery > ⚥
Xerjoff > 2008 > Irisss > ♀
Xerjoff > 2008 > XXY > ⚥
Xerjoff > 2009 > Casamorati 1888: Fiore d'ulivo > ♀
Xerjoff > 2009 > Casamorati 1888: Mefisto > ♂
Xerjoff > 2009 > Dhajala > ♀
Xerjoff > 2009 > Dhofar > ♂
Xerjoff > 2009 > Esquel > ♀
Xerjoff > 2009 > Ibitira > ♀
Xerjoff > 2009 > Kobe > ♂
Xerjoff > 2009 > Lua > ♀
Xerjoff > 2009 > Modoc > ♂
Xerjoff > 2009 > Nio > ♂
Xerjoff > 2009 > Oroville > ♂
Xerjoff > 2009 > Shingl > ♀
Xerjoff > 2009 > Uden > ♂
Xerjoff > 2010 > Casamorati 1888: Bouquet Ideale > ♀
Xerjoff > 2010 > Casamorati 1888: Fiero > ♂
Xerjoff > 2010 > Damarose > ♀
Xerjoff > 2010 > Oesel > ♂
Xerjoff > 2010 > Richwood > ♂
Xerjoff > 2011 > Casamorati 1888: Lira > ♀
Xerjoff > 2011 > Casamorati 1888: Regio > ⚥
Xerjoff > 2011 > Renaissance > ♀
Xerjoff > 2012 > Black Sukar > ⚥
Xerjoff > 2012 > Casamorati 1888: Dama Bianca > ♀
Xerjoff > 2012 > Java Blossom > ⚥
Xerjoff > 2012 > Join the Club: 40 Knots > ♂
Xerjoff > 2012 > Join the Club: Ascot Moon > ⚥
Xerjoff > 2012 > Join the Club: Birdie > ⚥
Xerjoff > 2012 > Join the Club: Comandante > ♂
Xerjoff > 2012 > Join the Club: Fatal Charme > ⚥
Xerjoff > 2012 > Join the Club: Ivory Route > ⚥
Xerjoff > 2012 > Join the Club: Kind Of Blue > ⚥
Xerjoff > 2012 > Join the Club: Marquee > ⚥
Xerjoff > 2012 > Join the Club: More Than Words > ⚥
Xerjoff > 2012 > Join the Club: Shunkoin > ⚥
Xerjoff > 2012 > Kampuchea Noir > ⚥
Xerjoff > 2012 > King Masarat > ⚥
Xerjoff > 2012 > Oud Luban > ⚥
Xerjoff > 2012 > Oud Stars: Al Khat > ⚥
Xerjoff > 2012 > Oud Stars: Alexandria II > ⚥
Xerjoff > 2012 > Oud Stars: Fars > ⚥
Xerjoff > 2012 > Oud Stars: Gao > ⚥
Xerjoff > 2012 > Oud Stars: Mamluk > ⚥
Xerjoff > 2012 > Oud Stars: Zafar > ⚥
Xerjoff > 2012 > Oud Stars: Zanzibar (Najaf) > ⚥

Xerjoff > 2012 > Warda Al Oud > ♀
Xerjoff > 2012 > Murano Collection: Damarose Perfume Extract > ♀
Xerjoff > 2012 > Murano Collection: Elle Perfume Extract > ♀
Xerjoff > 2012 > Murano Collection: Irisss Perfume Extract > ♀
Xerjoff > 2012 > Murano Collection: Richwood Perfume Extract > ♀
Xerjoff > 2012 > Murano Collection: XXY Perfume Extract > ⚥
Xerjoff > 2012 > Murano Collection: Homme Perfume Extract > ♂
Xerjoff > 2013 > Amber Star > ♂
Xerjoff > 2013 > Casamorati 1888: 1888 > ⚥
Xerjoff > 2013 > Casamorati 1888: Gran Ballo > ♀
Xerjoff > 2013 > Join The Club: Don > ♂
Xerjoff > 2013 > Star Musk > ⚥
Xerjoff > 2013 > Wabar > ♀
Xerjoff > 2013/2019 > Oud Stars: Indochine > ⚥
Xerjoff > 2014 > Blue Hope > ♀
Xerjoff > 2014 > Harrod's Emerald Star > ⚥
Xerjoff > 2014 > Oud Stars: Malesia > ⚥
Xerjoff > 2014 > Red Hoba > ⚥
Xerjoff > 2015 > Begum > ⚥
Xerjoff > 2015 > Casamorati 1888: La Tosca > ♀
Xerjoff > 2015 > Cruz del Sur > ⚥
Xerjoff > 2015 > Jebel > ⚥
Xerjoff > 2015 > Naxos > ⚥
Xerjoff > 2015 > Symphonium > ⚥
Xerjoff > 2015 > Zefiro > ⚥
Xerjoff > 2015/2018 > Pikovaya Dama > ⚥
Xerjoff > 2016 > Casamorati 1888: Italica > ⚥
Xerjoff > 2016 > Oud Stars: Alexandria Orientale > ⚥
Xerjoff > 2017 > Aubres > ⚥
Xerjoff > 2017 > Casamorati 1888: Dolce Amalfi > ⚥
Xerjoff > 2017 > Cavour I > ⚥
Xerjoff > 2017 > Cruz del Sur I > ⚥
Xerjoff > 2017 > Cruz del Sur II > ⚥
Xerjoff > 2017 > Oud Stars: Alexandria Imperiale > ⚥
Xerjoff > 2017 > Oud Stars: Ceylon > ⚥
Xerjoff > 2018 > Alexandria III Extrait Oil > ⚥
Xerjoff > 2018 > Allende > ⚥
Xerjoff > 2018 > Amber Gold > ⚥
Xerjoff > 2018 > Casamorati 1888: Corallo > ♀
Xerjoff > 2018 > Casamorati 1888: Mefisto Gentiluomo > ♂
Xerjoff > 2018 > Golden Dallah > ⚥
Xerjoff > 2018 > Golden Moka > ⚥
Xerjoff > 2018 > Join The Club: Jtc 400 > ⚥
Xerjoff > 2018 > Rose Gold > ⚥
Xerjoff > 2018 > Uden Overdose > ⚥
Xerjoff > 2019 > Accento > ⚥
Xerjoff > 2019 > Accento Overdose > ⚥
Xerjoff > 2019 > Apollonia > ⚥
Xerjoff > 2019 > Aubres (The Fortnum & Mason Exclusive) > ⚥
Xerjoff > 2019 > Coro - Selfridges Exclusive > ⚥
Xerjoff > 2019 > Erba Pura > ⚥
Xerjoff > 2019 > Join The Club: K'bridge Club > ⚥
Xerjoff > 2019 > La Capitale > ⚥
Xerjoff > 2019 > Laylati > ⚥
Xerjoff > 2019 > Muse > ⚥
Xerjoff > 2019 > Opera > ⚥
Xerjoff > 2019 > Oud Stars: Alexandria III > ⚥
Xerjoff > 2019 > Oud Stars: Alexandria III By Kostas Harrod's Exclusive > ⚥
Xerjoff > 2019 > Ouverture > ⚥
Xerjoff > 2019 > Soprano > ⚥
Xerjoff > 2019 > Starlight > ⚥
Xerjoff > 2019 > Wardasina > ⚥
Xerjoff > 2020 > Oud Stars: Luxor > ⚥
You First Pura Rinascita > 2015 > Fig Poudre Edp > ⚥
You First Pura Rinascita > 2015 > Spices Bouquet > ⚥
You First Pura Rinascita > 2015 > Velvet Woods > ⚥
You First Pura Rinascita > 2017 > Tomato Leaves and Orange Blossoms > ⚥
Zeromolecole > 2010 > Dudù > ⚥
Zeromolecole > 2010 > Iaia > ⚥
Zeromolecole > 2010 > Nuvole > ⚥
Zeromolecole > 2010 > Stromboli > ⚥
Zeromolecole > 2011 > Biancolatte > ⚥
Zeromolecole > 2011 > Bollicine > ⚥
Zeromolecole > 2011 > Neh?! > ⚥
Zeromolecole > 2011 > Nerocacao > ⚥
Zeromolecole > 2012 > Geco > ⚥
Zeromolecole > 2012 > Lalao > ⚥
Zeromolecole > 2014 > Osa > ⚥
Zeromolecole > 2015 > Amame > ⚥
Zeromolecole > 2018 > Tredici > ⚥
Zeromolecole > 2019 > Clori > ⚥
Zeromolecole > 2019 > Oscuro > ⚥

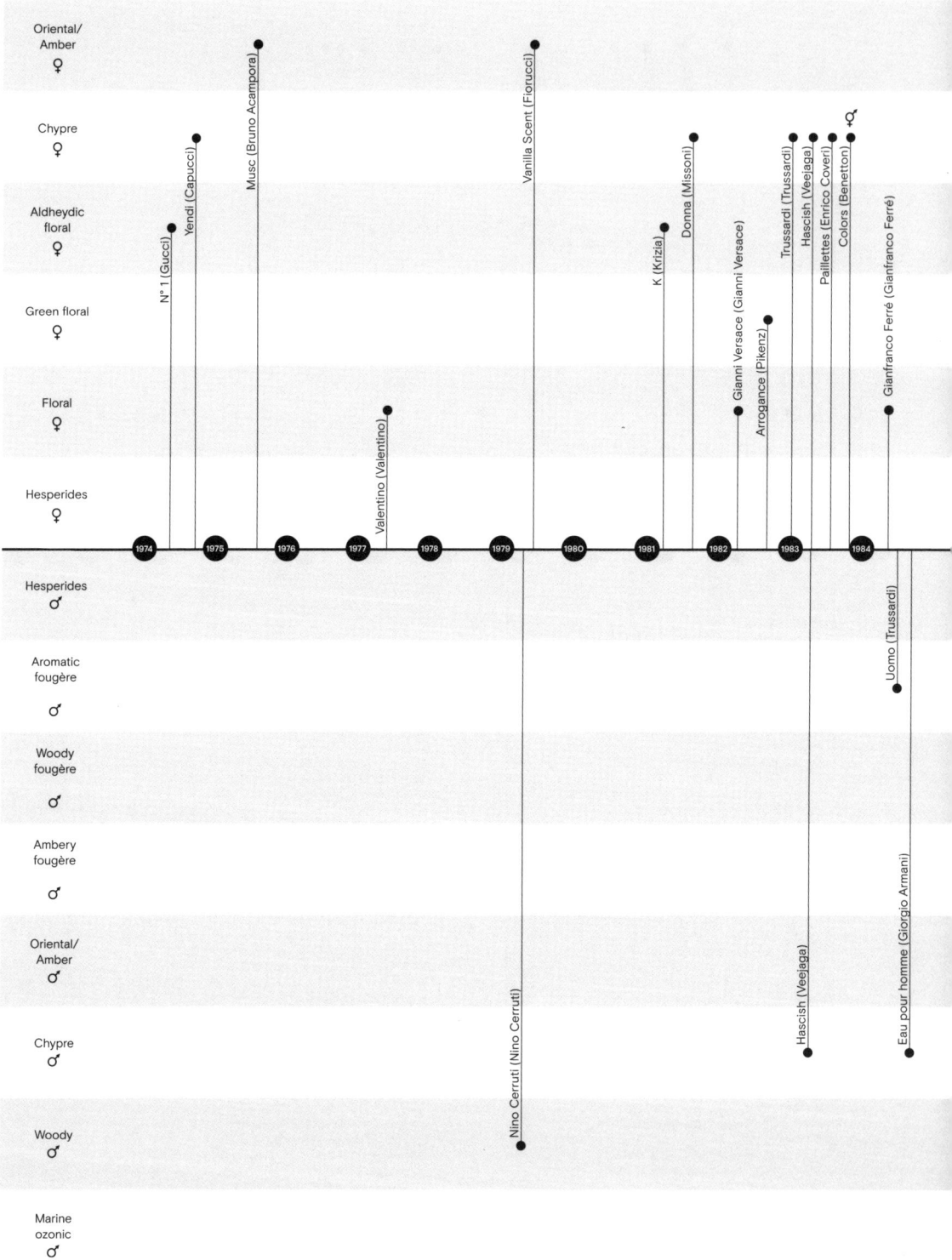

Chronology

Oriental/Amber ♀

Chypre ♀

Aldheydic floral ♀

Green floral ♀

Floral ♀

Hesperides ♀

Hesperides ♂

Aromatic fougère ♂

Woody fougère ♂

Ambery fougère ♂

Oriental/Amber ♂

Chypre ♂

Woody ♂

Marine ozonic ♂

1974 · 1975 · 1976 · 1977 · 1978 · 1979 · 1980 · 1981 · 1982 · 1983 · 1984

N° 1 (Gucci)
Yendi (Capucci)
Musc (Bruno Acampora)
Valentino (Valentino)
Vanilla Scent (Fiorucci)
K (Krizia)
Donna (Missoni)
Gianni Versace (Gianni Versace)
Arrogance (Pikenz)
Trussardi (Trussardi)
Hascish (Veejaga)
Paillettes (Enrico Coveri)
Colors (Benetton) ♂
Gianfranco Ferré (Gianfranco Ferré)
Uomo (Trussardi)
Hascish (Veejaga)
Eau pour homme (Giorgio Armani)
Nino Cerruti (Nino Cerruti)

352

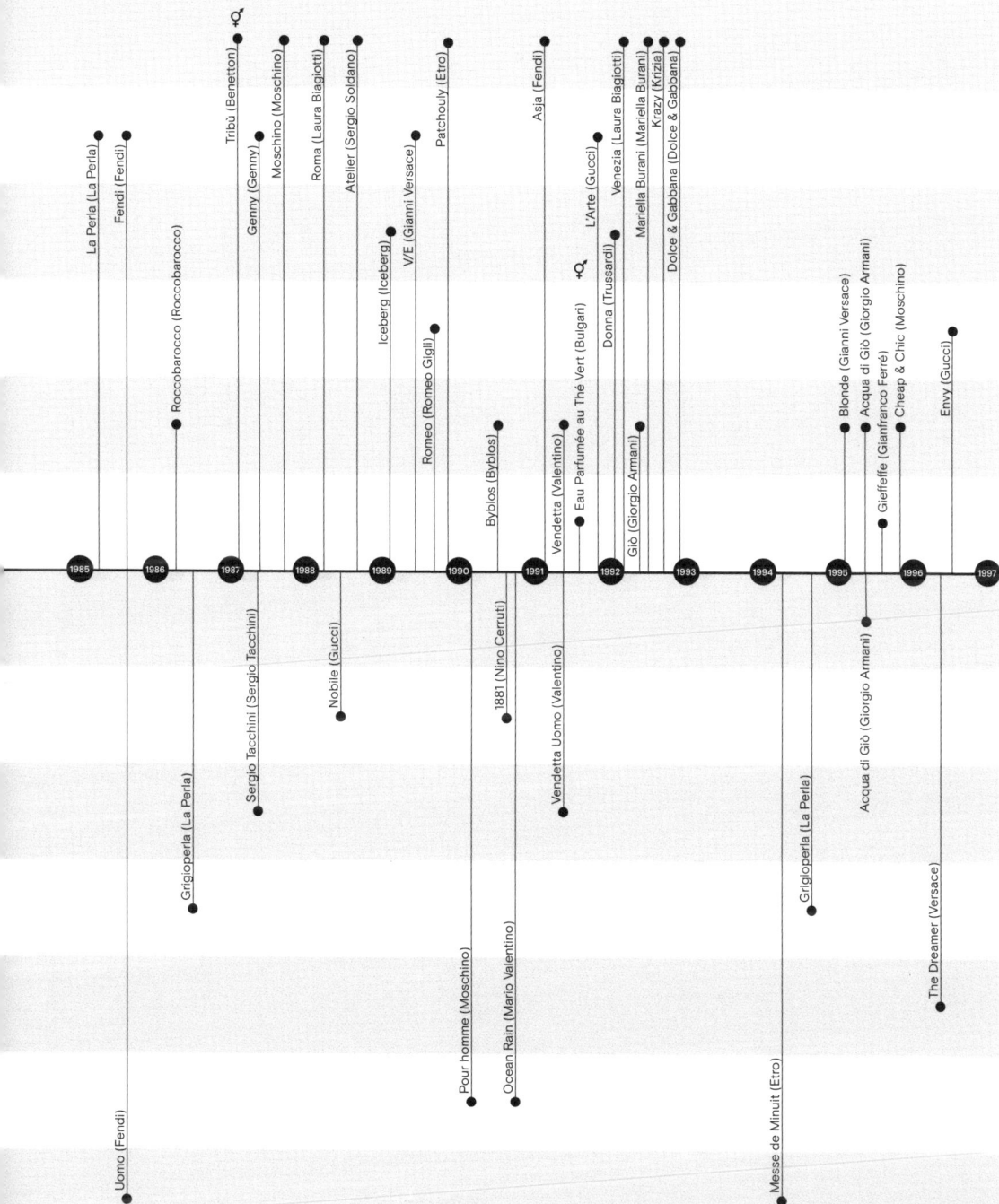

Uomo (Fendi)

La Perla (La Perla)
Fendi (Fendi)

Grigioperla (La Perla)

Roccobarocco (Roccobarocco)

Sergio Tacchini (Sergio Tacchini)

♀♂ Tribù (Benetton)
Genny (Genny)
Moschino (Moschino)
Roma (Laura Biagiotti)
Atelier (Sergio Soldano)
Patchouly (Etro)

Nobile (Gucci)

Iceberg (Iceberg)
V/E (Gianni Versace)
Romeo (Romeo Gigli)

Byblos (Byblos)

Pour homme (Moschino)

1881 (Nino Cerruti)
Ocean Rain (Mario Valentino)

Asja (Fendi)
L'Arte (Gucci)
♀♂ Donna (Trussardi)
Venezia (Laura Biagiotti)
Mariella Burani (Mariella Burani)
Krazy (Krizia)
Dolce & Gabbana (Dolce & Gabbana)

Vendetta (Valentino)
Eau Parfumée au Thé Vert (Bulgari)
Giò (Giorgio Armani)

Vendetta Uomo (Valentino)

Blonde (Gianni Versace)
Acqua di Giò (Giorgio Armani)
Gieffeffe (Gianfranco Ferré)
Cheap & Chic (Moschino)
Envy (Gucci)

Acqua di Giò (Giorgio Armani)

Grigioperla (La Perla)

Messe de Minuit (Etro)

The Dreamer (Versace)

1985 1986 1987 1988 1989 1990 1991 1992 1993 1994 1995 1996 1997

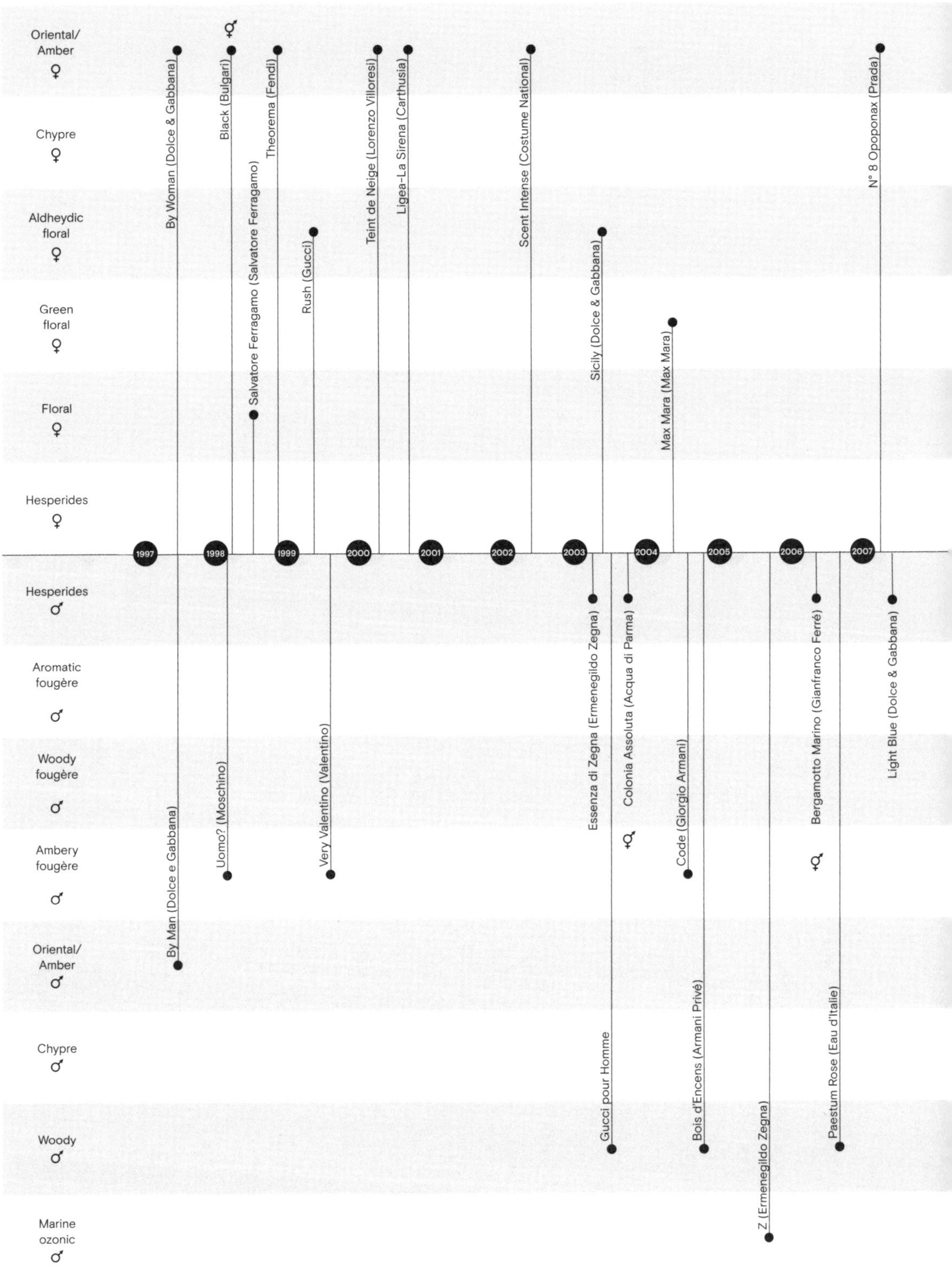

Oriental/ Amber ♀
Chypre ♀
Aldheydic floral ♀
Green floral ♀
Floral ♀
Hesperides ♀
Hesperides ♂
Aromatic fougère ♂
Woody fougère ♂
Ambery fougère ♂
Oriental/ Amber ♂
Chypre ♂
Woody ♂
Marine ozonic ♂
1997
1998
1999
2000
2001
2002
2003
2004
2005
2006
2007
By Woman (Dolce & Gabbana)
Black (Bulgari)
Salvatore Ferragamo (Salvatore Ferragamo)
Theorema (Fendi)
Rush (Gucci)
Teint de Neige (Lorenzo Villoresi)
Ligea-La Sirena (Carthusia)
Scent Intense (Costume National)
Sicily (Dolce & Gabbana)
Max Mara (Max Mara)
N° 8 Opoponax (Prada)
By Man (Dolce e Gabbana)
Uomo? (Moschino)
Very Valentino (Valentino)
Essenza di Zegna (Ermenegildo Zegna)
Gucci pour Homme
Colonia Assoluta (Acqua di Parma)
Code (Giorgio Armani)
Bois d'Encens (Armani Privé)
Z (Ermenegildo Zegna)
Bergamotto Marino (Gianfranco Ferré)
Paestum Rose (Eau d'Italie)
Light Blue (Dolce & Gabbana)

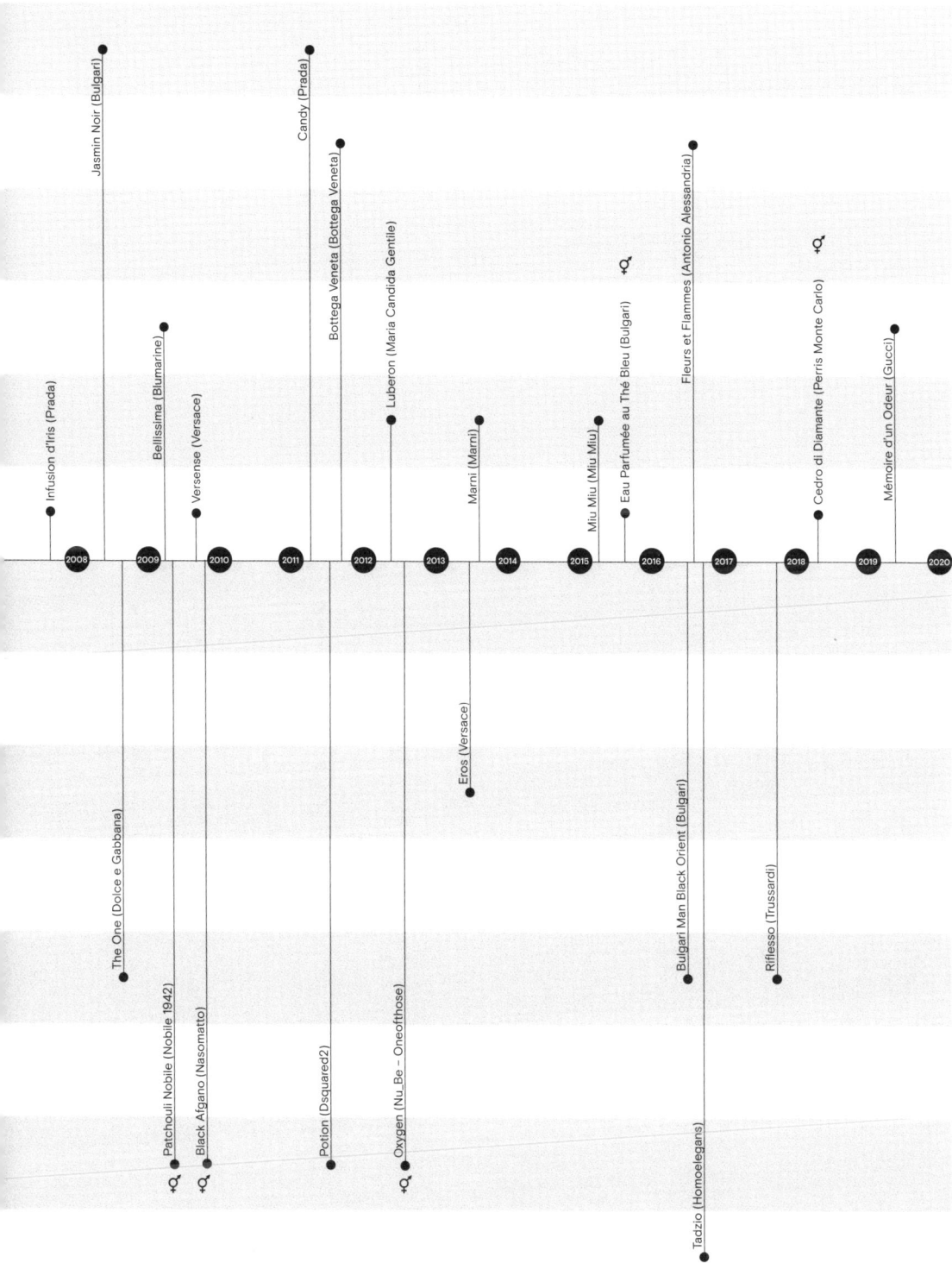

Infusion d'Iris (Prada)

Jasmin Noir (Bulgari)

Candy (Prada)

Bellissima (Blumarine)

Bottega Veneta (Bottega Veneta)

Versense (Versace)

Luberon (Maria Candida Gentile)

Marni (Marni)

Fleurs et Flammes (Antonio Alessandria)

Miu Miu (Miu Miu)

Eau Parfumée au Thé Bleu (Bulgari)

Cedro di Diamante (Perris Monte Carlo)

Mémoire d'un Odeur (Gucci)

2008 2009 2010 2011 2012 2013 2014 2015 2016 2017 2018 2019 2020

The One (Dolce e Gabbana)

Patchouli Nobile (Nobile 1942)

Black Afgano (Nasomatto)

Potion (Dsquared2)

Oxygen (Nu_Be – Oneofthose)

Eros (Versace)

Bulgari Man Black Orient (Bulgari)

Riflesso (Trussardi)

Tadzio (Homoelegans)

355

Bibliography

Webgraphy

Resources helpful for learning to smell perfumes:
Marika Vecchiattini, *Knowing Perfumes* (available on Amazon)
Mandy Aftel - *Essence and Alchemy, a natural history of perfume*; Garzanti Turin 2006
Steven Van Toller, George H. Dodd, *Perfumery: psychology & biology of fragrance*; Aporie, Rome 1998

History of perfumery
Profumo. Origini, Storie, Confezioni, edited by Cristina Maritano *et alii*, exhibition catalogue *Pro-Fumum* (Turin, Palazzo Madama, 15 February – 21 May 2018); Silvana Editoriale, Cinisello Balsamo 2018
Michael Edwards, *Parfums de Legende. Un siècle de Créations Francaises*, HM Editions, 1998
Annick Le Guérer, *Le Parfum. Des origines à nos jours*, Odile Jacob, Paris 2005
Marie Christine Grasse, *Perfume: a global history from the origins to today*, Museo della Profumeria di Grasse in collaboration with Somogy Art Publishers, Paris 2007

Blogs on perfumes
http://bergamottoebenzoino.blogspot.com The blog (in Italian and English) I began 13 years ago now, with reviews of perfumes and interviews with composers.
http://www.nstperfume.com/
http://perfumeshrine.blogspot.com/
http://www.mimifroufrou.com/scentedsalamander/
https://boisdejasmin.com

Sites and Forums
http://www.adjiumi.it/adjnpforum/ The Italian perfume community, with a Facebook page visited by thousands of fans.
http://www.basenotes.net/ The world's largest community of perfume lovers.
http://www.fragrantica.com/ A portal offering information on both traditional and artistic perfumery, in several languages.
https://www.perfumeintelligence.co.uk/library/ An extraordinary, exceptionally detailed web-encyclopaedia on perfume.
http://www.accademiadelprofumo.it/ Accademia del Profumo promotes the historical, cultural, artistic and social values of Italian perfumery. The cosmetic companies belonging to the Unipro (Italian Association of Cosmetic Companies) form part of it. The website is a good place to start to explore the world of perfumery.
http://www.ifraorg.org/ The website of the IFRA, the supervisory body that controls the raw materials used in perfumery.
https://olfatheque.com/ The educational website of Cinquième Sens (and its Italian partner, Mouillettes & Co.), with information and interviews.

Acknowledgements

This book has benefited from the contribution of many people.

The first I have to thank are my parents, Marco and Simone, who have helped me in more ways than I could ever mention.

Thanks to Accademia del Profumo for the precious patronage. And in particular Ambra Martone, Corinna Parisi and Valentina Rosina for their support in finding photos and useful information.

Thank you to all those splendid people whose interviews appear in the book: first and foremost, Emanuela Rupi, President of Mouillettes&Co., who devoted a great deal of time and energy to me, offering me information that would otherwise have been extremely difficult to track down. In addition, Emanuela and Sara Ravo opened the doors of Mouillettes & Co. to me, leaving me free to explore their archives: this is a privilege I will never forget.

The Bormioli Luigi company had an important role in finding vintage bottles; in particular, Federico Montali allowed me, photographing them all, to view the historical bottles produced by the company in order to ask for some of them for the photo shoot.

The information generously supplied by Ambra Martone of ICR gave me a better understanding of a number of issues; she also gave me contacts that proved of prime importance for writing the book.

Ing. Valerio Tateo of Moellhausen was among the first to believe in this volume, investing time and energy to ensure the success of the interview with Dr. Anthony Moellhausen and to promoting the book.

Gianfranco Capua offered me his vision of perfumery, vastly expanding my love for citrus raw materials.
Maurizio Cerizza, Carlo Pioli (Parma Color Viola), Stefania Giannino and Massimo Nobile (Nobile 1942) have a contagious passion for what they do: I am grateful to them for sharing it with me and with readers.

The precious support of Loredana Linati of the "Imagine" magazine allowed me to give completeness and precision to the list of Italian perfumes 1970-2019 which is found at the end of the volume.

Thanks also to Marco Beck Peccoz, whose talent and enthusiasm have allowed the bottles to show their best side, doing justice to their beauty, their innovation and their stories.

Thanks to the Gianfranco Ferré Foundation for the picture of page 223.
Picture at page 189 is by Nicholas Prahin.

Thanks also to Paola Leoni (Studio Leoni Genova), author of the beautiful pictures of pages 57, 191, 227, 235, 243, 261.

Giancarlo Gonizzi, Livio Radin, Alda Rapo and Franco Miglino, Maurizio Mugnano, Dionigi Zanchetti, Alessia Mangoni, Luigi Mancini have allowed me to acquire bottles, samples and interesting details on some vintage perfumes. The pictures at pages 71, 179 e 181 are by Dionigi Zanchetti, the picture at page 61 is by Luigi Mancini.
Alda and Franco are also authors of the picture of page 183.

Cristian Cavagna, founder, heart and soul of the Adjiumi community is an endless source of projects, food for thought and laughter. Thanks for sharing this all with me.

I owe to Paola Ottonello and Alda Motta my tranquility while I was writing this book.

Thanks also to my editor Dario Cimorelli of Silvana Editoriale, who supported me and this volume with his culture and intelligence. Together with Giacomo Merli, Sergio Di Stefano, Denise Castelnovo, Lorena Ansani and the other people who work in Silvana Editoriale, Dario has pushed my research work far beyond what I had planned, in an attempt to offer the reader as much completeness as possible. Working with such brilliant professionals cuts the effort in half and doubles the satisfaction with the final result.

Thank you to Italo Calvino, author of "Sotto il Sole Giaguaro" and Patrick Suskind, author of "Perfume – History of a murderer", among the first to have understood the power of the sense of smell, and to have illustrated it in such magnificent prose, inspiring at least two generations to study perfumery in depth.

Thanks to Elena and Marco; Sara and Nicola; Isa and Vito – they know why – and to E.

The world of perfume is able to spark passion in anyone who comes close to it: heartfelt thanks to the wonderful readers of my blog, "Bergamotto e Benzoino", of my FB page, and to all the people I've encountered over the years for transmitting a never- ending flow of emotions, reflections and issues that have enriched my ideas and my life. I feel extremely lucky.

And finally, I bow down before the God of Perfume.

"The golden age of perfumery is not behind us: it lies ahead of us" (Edmond Roudnitska)

Silvana Editoriale

Direction
Dario Cimorelli

Art Director
Giacomo Merli

Editorial Coordinator
Sergio Di Stefano

Copy Editor
Lorena Ansani

Layout
Denise Castelnovo

Production Coordinator
Antonio Micelli

Editorial Assistant
Ondina Granato

Photo Editor
Alessandra Olivari, Silvia Sala

Press Office
Lidia Masolini, press@silvanaeditoriale.it

Available through ARTBOOK | D.A.P.
155 Sixth Avenue, 2nd Floor, New York, N.Y. 10013
Tel: (212) 627-1999 Fax: (212) 627-9484

Silvana Editoriale S.p.A.
via dei Lavoratori, 78
20092 Cinisello Balsamo, Milano
tel. 02 453 951 01
fax 02 453 951 51
www.silvanaeditoriale.it

Reproductions, printing and binding in Italy
Printed by Tipo Stampa S.r.l.,
Moncalieri (To)
Printed September 2020